CHILD PSYCHIATRIC TECHNIQUES

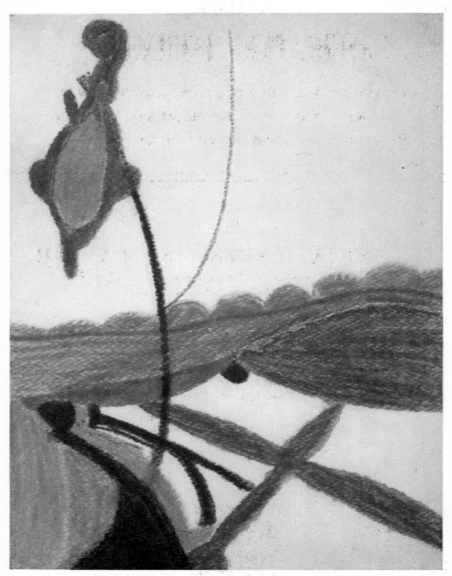

"Aeroplane" Abstraction by Francine (*Crayon*).

CHILD
PSYCHIATRIC TECHNIQUES

Diagnostic and Therapeutic Approach to Normal and Abnormal Development Through Patterned, Expressive, and Group Behavior

By

LAURETTA BENDER, B.S., M.A., M.D.

Professor of Clinical Psychiatry
New York University College of Medicine

Associate Attending Psychiatrist
New York University Bellevue Medical Center

Senior Psychiatrist in Charge of
Children's Service of the Psychiatric Division
Bellevue Hospital
New York, New York

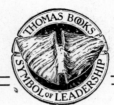

CHARLES C THOMAS · PUBLISHER
Springfield · Illinois · U.S.A.

NO LONGER THE PROPERTY
OF THE
UNIVERSITY OF R. I. LIBRARY

CHARLES C THOMAS · PUBLISHER

BANNERSTONE HOUSE
301-327 EAST LAWRENCE AVENUE, SPRINGFIELD, ILLINOIS

Published simultaneously in the British Commonwealth of Nations by
BLACKWELL SCIENTIFIC PUBLICATIONS, LTD., OXFORD, ENGLAND

Published simultaneously in Canada by
THE RYERSON PRESS, TORONTO

Printed in the United States of America

FOREWORD

THIS BOOK consists of a collection of papers written by Paul Schilder, Lauretta Bender, and a number of our associates at Bellevue Hospital during the past 15 years. The papers all deal with our experience in the care, treatment, observation and in many cases the re-examination of thousands of children with problems, in the children's ward of the Psychiatric Division of Bellevue Hospital. This group of papers is concerned with the techniques (especially those related to the expressive arts, patterned behavior and group activities) which were found useful in the residential care, observation, understanding, diagnosis, and therapy of this large number of deviate, disturbed and unhappy problem children.

In not a single instance is any one of these contributions the product of the editing author alone. Dr. Paul Schilder (1886-1940), who was for a short part of this period also my husband, was the originator of most of the concepts, attitudes, and resulting philosophies expressed in all of these papers, as will be readily recognized by those familiar with his work. He was also the author of Chapters VI, VII, IX and XIX which were parts of a book on *Art and the Problem Child* which we two prepared in collaboration but which was never published. He was also co-author of several other chapters (indicated in each instance), and the major influence in the conception of the remainder.

The thousands of New York City children who over the past 15 years have come to the children's ward of the Psychiatric Division of Bellevue Hospital, with their multiplicity of ungratified needs and their unexplored capacities for projective expression in creative, patterned, and group activities, have been the chief source of the data and inspiration which have made possible this volume and the others to follow.

By emphasizing problems of retardation in personality development, mental deficiency and regressive behavior in much of the illustrative clinical material, we have tried to give unity to the book. An effort has also been made to give a longitudinal picture of many children who were first observed by us when they were young and who have now reached young adulthood. The book does not aim at being comprehensive but seeks rather to bring together formulations of observations which have interested us over this period of years.

Many of the workers in the field associated with Paul Schilder and the author, including psychiatrists, psychologists, teachers, artists, and art teachers, have helped to observe, evaluate, and treat the children, and to develop the techniques and ideas which are here described and illustrated. Often they were responsible for a major part of the formulation of individual chapters and they are in every instance given appropriate credit. Franziska Boas, Allison Montague, Jack Rapoport, William Q. Wolfson, Adolf G. Woltmann, and Wanda Wright have all made invaluable contributions. Allison Montague has in addition been my principal aide in the planning and preparation of the material, and in the laborious task of final editing of the manuscript.

Following this volume on the projective, creative, configurational and group behavior of the children in the children's ward of Bellevue's Psychiatric Division, there will appear a volume on the psychopathology of childhood based on the same source material, and later a third volume dealing with the clinical psychiatric syndromes of childhood. The three books are similarly written by the same staff, the individual members of which have changed from time to time, and they deal with the same group of children. They have the same general point of view and tend to complement each other.

LAURETTA BENDER, M.D.

ACKNOWLEDGMENTS

THANKS are hereby expressed to all the publishers of books and journals who granted permission for the use of such of our material as had already been published and which has been, in part, rewritten to meet the particular needs of this volume. My monograph on *A Visual Motor Gestalt Test and Its Clinical Use* was published in 1938, and reprinted in 1948 by the American Orthopsychiatric Association. *The Manual for the Instructions and Test Cards for the Visual Motor Gestalt Test* was published in 1946. Chapters IV and V have been largely constructed from the above publications. Many of the illustrations from these chapters have also been reproduced from the monograph. Chapters X, XI, XIV, XV and XVI, including the illustrations, have also been reproduced from the *Journal of the American Orthopsychiatric Association*. Chapter I has been rewritten from a chapter with the same title in *Current Therapies in Personality Disorders,* edited by Bernard Glueck, New York, Grune and Stratton, 1945. Chapters II and III, including the illustrations in Chapter III, have been reproduced from the *Pedagogical Seminar* and *Journal of Genetic Psychology.* The first part of Chapter VII with its illustrations, Chapter VIII and its illustrations, as well as Chapter XIII and some of its illustrations have been reproduced in part from the *Journal of Nervous and Mental Disease.* Chapter XII has been rewritten from the *American Journal of Psychiatry.* Chapter XVIII has been reproduced from the *College Art Journal* with the addition of some material, including the color plate. Part of Chapter XVI has been rewritten from the *Journal of Esthetics and Art Criticism.* Specific reference to the source of each of these contributions is made at the beginning of each chapter.

L. B.

CONTENTS

CONTENTS

CHILD PSYCHIATRIC TECHNIQUES

TECHNIQUES IN CHILD PSYCHIATRY—
A SURVEY[1]

TECHNIQUES in child psychiatry are derived from the arts, the human-
ities, and the sciences. They are used for the examination, evaluation,
training and therapy of the normal child, as well as the child with a developmental, behavior, psychiatric or neurological problem. Child study has contributed to these techniques in all areas of psychology—behaviorism, gestalt,
clinical, physiological, educational, and academic psychology. The medical
sciences—psychiatry, psychoanalysis, and neurology—have become specialized
for dealing with the period of childhood. More recently, adaptations have also
been made in the fields of sociology and anthropology to include the study
of the child in every culture, remote and familiar. Accordingly, the history
of childhood psychiatry does not run parallel with that of adult psychiatry.

In the field of child psychiatry, the emphasis has been on the child's needs,
strivings and growth tendencies in a social and cultural background, and on
the variants and deviations in any of these areas which create problems for
the child. This survey will consider the contributions from the various
fields which help in evaluating the special needs of the problem child; and
the deviations which occur in child behavior because these needs have not
been satisfied. It will also consider how these needs can best be met. The
application of the various techniques may be diagnostic or therapeutic and,
not infrequently, both.

I. THE DIAGNOSIS AND CARE AND TRAINING OF THE
MENTAL DEFECTIVE CHILD

An historical survey of child psychiatry such as that made by Lawson G.
Lowrey (1945)[2] shows that the period of child psychiatry before 1909 concerned itself with the institutional care and training of defective children.

At the turn of the century, in France, J. M. G. Itard first tried to study
and train an "idiot" child, "the wild boy of Aveyron" and wrote a scientific
thesis on his experiences. Edouard Seguin established the first training
school for defective children in France. Two years later he came to America

---

[1] This chapter is rewritten from Bender, Lauretta: Techniques in Child Psychiatry, Chap. IV
in: *Current Therapies of Personality Disorders*, 1945; with considerable new material added.

[2] Lowrey, Lawson G.: *Psychiatry for Children*. For references to authors, see Bibliography.

to be superintendent of the first training school in this country which later became known for the work of Walter E. Fernald.[3] Meanwhile, in France, the same trend led to the psychometric tests of A. Binet and T. Simon who attempted to evaluate the intelligence of the defective children in the institutions. These tests have since developed into the whole field of psychometry and clinical psychology. In 1946[4] Florence Goodenough surveyed these tests for children. Psychometrics are no longer considered as being useful in the diagnosis of mental deficiency only. Batteries of tests by trained psychologists form a necessary part of the study of any child who needs educational or psychiatric evaluation, training or therapy. They have also become an essential part of the neurological examination of a child with a developmental deviation or pathology in the central nervous system.[5] The most recent and useful psychometric test for children is the *Wechsler Intelligence Scale for Children* (WISC 1949).

Walter E. Fernald was active in organizing institutions for the care, training, and education of feeble-minded children and in sponsoring laws for their welfare. He also established the first scientific association for the study of feeble-minded children, and stimulated workers investigating the problem of the feeble-minded child. In "ten fields of inquiry" he championed the cause of the feeble-minded child and its right to be understood and treated according to its needs rather than to be classified and segregated as feeble-minded on the sole basis of an intelligence quotient.

The findings of a low I. Q. still leaves the obligation to determine etiological factors, to make a clinical diagnosis, and to seek educational and therapeutic approaches suitable for each individual child. It is necessary to determine the area of dysfunction in order to consider the possibilities of compensation in other fields; the possibility of accelerated development or self-healing; and the responses to remedial training and psychotherapy directed at the personality or to a new environmental adjustment. Much is yet to be accomplished by a careful evaluation of so-called defective, retarded, exceptional, and deviate children. Up to the present, special techniques of examining and treating these children have made it possible to differentiate several groups:

1. The child with language disabilities, first emphasized in this country by Samuel T. Orton (1925) as a neurological and psychiatric entity. The developmental aphasias and alexias (reading disabilities) are congenital developmental lags in the language field occurring in children at all levels of intelligence. They are disabilities often associated with varying discrepancies

---

[3] For an evaluation of Fernald's work, see Baker, B. W.: *The History of the Care of the Feeble-minded.*

[4] Goodenough, Florence: The measurement of Mental Growth in Childhood, Chap. IX in: *The Manual of Child Psychology*, 1946.

[5] Gesell, Arnold and Amatruda, Catherine S.: *Developmental Diagnosis*, 1947.

in development of the total patterned behavior, as Stella Chess has shown in a study of such children on the children's ward of the Psychiatric Division of Bellevue Hospital. In a competitive culture in which a premium is placed on language, especially written language, such a disability proves a serious frustration in the development of the child. A clearly defined syndrome can be delineated with a battery of psychometric and educational tests, motility tests, tests for cortical dominance, observation of behavior, a familial history of cortical dominance and language problems, developmental and school history, and psychiatric evaluation of the personality responses. The indicated program consists of specific technical remedial training and a manipulation of the environment to allow for a compensatory program in fields of work and play where the individual can function constructively. If the language defect has struck so early or so deeply or has been sufficiently neglected as to interfere with the early personality development (especially in relation to social concepts), play or other projective techniques together with a free expression of the fantasy life may also be used to help. Although language disabilities always tend to retard the early development to some extent, this is not always so marked as to suggest mental deficiency.

2. The intellectually inhibited[6] or blocked child, also referred to often by such terms as psychogenic mutism or "pseudo-imbecility," suffers from a neurosis due to a disorder in the child-parent relationship, occurring before or during the period of rapid speech acquisition. Such a child may be successfully treated by psychotherapy using psychoanalytic principles, including relationship, projection, release, and insight. The latter may be supplemented by hypnosis, the use of projective techniques, or play therapies in group situations which encourage the child to be articulate in areas other than language. The treatment process may be hastened by special techniques directed specifically at the problem, including music, drama, or puppets. Chemotherapy, using sodium amytal[7] or benzedrine,[8] may also be used when indicated. The close relationship between diagnostic and therapeutic techniques is shown by the fact that the differential diagnosis of retardation due to psychogenic inhibition, organic defect, or schizophrenia, is not always easy to make until treatment is under way. In such cases, the response to therapy helps to determine the diagnosis.[9]

3. Schizophrenic children have often gone unrecognized in state schools

---

[6] See Klein, Melanie: *A Contribution to the Theory of Intellectual Inhibition,* 1931.

[7] This refers to sodium amytal injection or pentothal narcosis which often helps to break into the mutism and facilitates the child's impulse to speak.

[8] For the procedure of benzedrine treatment in children see Bender, Lauretta and Cottington, Frances: *The Use of Amphetamine Sulphate (Benzedrine) in Child Psychiatry.* Chapter XVIII shows the application of this drug in the therapy of a child.

[9] Jules, Henry has reported an interesting case of a child in Bali with this problem.

for defectives in cases where retardation is co-existent with the psychosis or secondary to the psychotic process. Howard Potter called attention to this in 1933. Melanie Klein has described the psychotic child who early defends himself from the schizophrenic process by withdrawing into a narcissistic position with resulting retardation. She has shown that the inhibiting effect upon the intellectual development may become irreversible and unmodifiable by treatment. At the present time childhood schizophrenia may be recognized early[10] and permits a treatment program which is aimed first at relieving the child of the terrifying anxiety which tends to disorganize the personality, and calls out defense mechanisms which may prove to be non-constructive for the development of the child. Treatment consists of socializing activities away from the home, which becomes the center of conflict; reassuring and interpretive psychotherapy dealing with the special psychological problems of the schizophrenic; any supportive and educational procedures which are needed.[11] Shock therapy helps to relieve the anxiety and seems to aid in re-establishing a pattern of biological behavior in spite of the disorganizing tendencies of the disease process. In retarded schizophrenic children development is frequently accelerated by such a treatment program. It must be remembered, however, that not all schizophrenic children are retarded or regressed; many are even precocious.

4. The emotionally deprived psychopathic personalities, especially those reared in institutions during infancy,[12] appear to be retarded in every field of personality development as well as in intellectual functioning. William Goldfarb has made a series of studies on the nature and extent of the retardation in such children. His conclusion is that the only corrective treatment is preventive; infants should not be raised in institutions. Otherwise the best therapeutic procedure is one directed at social imitation after the age of eight years in a well-organized institution where no personal responsibility for action is expected. This has been learned from repeated observation of these children in a controlled situation at Bellevue and in follow-up studies by Lauretta Bender, Maizie Becker, René Spitz, and William Goldfarb.

Efforts to study the retarded or defective child bring us towards a solution of many of the neuropsychiatric problems of childhood, since developmental discrepancies, inhibitions, blockings, infantile fixations, and regressions are among the more common ways for children to react to frustration whether from social, psychological, or organic pathology.

---

[10] Bender, Lauretta: *Childhood Schizophrenia,* 1947.

[11] Bender, Lauretta: *One Hundred Cases of Childhood Schizophrenia Treated with Electric Shock,* 1947.

[12] Arnold Gesell speaks of these conditions as "environmental retardations" in *Developmental Diagnosis,* 1947.

II. CLINICS AND INSTITUTIONS FOR THE STUDY AND CARE OF THE DELINQUENT CHILD

The problem child may respond with aggression and antisocial behavior. A new era began in American child psychiatry in 1909, according to Lawson G. Lowrey, when it began to show an interest in the delinquent child, with the kind of concern that had previously been focused on the defective child. In that year William Healy began his work at the Chicago Juvenile Psychopathic Institute in connection with the Juvenile Court, basing his work on the case study of the individual offender and on his own concept of the essential dynamic character of the human personality. In 1909, too, the National Committee for Mental Hygiene was established. In 1912, E. E. Southard opened the Boston Psychopathic Hospital, and in 1913 Adolph Meyer opened the Phipps Clinic at the Johns Hopkins Hospital after having already published the principles underlying his school of psychobiology. Several state bureaus for juvenile research were established in rapid succession (Ohio, California, Michigan) mainly in connection with state programs for the care of mental defectives. One of these was the Judge Baker Foundation in Boston. Douglas C. Thom (1920) established a clinic for the younger difficult child in Boston, and Ira S. Wile had a similar clinic in New York.

Subsequently the delinquent child has been studied wherever he has been found or wherever there have been facilities and interested workers. Study homes or institutions have often given opportunities for important contributions similar to August Aichorn's early contribution. More recently the tendency has been to recognize that the delinquent child is a mentally disturbed child, and should be studied with the view of arriving at a diagnosis of his condition, and with implications for a therapeutic rather than a disciplinary or correctional program. The delinquent child may be defective or retarded at least to a dull level, making competition difficult. Several studies of delinquency have shown that reading disabilities have been significant contributing factors. Although frequently neurotic, the delinquent child may be psychopathic or schizophrenic. He must therefore have adequate psychiatric, neurological, psychometric, and educational evaluation. Social factors—broken homes, deprived economic status, and large families— as well as retardation have been emphasized by William Healy and Augusta Bronner, Bernard Glueck, John Bowlby, and Maud Merril.

The psychoanalytic approach, beginning with August Aichorn's early study, has given both an understanding of the dynamics of the delinquent or antisocial child, as well as a technique for therapy[13] (however much it may have to be modified).

---

[13] Dr. Denis Carrol, of the Institute for the Study and Treatment of Delinquency of the National Health Service in England and the International Criminological Society has developed short-term psychoanalytic treatment techniques for delinquents.

III. THE CHILD GUIDANCE MOVEMENT

Since 1919, the Child Guidance movement sponsored by the National Committee for Mental Hygiene and the Commonwealth Fund has helped to organize clinics for children as independent units in connection with social agencies, schools, children's courts, and state departments of mental hygiene.[14] These clinics attempted to get away from medical and psychiatric concepts and to deal with children's problems by offering guidance to the adults concerned with them. They did not want to be too closely identified with any one social agency, as for example with a children's court which dealt with "bad" or delinquent children. They wished to become community centers cooperating with all community agencies and coordinating all those services needed in the interest of the child; especially those to be made available to the parents. Emphasis was put on E. E. Southard's concept of the clinical team made up of psychologist, psychiatric social worker, and psychiatrist, which functioned through conferences based on records. The child did not appear; it was not uncommon for the psychiatrist never to see the child and the child was not always the direct recipient of the treatment program. Social diagnosis and milieu therapy were the chief concern rather than the delineation of clinical syndromes and specific individual therapy.

Psychobiology, a school of thought originated and taught by Adolf Meyer, is historically related to the child guidance movement. The latter, too, was an offspring of the concepts of Adolf Meyer who is frequently regarded as the "father" of American psychiatry. The psychobiologists put their emphasis on environmental influences. The therapeutic technique which they use is referred to by them as distributive analysis; it is rather non-specific in nature.[15] Orthopsychiatry has been defined by Lawson G. Lowrey, until 1949 editor of the *Journal of Orthopsychiatry,* as "the science and art of prevention by therapy." The American Orthopsychiatric Association sponsors the concept of the three unit team of psychiatrist-psychologist-social worker. Its membership through its *Journal* and scientific meetings have made contributions in every field of human activity concerning itself with the prevention and correction of behavior disorders in childhood, adulthood, and senility. The work of the Association rests upon scientific findings in the fields of neuropsychiatry, clinical psychology, social work, sociology, anthropology, education, criminology, and psychoanalysis.

---

[14] An excellent, concise survey of the development of child guidance clinics appears in the introduction of Witmer, Helen L.: *Psychiatric Interviews with Children,* 1946.

See also, Witmer, Helen L.: *Psychiatric Clinics for Children,* 1940, for history of the development of child guidance clinics and the philosophy behind them.

[15] See Lief, Alfred (editor): *The Commonsense Psychiatry of Adolf Meyer;* Muncie, Wendell: *Psychobiology and Psychiatry;* and Schilder, Paul: *Psychotherapy,* for a discussion of various other therapeutic procedures, including distributive analysis.

IV. THE AMERICAN SCHOOL OF CHILD PSYCHOTHERAPY

In America, child psychotherapy has evolved and developed from the influence of Adolf Meyer, psychobiology, the child guidance movement, and psychoanalysis. Perhaps the most representative American in the field of child psychotherapy has been David M. Levy. His work has been directed toward the problems of sibling rivalry, maternal rejection, hostile aggression, affect hunger. The techniques of therapy described by him include milieu therapy, environmental, attitude, and manipulative therapy in which social workers play an important role. For individual therapy, he describes affect therapy, insight therapy, and release therapy; psychoanalytic principles and play techniques are also utilized. Dr. Levy has referred to psychoanalytic therapy as the "most highly evolved insight and affect therapy which in children is a form of free-play interpretative therapy."

Frederick H. Allen has been the most representative advocate of relationship therapy; Carl R. Rogers has advanced the technique of non-directive individual and group therapy. Helen L. Witmer's *Psychiatric Interviews with Children,* gives examples from each of the various schools illustrating the techniques of psychotherapy utilized, and includes detailed reports.

V. EDUCATIONAL PSYCHOLOGY

A survey of educational psychology reveals a wealth of techniques for studying the child, of psychological and psychopathological data, and of educational procedures and suggestions for psychotherapeutic techniques.

At the turn of the century, G. Stanley Hall represented the modern pedagogical psychologist in America with his emphasis on methods of study and his evolutionary or recapitulation theory. The biographical method, where biographical records were included, preceded him, with the German physiologist Wilhelm Preyer using experimental physiological approaches on his own two children. Elaborations upon these techniques together with other approaches—questionnaires, interviews, studies on learning processes, and direct observations—were made by William Stern, Heinz Werner, Jean Piaget, Karl and Charlotte Buehler, and many others. These studies were mainly concerned with developmental levels, formal aspects of behavior, thinking, learning, and language development.[16]

In the field of educational psychology, G. Stanley Hall was preceded by Jean Jacques Rousseau, Friedrich Froebel, and Karl Groos; he himself however came closest to representing the present clinical view. He paved the way

---

[16] Anderson, John E.: Methods in Child Psychiatry, in Carmichael, Leonard (editor): *Manual of Child Psychiatry,* 1946. This is an encyclopedic presentation of the subject. Dennis, Wayne: *The Historical Beginnings of Child Psychology,* 1949, has reviewed the earliest available reports or notes on the development and behavior of normal children, and furnishes a full biography.

for dynamic insight into deviating behavior with a new emphasis on methods for studying the individual child. More recently John Dewey, founder of the progressive education movement, with emphasis on the needs of the individual and the individual's capacity for self expression and self direction in the educational process, has come nearest to a dynamic clinical understanding of the normal individual, and has opened the way for the understanding of the problem child as a deviant from the normal. Herbert Read,[17] following the teachings of Plato that art should be the basis of education, has developed a philosophy of education in a democracy based on the development of freedom in self expression through art expressions.

The trends towards convergence of the observation of behavior, the encouragement of the creative impulses, and the psychoanalytic analysis of the fantasy life have led to the use of the projective technique in relation to personality studies. Also related to the latter are the gestalt concepts derived from child-in-a-field studies in nursery schools associated with colleges and universities.

In the *Sarah Lawrence College Nursery School Studies* a special effort has been made to develop techniques for the study of the personality of the nursery school child, through the use and coordination of modern methods in psychology. Lois B. Murphy and Eugene Lerner have formulated the results: "The basic point of view which emerges from consideration of contemporary work on the development of children is as follows: Personality development during the childhood period can be understood completely only when we consider the basic experience of the child in relation not only to his particular parents and to the universal discovery of sex differences, but to his individual pattern of physical and mental growth, the specific range of constitutional tendencies, abilities and effective responses and the total field of family and neighborhood in a given structure in which he is growing."[18] The techniques that are utilized in this situation are the usual ones emphasized in nursery schools: observation play techniques with raw materials and miniature toys, the group situation, and spontaneous art.

Werner Wolff has studied the personality of the pre-school child by applying the projective methods to bring forth the expressive behavior of the child, and has analyzed his observations by utilizing the methods of the gestalt school. His observational and experimental studies were made over a fifteen year period in nursery schools and children's homes in Germany, Spain and United States of America. Most of his American experience was in

---

[17] Read, Herbert: *Education Through Art.* This book is scholarly, readable, an artistic production itself; its thesis is very convincing.

[18] Lerner, Eugene and Murphy, Lois B.: *Methods for the Study of Personality in Young Children,* 1941.

the Department of Child Study and the Nursery School of Sarah Lawrence College; material from Bard College and Vassar College was also used. He analyzed the expressive behavior of children in their static posture as well as when engaged in bodily movements. He also studied their finger painting and especially their graphic art drawing and scribbling.

Susan Isaacs[19] in London studied the social development of the child by observing daily behavior in nursery schools and analyzing her observations from the psychoanalytic viewpoint. Some of the earliest observations of children in nursery schools were made by nursery school teachers themselves. One of the latter, Harriet M. Johnson, recorded her studies in the nursery school bearing her name.[20] Barbara Biber and her co-workers felt the need to observe the seven-year-olds, using a variety of projective techniques as well as day-by-day observation in the school room.[21] J. Louise Despert working as an observing child psychiatrist in the Nursery School of the New York Hospital analyzed the play of children with miniature toys in group situations and in the child-doctor relationship.

VI. BEHAVIORISM

Watson's school of behaviorism opened up a new approach to development, learning and therapy. Many universities have established centers for child study which have made important contributions at a behavioristic level. Of the latter, Arnold Gesell's studies are the best known. The center which he led at Yale University has been called the school of "developmentalism." Here the emphasis is on maturation as a biological process in a cultural setting. Test procedures, especially for infants and children up to the age of five years, have been standardized and followed longitudinally. Levels of behavior are determined with a wide range of deviation which makes the standards particularly useful for non-professional but well informed parents and teachers. There is little concern with interpretation of the inner life of the child. The five to ten year level has been largely obtained from reports of mothers. However the concept of a genetic and developmental view is based on the wide knowledge of the Yale group of scientists. Each level of development is derived from the preceding one and discussed in terms of the inherent biological maturation tendencies and patterns in a cultural setting. There are studies on the environmental effects of intellectual development from the State University of Iowa; and longitudinal studies from the University of California and the University of Colorado.

---

[19] Isaacs, Susan: *Social Development in Young Children,* 1933.

[20] Johnson, Harriet M.: *School Begins at Two,* 1936.

[21] Biber, Barbara, *et al.: Child Life in School,* 1942.

VII. PROJECTIVE TECHNIQUES—PLAY WITH MINIATURE TOYS

Play techniques with miniature toys have developed from a number of sources. The child analysts, Melanie Klein and Anna Freud, have used this procedure combined with varying degrees of interpretation in place of free association and dream analysis as employed in the analysis of adults. Susan Isaacs has used the free play of the nursery school type—observing, recording, and analyzing the behavior and her interpretations. The world pictures of disturbed children, formed by miniature toys in a standard setting, have been studied by Margaret Lowenfeld at the Institute of Child Psychology in London. Charlotte Buehler has studied the world pictures of normal children at different age levels.[22] Many modifications of the miniature toy techniques are now used wherever children are studied.

Through play the child experiments with reality in the physical, social, and emotional world. There have been many other definitions of play[23] but this is the most valuable at the present time especially where play is utilized psychotherapeutically.

Jean Jacques Rousseau, who stressed the pragmatic value of play, and Friedrich Froebel who emphasized its symbolic components, were among the first to give special attention to play activities. Through the practical applications of his "method," Froebel called attention also to the educational values of the inherent socializing factors in play. By attacking the complex problem of play and play activities from a speculative, philosophical point of view, Herbert Spencer was satisfied in considering "surplus energy" as the basis for all discharges called play.

By comparing play activities of young animals and children, Karl Groos came to the conclusion that play is a biological function which provides the necessary practice for maturing organs. To this "practice" theory he later added the concept of play as a catharsis, explaining that play very often is a kind of safety valve for the expression of pent-up emotions.

In approaching play activities from the anthropological point of view, G. Stanley Hall formed his theory around the assumption that the phylogenetic development of mankind is repeated by each child in an ontogenetic manner. In studying the play activities of adult savages and civilized children, Estelle Appleton found that great similarity does not exist between the two. According to her, play is not a recapitulation of phylogenetic factors but a biological instinct present in both primitive and civilized man. Modern psychology

---

[22] Lowenfeld, Margaret: *The World Picture of Children, A Method of Recording and Studying Them,* 1939.

Buehler, Charlotte, Kelly, Lumry G. and Carrol, H.: *World Test Standardization Studies,* 1949.

[23] Mitchell, Elmer D. and Mason, Bernard S.: *The Theory of Play,* 1934.

tends to follow John H. Dewey who states that "all organic beings are naturally active. Therefore it is unnecessary to seek any further explanation for the fact that they are active than the fact that they are alive . . . the only thing necessary is to state the conditions under which the organic activity takes place."[24]

Sigmund Freud was able to explain much of children's play on the basis of the gratification of pleasure principle. "In the play of children we seem to arrive at the conclusion that the child repeats even the unpleasant experiences because through his own activity he gains a far more thorough mastery of the strong impression than was possible by mere passive experience. Every fresh repetition seems to strengthen this mastery for which the child tries."[25]

Robert Waelder says: "Play may be a process like a repetition compulsion by which excessive experiences are divided into small quantities, re-attempted and assimilated in play."[26]

M. N. Searle defines play as the activity of the child which links non-reality to reality, or better, which links psychic reality to the external reality.

In the opinion of Margaret Lowenfeld "Play in children is the expression of the child's relation to the whole of life and no theory of play is possible which is not also a theory which will cover the whole of a child's relation to life. Play in this sense, therefore, is taken as applying to all activities in children that are spontaneous and self-generated, that are ends in themselves, and that are unrelated to 'lessons' or to the normal physiological needs of a child's own day."[27] Play serves as the child's means of making contact with his environment. It forms the bridge between the child's consciousness and his emotional experiences and so fulfills the role that conversation, introspection, philosophy, and religion fill for the adult. To the child play represents the externalized expression of his emotional life and serves for him the function assumed by art in adult life.

Lawrence K. Frank, in his first article on the projective methods for the study of personality states that "The task calls for an application of a multiplicity of methods and procedures which will reveal the many facets of the personality and show how the individual 'structuralizes his life span' or organizes experiences to meet his personal needs in various media." The criteria for the value of a medium or a method lie in the ability of the subject to "project similar patterns or configurations, upon widely different materials and reveal in his life history the sequence of experiences that make these projections psychologically meaningful for his personality. . . ." This contri-

---

[24] Dewey, John H.: Art in Education in *The Encyclopedia of Education,* 1925.
[25] Freud, Sigmund: *Beyond the Pleasure Principle,* 1924, p. 43.
[26] Waelder, Robert: *The Psychoanalytic Theory of Play,* 1933.
[27] Lowenfeld, Margaret: *Play in Childhood,* 1935.

bution of Lawrence Frank's was the origin of the term "projective techniques."[28]

Max Gitelson found that direct psychotherapy of children is not a self-sufficient procedure and that the therapist must deal with the external factors in terms of the social situation, of the emotional problems of other members of the family, and of the specific educational defects.[29]

Psychotherapy is not merely "free play" but must include a complete understanding on the part of the therapist of the dynamic forces which enter into the relationship between the child and the therapist (transference), and the psychological processes which take place in the child in the course of psychotherapy by play. Surveys on psychoanalytic techniques have been written by Margaret Gerard and Mary O'Neal Hawkins. H. Whitman Newell and William M. Cameron have written on other methods of play therapy.

Edward Liss emphasizes the synthetic value of play in sublimation and suggests that it be used in psychoanalysis both for improving the transference relation and in furnishing data from the unconscious. With these two aims kept clearly in view there is practically no limit as to the materials or techniques that can be used. What to do can best be learned by watching the child at play with all sorts of symbolic images and raw materials.

David M. Levy has employed a carefully worked-out play technique with which he approaches the problems of sibling rivalry in children, for its experimental and therapeutic values. He creates a specific situation in which the child is placed before an "amputation doll," representing the mother. This is a doll which can readily be taken apart. It is suggested that breasts be made of clay and attached to the mother doll. A baby doll may then be put to the breast. A brother or sister doll representing the child under investigation or treatment is added to the play setup. The child is encouraged to destroy the baby at the breast, the breasts, and also the mother. The patient may also punish the brother or sister doll.

J. Louise Despert has utilized a number of techniques in studying aggression in children. She includes story telling and a specifically delimited situation, in which the child is encouraged to phantasy while he is using a sharp knife for cutting up pasteboard. Later he is encouraged to re-synthesize by forming a clay-like material, made from the pasteboard shavings mixed with glue and water, or to use a substitute in the form of clay. Thus she emphasizes the constructive tendencies which follow destructive behavior.

Margaret E. Fries has used play activities as a group project for studying the child's adjustment to companions of his own age, to a person of authority, and to his own deprivations and indulgences. From these data she has also gained insight into the validity of the mother's report about the child;

[28] Frank, Lawrence K.: *Projective Methods for the Study of Personality*, 1939.
[29] Gitelson, Max: *Direct Psychotherapy of Children*.

finally, through group work, some therapeutic results have been accomplished.

Jacob H. Conn of the Baltimore School has re-investigated many of the play techniques, using psychobiological interpretations as a contrast to the psychoanalytic.[30] The results seem to be comparable in similar situations, if somewhat more superficial. The psychoanalytic literature which deals with the problems of childhood takes these techniques for granted and uses them to explore and treat unconscious and past emotional factors as well as conscious and present problems.[31]

These techniques bring about a view of psychotherapy which entails an understanding of the child as a social individual in a society and in his own family. Such psychotherapy must deal with his emotional problems as they develop in a new emotional (therapeutic) situation. He must be considered also as a growing individual with maturation levels which need to be understood and dealt with as they arise (sometimes with special intellectual or motor disabilities that require special training). He must likewise be regarded as an integrated individual capable of expressing himself creatively in different media or play situations by a repetition of meaningful and revealing patterns. The final effort is to bring him to where he is capable of arriving at a new level of social adaptation, biological maturation and integrated behavior due to new experiences and insight permitting greater self-fulfillment.

VIII. GRAPHIC ART

Florence Goodenough in 1926 published her monograph on *The Measurement of Intelligence by Drawings*. This is the "drawing-of-a-man" test which she standardized as an intelligence test for children. The first chapter is a historical survey of studies of children's art and its relationship to child development. Following Florence Goodenough's work, children's art has been extensively used to investigate intellectual maturation, personality factors, fantasy, and symbolism, and as an adjunct to psychotherapy. John Levy (1934) was among the first to use art in child psychotherapy to help overcome resistance and to handle material below the level of consciousness. He believed that the value of the method came from re-interpretation to the child of his own interpretation of his art production.

Paula Elkisch in 1945 and Trude S. Waehner in 1946 studied and interpreted children's art as a projection of the personality. Rose H. Alschuler and

---

[30] Conn, Jacob H.: *The Child Reveals Himself Through Play*, 1939; and *The Play Interview*, 1939.

[31] Similar studies have been made in other groups of young children, and in pediatric hospital wards. See Baruch, Dorothy W.; Burlingham, Susan; Horowitz, R.; Murphy, Lois B.; Richards, Susan S.; and Weiss-Frankl, Anni B.

LaBerta W. Hattwick in 1947 published a two-volume work on the graphic art of the pre-school child. They studied 150 children, two to four years of age in a nursery school and correlated each child's numerous art productions with daily observations of his behavior. They showed that "the meaningless daubs of the pre-school child are directly expressive of his inner life and the dynamic forces affecting him."[32] Study of the children's abstract treatment of color, space, line, and form led them to general conclusions regarding the value for interpretation of each of these aspects of painting. Color tends to reflect the nature and degree of intensity of the emotional life; line and form express energy output and control; space usage gives clues to the pattern of relationship with the environment. The significance of details in each of these areas is explored and the conclusions are for the most part impressive. While easel painting is found to be the most satisfactory medium for projection, crayons, block building, clay, and dramatic play are also used; and comparative analyses are reported.

Margaret Naumburg in 1947 collected into a monograph six of her previously published case studies in which art has been used as a means of diagnosis and therapy in children and adolescents. Most of the children described are pre-adolescent and present neurotic conduct disorders; treatment is carried out in a hospital children's ward. Each child is seen in individual art sessions in which a therapeutic relationship is fostered. The relationship is used to encourage progress in art work from routine tracing, through representational depicting of observations, to spontaneous or "free" expression of fantasy and unconscious material. There is no regard for technical proficiency; formal art lessons received in school tend to inhibit free expression.

The therapeutic value of the projective technique emerges clearly in these studies. It does not depend upon interpretation but rather on its function as "an image language of the unconscious." The technique is especially useful with children who are "closer than adults to primitive expression through images and play." In addition to its therapeutic value, spontaneous creative expression serves as a diagnostic aid; when interpreted, the child's art productions can serve as "a language of communication." The author discusses the psychodynamics of art work and the symbolic meaning of some aspects of abstract form and color. Through the therapeutic relationship the child comes to express in images what he cannot communicate in words and gives the therapist insight into the dynamic mechanisms at work.

Ruth Dunnett reported (1947) on her wide experience with art classes of boys in a wartime British residential school. The gradual progression from directed or representational productions to spontaneous free expression is accompanied by emotional release and gratification. The teaching methods used are ingenious and serve to stimulate the communication of unconscious

---

[32] Alschuler, Rose H. and Hattwick, LaBerta W.: *Painting and Personality*, 1947.

conflict material. This study illustrates again the value of free art expression in therapy and the role of esthetic appreciation in social identification.

Werner Wolff, largely through the medium of drawings of pre-school children, has developed a technique of expression analysis with gestalt concepts which brings him to an understanding of the personality, its growth tendencies and problems. He has developed a technique for determining a Rhythmic Quotient based on innate capacities for projecting spatial relationships in spontaneous drawings. He refers to this function in formal relations as a part of the unconscious sensing of relationships and as an innate personality factor. He regards the Rhythmic Quotient (RQ) as an indicator of the personality comparable to the Intelligence Quotient (IQ) as an indicator of the intelligence.

Herbert Read has developed a thesis which he ascribes to Plato that art should be the basis of education. His study is artistically and convincingly presented, and includes a scholarly review of the purpose of education and the meaning of art. He also develops the application of this thesis to the art of children. He attempts to classify the art of children on a principle of typology; since he himself admits that typology as applied to child personality is largely a myth, his results are not convincing. He endeavors to explain the evident expressive nature of children's art without any understanding of either projection as the American school has applied it to the projective techniques or of the concept of body image as it has been hitherto understood. Moreover he has not recognized Florence Goodenough's data concerning the maturation processes in the drawing of a man.

Madeleine L. Rambert has reviewed the use in psychoanalytic therapy of children's drawings and play with hand puppets as practiced in France. She gives us the significant references to the French literature on child analysis and the use of art expressions in the analytic procedure. She speaks especially of Sophie Morgenstern who concentrated on the study of the child's character as revealed in drawings.

Saul Gurewicz has studied children's drawings and analyzed them from the point of view of the Adlerian individual psychology, and has reviewed the German literature.

Karen Machover has used the drawings of the human figure as a projective technique for the investigation of the personality.

IX. PLASTIC ART

Plastic art of the child is best known in the form of clay modeling. It is a routine part of the activities of the modern nursery school. A number of German workers, noteworthy among them Otto Krautter, have made extensive studies in the analysis of the objective side of the creative function of children as it is expressed in their clay modeling. A number of psychotherapists have used clay modeling in one form or another as an adjunct to their psychotherapeutic technique for the individual child. In this connection we may refer to David M. Levy, J. Louise Despert, Berta Bornstein, and Steff Bornstein. Werner Wolff points to the use of clay as a medium for formative qualities and as an outlet for aggression. Herbert Read, also, has emphasized that plastic art belongs to the area of design or has adapted itself to formal patterning. Our experiences with clay have shown that it is particularly useful in dealing with body image problems, especially genital-anal ones, with consequent problems in social and interpersonal relationships.[33]

X. MUSIC AND DANCE[34]

Herbert Read emphasizes the importance of music and dance or eurhythmics in education. He amplifies the teachings of Emile Jacques Dalcroze who draws a parallel between music and life itself as being based on rhythm and time. Herbert Read also calls attention to the work of Heinz Werner in using music as a mode of free expression in education. He refers also to P. Lamparter who investigated the use of music as an index to the psychology of the child.

Music, in one form or another, is a recognized part of all school programs.

It also has long been acknowledged as a useful adjunct in all types of hospitals and institutions. Willem Van de Wall has given a detailed exposition of the use of music in institutions for the mentally sick, the mentally defective, delinquent adults, and children. The use of music in institutions for defective children is an organized and recognized means of recreation and social training.

XI. DRAMATIC PLAY

Susan Isaacs claims that in the free dramatic play of children they work out their inner conflicts in an external field, thereby lessening the pressure of conflict and diminishing feelings of guilt or anxiety. This dramatic play also makes it easier for the child to control his behavior and to accept the limitations of the real world, whereby the development of the ego and the sense of reality are furthered.

Melanie Klein in her psychoanalytic technique utilizes the child's spontaneous, dramatic play acting. The child may play by himself or with the analyst; he may use available toys and other objects for his make-believe play. One must read the whole of Melanie Klein's book on *The Psychoanalysis of*

---

[33] See Chapters 12 and 14 for our discussion of the use of clay modeling.

[34] Music and dance is discussed by Franziska Boas in Chapter 16.

Children to understand her psychoanalytic theory of the child's play acting. Even then it seems that she goes too far when she says "the theatre and performances of all kind have a universal symbolic significance for the coitus between the parents."[35]

Spontaneous play acting has been used by J. L. Moreno among institutionalized, delinquent girls as a means of personality development and resocialization. In his technique which he calls psychodrama a group of girls act out together various social situations. Through frequent changes each girl gets a chance to portray every character in the plot. Spontaneous dramatic play has also been used for both its socializing and therapeutic values on the adolescent boys' ward at the Psychiatric Division of Bellevue Hospital. Under the guidance of Frank J. Curran and a dramatic coach, the boys wrote their own plays, acted them out before the other patients on the ward, and afterwards participated in a group discussion under the leadership of the ward psychiatrist.

The psychotherapeutic qualities of dramatic play were described by Smith Ely Jeliffe in his study on psychoanalysis and the drama.

Puppets have been used extensively by us at Bellevue. Madeleine L. Rambert has also used them in psychoanalytic treatment with children in France.

XII. GESTALT PSYCHOLOGY

Since gestalt psychology deals essentially with the psychology of perception it has been highly significant in advancing the scientific understanding of the problems here dealt with. It has contributed largely to the data and concepts advanced in this book. The principles of form in perception and the concept of the "gute Gestalt" which were established by Max Wertheimer were essential, although our investigation led to different principles on the basis of the genesis of form perception in the developing child. Kurt Koffka in *The Growth of the Mind, an Introduction to Child Psychology,* has applied the principles of gestalt psychology to the developing mind of the child. Kurt Lewin, Heinz Werner, and Werner Wolff have applied gestalt psychology to the study of both the normal child and the deviate child.

Work on conceptual thinking and the configurations of emotions and memory has been done by David Rapaport and his co-workers. Werner Wolff has studied the personality of the pre-school child through drawings, using the concepts of gestalt psychology and emphasizing the importance of innate rhythmical perceptual experiences as a part of the dynamics in the growth of the personality. Herbert Read has recognized the significance of gestalt psychology for the concepts of esthetics, giving special cognizance to Wolfgang

---

[35] Klein, Melanie: Personification in the Play of Children, in *Contributions to Psychoanalysis,* 1948, p. 215.

Koehler's *The Place of Value in the World of Facts* in which he postulates a "psycho-physical isomorphism" to solve the problem of dualism versus monism, which is undoubtedly one of the most significant contributions of the gestalt psychology. Kurt Koffka also dealt with similar problems in the psychology of art.[36]

XIII. PERSONALITY TESTS

Personality tests of all types have been applied to the child. Ruth Bochner and Florence Halpern have analyzed and published children's Rorschach records for normal, defective, behavior problem, and psychotic children. Bruno Klopfer and M. A. Margulies have also described the Rorschach reactions in early childhood, and Mary Ford (1946) applied the Rorschach test to 123 normal children between the ages of three and eight years. Mary Leitch and Sarah Schafer have found that the Thematic Apperception Test is crucial for differentiating between psychotic and nonpsychotic illnesses in children. The psychotic responses tend to be characterized by incoherence, contradictions, queer ideas, verbalizations, overspecific statements, autistic logic, and overgeneralization.

Bruno Bettelheim claims that the Thematic Apperception Test is useful in diagnosis, education, and therapy because it frees association and helps to give the student insight into his defenses.

The use of batteries of personality tests is well exemplified in the work of William Goldfarb who studied children who had suffered from emotional deprivation by institutional care in infancy, comparing them with similar children raised in foster homes. His work throws considerable light on significant factors in personality development. Karen Machover has used the figure drawings as a personality test.

Werner Wolff's expression analysis of children's behavior and drawings is a personality exploration. Almost all of the projective techniques have been or may be used to explore personality. There are many applications of the various projective techniques to personality analysis in children.

XIV. PSYCHOANALYSIS

Psychoanalysis has brought techniques to child psychiatry from an entirely different source. The emphasis has been on the inner instinctual life and on unconscious mechanisms. In the beginning of Sigmund Freud's work many of the insights were, as they still are, derived from the psychoanalysis of adults. However, Freud's original *Three Contributions to the Theory of Sex* still hold with regard to the main principles in the development of children. The chief changes are that the beginnings of various stages of development

---

[36] *Bryn Mawr Symposium,* 1940.

must be placed further back at an earlier age. Thus, Melanie Klein has found evidences for superego development, anxiety, and aggressive drives against the mother's body, or the depressive position, well within the first year. But there has still not been a sufficient readiness to accept data so easily available from children, and there is still the tendency to try to take over interpretations from the memories of adults. In this way errors have been made which are hard to correct. Play techniques have shown that the classical free-association technique is not the only means of reaching into the unconscious.

The direct effects of different forms of relationship therapies, and the indirect evidences of the distortions of personality of children who have been without relationships in the early months of life clearly show that identifications and relationships are made within the first year of life. Such identifications and relationships can be used constructively or destructively for normal personality development, education, or therapy. Margaret Ribble's observations of infants show that the need for mothering, for sensory stimuli to skin and mucous surfaces, and for instinctual emotional gratification is present from the time of birth, and that the lack of such gratification may result in serious detriment to physical well-being and inhibition of personality development. The prescribing of such gratifications may well be looked upon as one of the psychotherapeutic techniques.

In 1940, the American Orthopsychiatric Association held a symposium with Goodwin Watson as chairman on Areas of Agreement in Psychotherapy. There was agreement as to objectives, in terms of "increasing the patient's capacity to deal with reality, to work, to love and to find meaning in life." There seemed also to be considerable agreement with the idea that the treatment should be directed at the structure of the personality and not at superficial symptoms. Melanie Klein in the last summarizing pages of her book on *The Psychoanalysis of Children,* speaks of the function of child analysis in terms of lessening anxiety and the pressure of the instinctual desires, of adjusting the superego, and of establishing an adequately strong ego. There has been well-known controversy between the two chief exponents of the field of child analysis, Melanie Klein and Anna Freud. Anna Freud tends to deviate from the Klein technique because she believes that the infantile ego is weak and that children do not develop a transference neurosis. She combines the analytic approach in which play techniques are utilized, with a general educational method.

Melanie Klein believes that a transference situation can be produced in children if the technique utilized is equivalent to an adult analysis; she avoids educational methods. She believes that her technique tends to strengthen the child's ego. Accordingly she places a strong emphasis upon early insistent interpretation of the child's play in psychosexual terms, stressing especially the primal scene or early observation of coitus between the parents. Play technique for children as a substitute for the free association and dream analysis used with adults, was apparently initiated by Melanie Klein. Nevertheless, Anna Freud made the most original contribution to the evolution of the personality, in her *The Ego and the Mechanisms of Defense*. During World War II in her reports from the Hempstead Nurseries she modified her approach to children's problems more and more realistically.

Susan Isaacs follows Melanie Klein but she takes psychoanalytic interpretations into the nursery school. They have all clung to certain of the original Freudian concepts that were deduced from adult analysis, and have continued to use the old terminology and concepts of instinctual psychology. These include the idea of an early sexual trauma or the primal scene of Melanie Klein, the idea of an aggressive (or death) instinct, of primary hostile aggression with instinctual anxiety, and the castration complex (especially as it refers to girls). A tendency to emphasize the negative emotions in children, and the failure to see the significance of form as well as symbolism in the normal development of children are some of the controversial issues.

Melanie Klein's contributions to psychoanalysis through the years 1920 to 1945 have been collected in one volume; the evolution of her theories provides a stimulating study. Her earlier formulations regarding superego development and the role of introjection are amplified and even more positively asserted. Basic to Mrs. Klein's philosophy is the concept that anxiety, guilt and depressive feeling are intrinsic elements of the child's emotional life, permeating all object relations to actual people as well as to their representatives in the inner world. From these introjected figures, the child's identification, the superego develops. The oedipus complex begins during the first year of life. The relationship to the mother's breast and later to the father's penis is taken as the starting point in this theory. In both sexes there is an inherent unconscious knowledge of the penis as well as of the vagina. From the beginning the infant introjects his objects, the primary imagos of his mother's breast and his father's penis. "Good" and "bad" breast and penis are introjected and represent protective and persecuting internal figures. Fear of the loss of the introjected loved object is seen as the core of infantile depressive feelings and the psychogenesis of depression in later life. Fear of internal attack and destruction by "bad" introjected figures is viewed as the psychogenesis of paranoia in the paranoid position at one and a half years.

A collection of Susan Isaacs' essays and clinical studies appeared in 1949. The point of view is very close to that of Melanie Klein. In the cases reported there is a great effort to reach the deep inner life of the child, and the technique used is described. Melanie Klein has written a summarizing article on the mechanisms of anxiety and guilt, and Susan Isaacs has written one on the mechanisms of phantasy in personality development. These articles tend to summarize the outstanding contributions that the two authors have made in regard to the deep inner life of the child, its genesis and evolution.

The Psychoanalytic Study of the Child, edited by Anna Freud, Heinz Hartmann and Ernst Kris, has appeared as a year-book since 1945, and now comprises five volumes. It has presented both theoretical considerations and the applications of various technical procedures to psychoanalytic practice in the understanding and treatment of the child.

A review of techniques of direct treatment of the child is given by Margaret Gerard in *Orthopsychiatry—1923 to 1948,* with concise descriptions of the methods of Melanie Klein, Anna Freud, August Aichorn, Max Gitelson, Frederick H. Allen, David M. Levy, and Lauretta Bender. Margaret Gerard's own approach, illustrated with case material, emphasizes the necessity for flexibility, a correct atmosphere, education, and in most cases an avoidance of direct interpretation in favor of indirect methods.

A review by Ernst Kris *On Psychoanalysis and Education* has brought together many of the significant concepts in psychoanalysis that bear on the development of the child's personality.

XV. PSYCHOSOMATIC STUDIES

Derived from psychoanalytic concepts, psychosomatic studies in many areas have been applied to the child. Hilde Bruch's studies of obesity in childhood are comprehensive and convincing. Hilde Bruch and Irma Hewlett have studied the diabetic child with less impressive results. The psychosomatic studies on fifty stuttering children (J. Louise Despert) were not convincing as far as the psychosomatic concepts were involved, although the application of the Ozeretsky motor test (Helen Kopp), the Rorschach study (Morris Krugman), and the analysis of the response on the revised Stanford-Binet (J. J. Carlson) were highly significant and gave a consistent picture of the personality and psychopathology of the stuttering child. Paul Deutschberger has made a report on the psychosomatic component in problem behavior which is also less convincing than M. F. Gates' comparative study of some problems of social and emotional adjustment of crippled and noncrippled boys and girls. Melitta Sperling has reported on the therapy of psychosomatic illness especially coeliac disease and ulcerative colitis. A very significant article by Therese Benedek discusses the psychosomatic implications of the symbiotic relationship between mother and child in pregnancy, birth, and the nursing period.

XVI. PEDIATRIC PSYCHIATRY

Psychoanalytic concepts and psychological studies have long been influencing pediatrics and the pediatrician's care of the infant. C. Anderson Aldrich and Mary M. Aldrich published their book *Babies Are Human Beings* in

1938. They defended the infant's right for gratification of its instinctive desires and needs.

Feeding disturbances in infants and children have been considered from a psychoanalytic point of view by Anna Freud.[37]

Feeding Behavior of Infants, a Pediatric Approach to Mental Hygiene of Early Life, by Arnold Gesell and Frances L. Ilg, is credited with making the change in child rearing from schedulized feeding, early conditioning in toilet training and repressive discipline to self-demand feeding, self-regulation in toilet training and permissive attitude toward maturation trends in behavior. Schedulized feeding methods tend to disturb the instinctual process of feeding and to dissociate the act from the powerful urge for pleasure with which it was originally associated. Because eating, more than any other bodily function, "is drawn into the circle of the child's emotional life and used as an outlet for libidinal and aggressive tendencies,"[38] it serves as fertile ground for neurotic superstructures. Considerate handling with a judicious amount of self-determination for the child will reduce vulnerability to neurotic development. D. W. Winnicott has discussed the early infant-mother relation with its implication for physical and mental health.

The transactions of the First Conference of the Macy Foundation on Problems of Early Infancy have been published, edited by Milton J. E. Senn. From the discussions of an authoritative group of contributors, four principal recommendations emerge: 1) anticipatory guidance for prospective parents; 2) the establishment of "rooming-in" projects for selected obstetrical cases; 3) a return to breast feeding; and 4) self-demand schedules. These can be considered as significant future trends for infant care.

Margaret E. Fries describes age-level tests for infants and children involving the presentation, removal and restoration of an object of gratification. The test for infants is oral, that for ages 1½ to 6 years, motor; older children are presented with a doll-family situation to encourage projective responses. The test conditions are designed to approximate life situations, and the results are considered an indication of the child's general mode of adjustment. The attempt to develop objective methods of study is a progressive step and points the way to further work. The close relationship between pediatric practice and child psychiatry is indicated and furthered in papers by C. Anderson Aldrich, Benjamin Spock, Edith B. Jackson, J. C. Montgomery, and L. H. Bartemeier in a symposium on pediatric psychiatry presented at the 1947 meeting of the American Orthopsychiatric Association. Hale F. Shirley published a *Psychiatry for Pediatricians,* 1948. There was a Commonwealth Fund Conference on the Mental Health Aspects of Pediatrics, the proceedings of which were edited (1948) by Helen L. Witmer.

---

[37] In *The Psychoanalytic Study of the Child,* Vol. II, 1947.
[38] Freud, Anna: Psychoanalytic Study of Infantile Feeding Disturbances, p. 119.

XVII. IN-PATIENT PSYCHIATRIC SERVICES

The first report on an in-patient service for children was by Howard Potter in 1935, when he described the psychiatric service for children at the New York State Psychiatric Institute.

In 1940 Frank J. Curran and Paul Schilder in a paper on *A Constructive Approach to the Problems of Childhood and Adolescence* made a survey of published studies for the preceding ten years from the children's and adolescent's wards in Bellevue Psychiatric Hospital. "In the course of a lengthy and extensive scientific program, the workers in Bellevue Psychiatric Hospital have acquired a general point of looking at problems of children and adolescents which might be of sufficient interest to others to be discussed in some detail."[39]

The survey described the various types of individual and group activities utilized on the children's and adolescent's wards of Bellevue Psychiatric Hospital. Detailed descriptions were given of organic problems, emotional problems, problems of the group, and the diverse forms of treatments utilized in the hospital. The correlation between the various theories of causation of emotional disorders and the treatment of the problems was pointed out, to show that theory and practice should go hand in hand. There should be close relationship between individual and group treatment. Group therapy in the form of puppet projects and dramatic activities is useful. Free expression of rhythmic patterns in perceptual, motor, and emotional fields is provided by dancing and music classes. Group discussions provide relief from the child's fears and anxieties by sharing of mutual experiences, and by the conviction of social approval. Intensive individual treatment, where it is indicated, progresses more rapidly on the background of organized group interests.

Lawson G. Lowrey, in *Psychiatry for Children—a Brief Historical Development* (1944), outlined the origins of the first institutions having in-patient services for children.

The number of in-patient psychiatric services for children is increasing steadily and there have been numerous reports on the organization of these services and on the kinds of program that they offer the children. These reports have come from the following sources: 1) J. Franklin Robinson, Children's Service Center of Wilkes-Barre, Pa.; 2) Kathleen K. Stewart, Pearl L. Axelrod, and S. A. Szurek, Langley Porter Clinic of San Francisco; 3) Wrenshall A. Oliver, Napa State Hospital of California; 4) Anne Benjamin and Howard Weatherly, Children's Ward, Psychiatric Division of the Illinois Neuropsychiatric Institute in collaboration with the Institute of Juvenile Research; 5) Helen A. Sutton, who presented some of the nursing

---

[39] From the Introduction to *A Constructive Approach to the Problems of Childhood and Adolescence*, p. 125, 1940. Portions of this paper are quoted here. Further sections will appear in full in this and subsequent volumes.

aspects on the same service; 6) Bruno Bettelheim and Emmy Sylvester, Orthogenic School, University of Chicago; 7) Charles Bradley, Emma Pendleton Bradley Home, East Providence, Rhode Island; and 8) Kenneth Cameron, Maudsley Hospital, London. Most of these reports concern themselves with the importance of the therapeutic tone of the school or hospital ward, the participation of the total staff, the beneficial effects of group living, and the opportunities for group therapy.

After 15 years of experience with some 8,000 problem children brought to the children's ward at the Psychiatric Division of Bellevue Hospital, we regard the behavior and development in the child as a continuous flow of patterned and patterning experiences within a relationship involving the inner life of the child and the outer world of people, objects, and concepts. Deviations occur at any point because of disturbances in the continuous flow in the patterning, or in the relationship.

XVIII. CLASSIFICATION OF PROBLEM CHILDREN

We have found that the problem children of New York City who have come to this service can be classified according to the following etiological factors:

1. An inadequate or distorted child-parent relationship during the critical infantile and early childhood period due to a) the absence of one or both parents; b) the presence of a seriously neurotic, psychopathic, alcoholic, or psychotic parent; c) parents who are otherwise antisocial, aggressive, or inadequate. These conditions result in neurotic behavior disorders or other psychoneurotic reactions.

2. A critical emotional-social deprivation during infancy with no continuous relationship to a mother figure, e.g., early institutional care or critical breaks in the continuity of mother-infant relationships so that normal identification processes for social conceptualization do not develop. This leads to the psychopathic behavior disorders.

3. Belonging to a minority social group with all that this implies in economic insecurity, conflicts in identification within one's own family group and with the larger social group of the accepted culture. Related factors are the greater instability in family structure, lack of privileges in social and educational experiences, discrepancies in social ideologies, and often in addition, a language problem.

4. Special language or intellectual problems such as retardation in the development of language (especially reading disabilities), or specific intellectual defects interfering with adequate identification and competition with the group. Cultural differences in language may function in the same way. When the language difficulty occurs at the early critical period of personality development it tends to distort the whole personality. Difficulties in pattern-

ing in all fields of behavior are usually coexistent with language disabilities.

5. The various organic pathological states which may interfere with normal intellectual and personality integration, thereby reducing the margin of adaptability, and creating more or less severe frustrations and consequent anxiety. These include all the encephalopathies—congenital, progressive inflammatory, and traumatic. Schizophrenia may also be included in this group. Except when an organic process is heredodegenerative, or the loss of tissue is great, or there is associated a progressive epilepsy; the response to treatment is more favorable than is generally realized, provided that one or more of the other factors do not also exist.

The children who are brought to Bellevue usually present a combination of two or more of the above factors. In general, children have a remarkable capacity to withstand difficult situations and disabilities, especially if they have the support of a sustaining relationship with some adult.

XIX. THERAPEUTIC NEEDS OF PROBLEM CHILDREN

When children with such problems come to the children's ward at Bellevue Hospital their therapeutic needs may be analyzed as follows:

1. A child-adult relationship on some realistic basis, i.e., with a psychiatrist, teacher, or nurse responsible for the ward routine. Through this relationship they may be able to work through, unconsciously or consciously, their identification problems. The relationship should run its normal course; there should be free and gratifying expression of affection and relationship appropriate to the level of personality development, i.e., good comradeship with hero identification in the latency or puberty period, accompanied by occasional mothering gestures, and a good deal of frank mothering (or fathering) for the more immature, infantile or childish levels of development, regardless of the chronological or mental age.

2. Group experiences with contemporaries, in which the individual personality finds its own place in an interchange of personality needs. There may be successful competition, a passive need for support from a stronger child-personality, means for mutual identification or rivalry, objects for social imitation, leadership, or punishment.

3. Opportunities for the projection, formulation, or living out of the inner fantasy life by means of projective or play techniques. This is what Lawrence K. Frank speaks of as "Multiplicity of methods and procedures which will reveal the many facets of the personality and show how the individual structuralizes his life span or organizes his experience to meet his personal needs in various media."[40] The children need the experience of experimenting by trial and error with new formulations of personality mechanism and of conflicts, by the use of various raw materials, and in controlled group situa-

---

[40] Frank, Lawrence K.: *Projective Methods for the Study of Personality.*

tions where they can check their experiences with those of others. They need opportunities to enrich their concepts and fantasy material from literature, folk lore, comics, and other fields, especially with data that is timely and appropriate to the human problems of the culture in which they are living.

4. Expansion of intellectual, motor, and language patterns; acquisition of new techniques of acting, thinking, feeling, and living from educational formulas and projects, organized games, and cultural patterns.

5. A well-established pattern of daily routine based on the child's biological rhythms and the cosmic, institutional and cultural pattern. This offers the best form of security and discipline through experiencing a readily anticipated flow of action on a recognizable background with a meaningful pattern.

6. An adequate specific evaluation by the hospital staff of all factors which interfere with normal development, which result in frustrations, and which prove to be the cause of deviate behavior. Also the correction of all remediable factors with appropriate treatment from any field of medicine or education including psychotherapy.

XX. PSYCHOTHERAPEUTIC TECHNIQUES TO MEET THE NEEDS OF PROBLEM CHILDREN

The various psychotherapeutic techniques or procedures which may be used to meet these needs in a general way include:

1. A well-organized psychiatric hospital ward,[41] study home or resident school in which the entire program for the children is organized in a realistic situation with school, recreational and ward routine or housekeeping activities. The staff of adults should be adequate in number, and especially trained in both their own field of activity (psychiatry, teaching, puppetry, dramatics, etc.) as well as in the general field of child psychology. They should expect to give themselves continually in a warm relationship to the children.

All activities should be group activities with an accepted adult to represent the leader, teacher or parent substitute, and with the acceptance of other children for identification or rivalry.

Group discussions of ideologies, especially those pertinent to the group, and the minority representatives in the group. These discussions should be timely. For example, during the war the special problem of the war and how it concerned one's own family problems and its relation to the general problem of aggression was brought up for discussion.

It should be emphasized that group therapy is not time conserving for the therapist. It is not easier, nor can the therapist treat more patients in less or the same time and get better results. Group therapy does not mean the loss

---

[41] See Chapter 12 for description of the specific experiences which we have had on the Children's Service of the Psychiatric Division of Bellevue Hospital.

of individual identifications in the group. On the contrary, group therapy is the most difficult form of therapy and is therefore seldom used in an adequate way. It entails many more relationships between each child and all the other children and the adult therapist. The therapist must participate in all of these relationships. Among problem children, spontaneous group phenomena are always developing. They need to be observed, understood, and allowed to take their time to develop into a total experience. Group therapy may be time conserving for the patient if it is adequately done; through it he may get more speedy relief from his disturbances. This is its chief justification since time is a most important factor in children where development proceeds so fast and regressions and infantile fixations quickly interfere with the demands of growth and the attainment of a new stage in maturity.

4. Projective techniques with all types of raw materials and with miniature toys may be included in various forms of play therapy, such as graphic and plastic art, music, puppets, drama, and as many other activities as anyone has the ingenuity to utilize. The therapist must clearly understand what children at each age level can do with each medium used, and in each cultural situation, and what any deviation from such normal patterns means. With the projective techniques, supplemented by the careful observation and preservation of fragments of behavior, one can build a picture of the total life pattern of the child, his problems and his progress in the therapeutic situation.[42] The adult definitely belongs to and is a part of this situation. Treatment techniques are not gadgets to be used merely as time, labor, and energy-saving devices for the therapist. Nor are they to be used as barriers between the child and the therapist. Unless the technique makes demands on the therapist, brings him into a closer relationship with the child, increases both his and the child's experiences, it should not be used.

5. Play therapy can be organized to follow any special plan or pattern, such as release therapy, insight or affect therapy.

6. Relationship therapy is of course the background of most of the techniques, but it may be especially emphasized in some situations by some therapists (Frederick H. Allen).

7. Hypnotherapy may be used to speed up therapeutic procedures by increasing the relationship and the expression of fantasy projection.

8. Chemotherapy, narcotherapy, and shock therapy are not ordinarily psychotherapeutic by themselves. They are adjuncts to treatment and in suitable cases shorten the time of treatment and facilitate relationships by relieving anxiety and aiding in the acquisition of new patterns of thinking, feeling and acting. All the other needs of the child have still to be met, and no program should be considered satisfactory which keeps the psychiatrist busy with mechanical procedures.

---

[42] See Chapter 18 on the therapy of an individual child utilizing the projective techniques, etc.

9. Remedial tutoring in reading, speech, or language is one of the most important factors in therapeutic approach to a large number of children who come to the attention of psychiatric clinics, hospitals or correctional schools.

10. Medical and psychosomatic therapies appropriate to the child's own condition are important and are a necessary part of any total therapy program.

11. Environmental therapies where one treats or otherwise modifies the attitudes, relationships, behavior, and programs of parents, teachers, and other adults in the child's life.

12. Conferences in which the child appears are a positive therapeutic factor, not sufficiently appreciated.[43] Staff conferences in which the child does not participate and which are based instead on long reports too often turn out to be therapeutic not to the child but only to the adults participating. They tend to take the adults away from the child for too large a part of the time.

Finally, the task for any child psychiatrist as a diagnostician and psychotherapist, whether he is functioning in an individual role as a private practitioner or in a group institutional setup, is to know the child who comes to him, his cultural background and the social ideologies of the group to which he belongs, the specific family problems important in the child's lifetime, the educational theories and techniques to which the child is exposed, his own group and interpersonal relationships. Then he must know how to evaluate the biological data on the child, his somatic equipment and total neurological functioning especially in terms of motility, impulse regulation, mannerisms, neurological deviations, and patterned functioning. He must know the child's intellectual level with any special disabilities and their meaning in the total picture and its special abilities or compensatory abilities. It is also necessary to evaluate discrepancies in functions and what they mean and be able to compare them through a battery of test situations in order to get a pattern or profile of functioning. The child's personality development and any discrepancies with other maturational functions, his fantasy life, handling of anxiety, identifications, striving and goals—all must be understood. Any deviation at any point must be traced through the total personality to seek out syndromes which may lead to a specific diagnosis, implying a course of treatment, an outcome, and a specific treatment program.[44] Diagnosis must be further checked with therapeutic tests and the final evaluation made in terms of the child's needs for treatment and his ability to use the treatment procedure available. The successful application of the therapeutic technique must be determined by the proper evaluation of the child's problems and needs and by the utilization of the particular technique to satisfy those needs and to solve those problems.

---

[43] See Bowman, Karl M.: *The Psychiatrist Looks at the Child Psychiatrist.*

[44] Special therapeutic procedures for specific syndromes or conditions will not be dealt with in this book.

FORM AS A PRINCIPLE IN
THE PLAY OF CHILDREN[1]

WHEN one watches children at play, one soon observes that there are certain principles that appear again and again. Children often take toys such as carts, trains, etc., and move them on the ground with outstretched arms in a curve or in a half circle, the center of which is the shoulder joint. The plane on which the play takes place appears to be one factor, the characteristics of the motor apparatus is another. Heinrich Kluever has observed drawings in monkeys which are determined by similar principles. In the next chapter it will be shown that motility is a factor in determining the form in children's sidewalk drawings and games. In hopscotch the curved form is drawn with outstretched arms with the body as a pivot, and the figure in which the play takes place is determined by the range of jumping on one leg. Rotation around the longitudinal axis is one of the basic forms of movements. Wolfgang Koehler has described whirling as a form of play in apes. The principle of rotation is demonstrated in the movements of the circular joints—the shoulder, the hip and to some degree also in the hand. In parietal lobe lesions with spontaneous turning on the longitudinal axis, Hans Hoff and Paul Schilder also observed a tendency for rotation in movements in the circular joints.[2]

Specific motor tendencies find an expression in the play of children. The motility adapts itself to the plane on which the play takes place. The formation of foreground and background is basic for the play of children. When a child gets a number of lead soldiers or other toys for play, the form of its play is partially determined by the form of the field in which the play takes place.

On the ward, Joey, aged 3½, put soldiers near to the border on the table and also on the bench. He also transferred them to the border of the wash

---

[1] Bender, Lauretta and Schilder, Paul: reprinted from *The Journal of Genetic Psychology,* 49:254-261, 1936.

[2] Subsequent to the writing of this paper, we developed the concept that the whirling on the longitudinal axis in childhood schizophrenia was the characteristic motility of the schizophrenic child, already suggested by Paul Schilder, and was in part, at least, the basis for body image problems, "ego boundary" problems and many other psychological problems. See Bender, Lauretta. *Childhood Schizophrenia,* 1947.

Joseph B. Teicher, with the assistance of Paul Schilder studied the motility of 200 children 4 to 13 years of age on our wards; he also reviewed the literature pertaining to motility of children.

basin. He put a horse in the center of a small desk calendar. He pressed the head of the horse against the cork of a closed ink bottle as if trying to push it in and said, "I push him in this." He even attempted to put the soldier parallel to the vertical wall and was disappointed when it did not stay in this position. The geometrical and physical qualities of a given field are determining factors in the play of children. The instance of the ink bottle shows that the form of the object is another determining factor. It becomes a symbol of something into which one can push something else. Later the more primitive geometrical forms will again be considered. This child liked clusters of three men around a horse. He arranged soldiers in a row. He put a soldier in each of three corners of the wash basin. He arranged soldiers and tongue depressors in forms of incomplete symmetry so that he got primitive arrangements of clusters, rows, or an irregular star.

The observation of this child attempting to place the toys against the wall makes it clear that experiments with gravitational qualities are factors which have to be considered in the play of children. This child at first did not understand the significance of gravity. For Nora, 4 years, and Rita, 3 years, pushing objects over or allowing them to fall in play was a great pleasure. These are instances of active experimentation with gravity.

There is no question but that the play of these children also had another meaning. Joey was continually giving commands to the toys which he put in specific places. In the play of the two little girls, their delight in asserting their power and aggressiveness was obvious. The formal elements are, of course, not isolated parts of psychic life but are parts of the biological orientation of children. Knocking toys down satisfied the aggressive impulses of the children but it also helped to a better handling of problems of physical laws connected with gravitation. Whether an object is to be upright or is to lie down is partially a moral problem (aggression and submission), but it is also a problem of physics and of the orientation of the individual with regard to gravity and the physical world. Orientation means (for man) not only perception and knowledge but includes also the motor side of the adaptation of the individual.

Larry, 4 years, and Russell, 5 years, showed a great interest in replacing into an upright position the dolls that had fallen down. Whenever the examiner pushed a doll down, Russell would stand it up again. Immediately after this play, Larry noticed a man cleaning the windows and said, "He will fall down."

In children's later development there is a tendency for clusters to develop into more symmetrical forms. The matching of objects plays a great part. Objects which are similar in shape and color are put into groups. This was shown, for example, by Vivian, 9 years. Her play with china toys consisted entirely in arranging them in different symmetrical forms on the table and in moving them from one form to the text, sometimes transporting them by means of tiny carts.

Mention has been made that Joey, 3½ years, showed a tendency to push the horse into the ink bottle. In older children, the tendency to put lead soldiers into carts, either lying down or standing, was found. They tried to pile in as many soldiers as possible, sometimes shoving the soldiers in rather roughly. It was a great satisfaction for them to have as many in the car as possible. If there were both bigger and smaller cars, the smaller cars were put into the larger cars as well. Emmanuel, 5 years old, for instance, puts one car in the other and says he will put them in the garage. The same principle can be observed in older children as will be noted from the following protocol from Charles, 11 years, a boy with average intelligence:

> They had a war—the Americans and Indians. I am on the side of the Americans because that is my nationality. (*What is the matter with the Indians?*)[3] They can't fight so good. I am only playing with them. Here is the battlefield (puts all the soldiers in carts and puts them in another position). Bang Bang. The guy is dead. (The Americans kill four Indians; one Indian knocks down an American.) They are having a war because they don't like Indians . . . (he puts the small racer in the big truck). That is the place where they carry things because they can't carry them with their hands; they are too big. (He lines all the vehicles up and lines the soldiers up along the edge of the table.) I am going to put some over here, too. (In a later course of the play he places vehicles in a series whereas they were parallel before. He likes to give orders to his lead soldiers. He always arranges the soldiers in groups.)

This protocol shows an elaboration of the same form principles which we found in the younger children. The elaboration partly consists in adding meaning to the formal situation. This tendency is already present in the younger children. They put a soldier, for instance, in a car "because he is dead" or "tired" or "he has gone home." One gets the impression that the formal principle of putting something in something is more basic and is merely exemplified by the meaning that is added.

Children are never satisfied with any form that is reached. One form is merely a transition to a chaos, that is, putting the toys into an unorganized heap. But new organization is immediately sought again. For the older children, the groups of the materials have a definite meaning as for instance a group of soldiers, pirates, or Indians. In younger children, however, grouping as such is the main purpose. Although the same principles reappear in the new groupings, the new grouping is never completely identical with the previous one. Joey, 3½ years old, brought soldiers and tongue depressors together in a symmetrical form without comment, the older children usually gave some definite meaning to their groupings. It is as if they were trying to

---

[3] Questions by the psychiatrist to the child are italicized.

adapt the formal principles better to the total situation and to its meaning. In this respect it is particularly interesting to follow the development of a situation which we have called the automobile test.[4] A man is put between three cars which are so placed that the front ends are all pointing towards the man. In the younger children the man and the cars are pushed about without much regard for the inner quality and meaning of the objects. Children start to move the car, or at any rate to imagine a movement which corresponds to the structure and position of the cars. In such an experiment where James, 7 years, and Dorothy, 9 years, are present, the girl starts running the car, the boy runs the man down with a car and puts him into another car. (*What did you do?*) "I knocked him down, he was run over, the guy was carrying him." (*Why did you stand him up again?*) "He will be run over again," said Dorothy. "The car will run over him and he will be dead." In the midst of a discussion about death, Dorothy kisses the smaller car and says, "Because it is so little." She puts it in another car and says, " I don't want it to get knocked over." The car with its momentum needs to be played with, according to its structure. It carries with it an immediate pattern for aggressiveness but only older children are able to grasp this situation. The younger ones express aggression by merely knocking over. Of course a complicated object like a car does not merely carry the meaning of aggression in it, but it is also, as mentioned before, a vessel and a container. The definite meaning of an object, of course, depends on the total situation.

The following protocol of Emmanuel, 5 years old, is given as an example of this discussion:

(A cowboy is placed between two cars in front of Emmanuel.) He says: It bumps him. He better watch out—because—he is dead. (He knocks down the car.) Fall down car. (Several other cars are now put at his disposal and he piles up the cars.) I am making something. Put this one on top because it fell down. Goes slow because it is broke. (He lines up the little cars against the wall.) It will crack. (Knocks a big car against a little one.) Now it cracks. (Piles them up again.) Now I make a car. (He puts a little car in a big one.) It is broke— I tell you so many times. It broke itself, I say. All the cars broke. Put it in the garage and get it fixed. I bring it back. (Gets men and puts them in the larger car.) They are garage men to fix the car. (The next day he gets a set of lead soldiers with carts and wooden toys representing the various members of a circus. He puts all the toys in the largest cart including the smaller carts. He looks all over the floor for more toys.) This is the march. (He lines all of the circus toys on one side and the lead soldiers on the other side and knocks over the circus toys and then the lead soldiers.) They knock down, they go to sleep. I fix them all over. (He puts all the lead toys and the circus toys in the cart again. He puts small autos, soldiers, elephants, etc., all in the larger cart. Then he knocks them all out again.) They are dead. They got run over.

---

[4] See also Bender, Lauretta and Schilder, Paul: *Studies in Aggression,* 1936, p. 423.

In a little older age group, the consideration for the actual meaning of the toys is greater. The following is the protocol of a play session with Amad, age 9 years, and Leon, age 7 years:

Leon: (Two cars and a man.) The car is going to run the good guy over. He will die.

Amad: He don't die. He will get hurt and they bring him to the hospital and he will get better and when he sees that truck again he gets that man and kills him.

Leon: That man is going to break the car up and burn the man in the car so it won't run over him no more. (*How can he if he is dead?*) The car got electric and burns him up. The car could fall. The feet must go on the electric and then the car could fall. This car was coming and he was strong, and he went back that way, then that car comes and he don't see it and he gets hurt and they bring him to the hospital. He gets better, sees the truck, burns it up, puts it on fire and brings it in the river, makes the motor go.

Amad: He puts dynamite under it, then ran away.

Leon: The car is coming and the man is going across and the car got the man run over, and the man got hurt. The car went right on the man's foot and the man got a broken foot. They bring him to the hospital. They gave him a stick and a foot to walk. When he sees the car he is going to take the wheels off and the motor off and put it on his car, and break that car and put it in the river.

Leon: (Presented with an irregular arrangement of several figures with a small car.) This is a good guy. This is a bad guy. This guy is going to kill this guy with a knife, so that he comes with all the guns and he is going to shoot that guy. (The play becomes increasingly violent and many more of the lead soldiers are considered as dead and piled into the car.)

The purely formal elements are decidedly subordinated and integrated to the mental content. Only when the play progresses do the more primitive form elements come more and more into the foreground. The play satisfied those instinctual tendencies of the children which correspond to the form of the play. In the instances given the aggressiveness of the children is able to express itself in play.

It is characteristic of the children never to be satisfied with any less than all the playthings which are available. They want to get everything that is to be had, otherwise they are restless and dissatisfied. The child is only temporarily satisfied when he has got everything that is in the room. The children often ask where the toys come from and whether we could not buy all the toys in the store for them. The following protocol is very characteristic:

Russell, 5 years old, was an aggressive, overactive child with inferior intelligence (IQ 71) and Larry, 4 years old, average intelligence, was usually shy and quiet in the hospital but had come in with a history of temper tantrums at home. The examiner knocks a doll over in the presence of the children.

Larry: Take another one.

Russell: Me take another one.

Larry: Look at the two here.

Russell: Me throw it down. Stand it up. One doll. Two dolls. Stand up one doll. (When the doll falls down very easily, the chief interest of the children is to get it into an upright position. Whenever the examiner pushes the doll down, Russell stands it up again and takes it in his hand. He is rather petulant. Larry takes the dolls in his hand in a protective way. He picks up the lead soldiers and looks at them very carefully. Russell wants everything immediately. He insists on it.) Give me all the mans. (When the toys are taken out of the drawer he does not want the toys which are given to him but tries to take other toys out of the examiner's pocket. Larry does not show any constructive effort to play. He merely takes everything to himself in a rather protective manner and only lets a car run slowly over the table. He is careful not to let the cars collide. Russell, meanwhile, had apparently forgotten that he wanted dolls out of the examiner's pocket, but he is readily reminded of it. He puts his hand in the examiner's pocket and says, "No more, only matches." He appears to be disappointed. Larry asks for the horse, "Let's see the horse." Russell immediately loses interest in what he has. Russell has a definite reaction pattern in that he wants everything and once he has it he is not interested in it any more.)

Russell: The bad boy won't give me the cars. Russell is somewhat dominated by the idea that something is being withheld from him. In order to get the cars he takes two pieces of paper and gives them to Larry. When Larry finally gives him the things he has no more interest in what he has asked for. Russell offers Larry the broken legs of a doll. The interest in getting something he hasn't got makes active play for him completely impossible. He wants to get the last thing that the other boy has. When something is given to Larry, Russell immediately becomes excited. Finally he gives Larry the broken legs of the doll again with a great gesture of generosity. Larry could be induced to give the other boy everything.

In play Larry seems to put the lead soldiers together without putting them in any action. He is careful to avoid knocking any of the figures over. He does not protest when one toy after another is taken away. He takes two trucks and when given a doll which is named Doris, his sister's name, he makes a noise with his mouth, plays with the larger car and tries to put the doll in the car. He is shy and does not even dare to take off the doll's hat. When the examiner pushes the doll over, he heaps the two cars upon her abdomen and face and he continues to play, covering the dolls with cars. Finally he brings the car near the doll, which is now standing, but does not push her down. He brings it as near as he can. The examiner pushes the doll down with the car, and he repeats it. He lets the doll fall down rather carefully. When he plays he is careful not to come too near the doll. He frequently covers the doll up with the cars.

He sees a man cleaning windows and says, "He will fall down." This is a child who restricts himself in movements to small and rhythmic expressions. He is not very active in play. After he left the room, he had a severe temper tantrum in the nursery. Later when he was sought out he was found smeared with his feces.

It is evident that the emotional problems and the formal problems cannot be completely separated. The child's experimentation with form and configuration is an expression of its tendencies to come to a better handling of objects by action. By trial and error the child comes to an insight into the structure of objects. To the structure of the objects belong also the general spatial qualities, the law of gravitation, push and momentum. The child has to learn about lines, series, and groups. Furthermore, when something can be put into something else the child is learning about form in general. It is remarkable that the same gestalt rules apply to the play of children as we have found in spontaneous drawings and sidewalk games[5] and also in the visual motor gestalt experiences.[6] These form problems lead to emotional problems—problems of destruction, preservation and protection. We are of the opinion that the emotional problems and the so called form problems are in essence identical. One could consider the problems of impact and putting one thing into another as specifically sexual problems as, for example, Melanie Klein has done. She sees every collision in the play of children as a symbolic reference to parental intercourse. If one puts emphasis merely on the sexual interpretation, one neglects biological connections which are at least as important as the sexual. One could with some justification consider the child's interest concerning parental intercourse as an application of its general interest in impact and in putting one thing inside of another. In the children in our group in which this play method could be used (under 10 years of age) we found no difference between boys and girls in this respect. The specific life history of the individual child often determined the particular formal principles which were used. In one of our children the motif of attacking from behind was conspicuous. In some children the impact problem plays the greater part; in others the tendency to put things into other things. In other words there is a general trend of psychophysiological organization which is not rigid but is rather a mode of procedure adaptable to the biological situation.

SUMMARY

The play of children is determined by the possible motor and perceptual patterns of the organism. Rotation of the body around its longitudinal axis and circular movements of outstretched limbs are of special importance. The motility adapts itself to the plane on which the play takes place. The play starts

---

[5] See Chapter 3.
[6] See Chapters 4 and 5.

with the formation of foreground and background. The child undertakes a continuous experimentation with regard to the geometrical qualities of lines, angles and clusters. In three-dimensional play the child is particularly interested in whether something can be put into something else. Further experimentation concerns gravitation, push, pull, and momentum. The experimentation with space and mass (geometry and physics) is based upon the instinctive drives of children and is accordingly dependent upon their individual problems. The definite form of the play is adaptable to the biological situation. Form principles reflect merely the general plan of psychophysiological organization.

~ 3 ~

FORM PRINCIPLES IN THE SIDEWALK DRAWINGS AND GAMES OF CHILDREN[1]

CHILDREN'S drawings have been studied extensively from many viewpoints, and these studies have thrown much light on the conceptual and intellectual development of the child. Florence Goodenough was able to standardize children's drawings of a man and thereby has produced a simple and satisfactory test for the child's intellectual level of development. Before her, however, James Sully in 1897 had made a valuable study of children's drawings at different developmental stages; he arrived at conclusions very similar to those established by Goodenough's more systematized study. He outlined three stages: 1) There is an early stage of vague formless scribblings as the result of an aimless to-and-fro swaying of the pencil producing a chaos of slightly curved lines. These scribblings are purely spontaneous and have no resemblance to any model presented. They may accidentally resemble some form and be given a name, or the child may make believe that they have meaning which is arbitrarily given. Wilhelm Preyer's child[2] in his second year said that he was "writing houses" while he was scribbling in this fashion. 2) There is a second stage of primitive circular design best characterized by lunar schemes of the human face. This is gradually evolved from the first stage as the curved lines become loops, and crudely placed dots indicate that the relationship of features is more important than their details. Trunk and limbs are entirely unimportant (see Fig. 3b). 3) In the third stage there is a more sophisticated treatment of the human form. James Sully makes the interesting observation that the early pictorial forms of human beings have an embryonic configuration. He concludes that the child as an artist is more of a symbolist than a naturalist.

The report of investigations the world over shows a remarkable constancy

---

[1] Rewritten from *The Pedagogical Seminar and Journal of Genetic Psychology*, **41**:192-210, 1932.

Since this paper was written in 1932, there have been noteworthy contributions in this field, especially Wolf, Werner: *The Personality of the Pre-school Child.* He studied expressive activity in young children in various areas of behavior but especially in their drawings, analyzed them on the basis of gestalt principles, and based his thesis of the development of the personality of the child on this material. Many of Kurt Lewin's students use children's drawings for their studies. See Chapter I, pp. 15-17.

[2] Preyer, Wilhelm: *Die Seele des Kindes*, 1882.

See Dennis, Wayne: *The Historical Beginnings of Child Psychology*, for the earliest studies pertinent to this subject.

in the order of development both in regard to the method of indicating separate items and their relationship to each other, and in regard to the order in which these items and relationships tend to appear. George S. Rouma (1912) made one of the most extensive studies and included the productions of subnormal children. He found that the drawings of these children were similar to those of younger children and were characterized by frequent regressions to the inferior stages with special emphasis on automatisms, flight of ideas, fragmentation, meticulousness, and frequent recurrences of the same form.

Careful studies of individual children were an important source of information in the early stages of research in this field. In 1913 J. M. Baldwin reported the course of his daughter's development in her ability to draw from the 19th to the 27th month. At the earliest age there was the "simplest and vaguest and most general imitation of the teacher's movements, not the tracing of the mental picture. There was no semblance of conformity between the child's drawing and the copy. She could not identify it herself."[3] He found that at the 19th month there were only sweeping, whole-arm movements from the shoulder. A few months later she began to flex the elbow and wrist and at 27 months she was able to manipulate her fingers. At that time her productions were made of loops in the clock-wise direction with an emphasis on the horizontal plane. In each new drawing there was a tendency to carry over a whole or a part of the previous drawing. The motor functions appeared to develop somewhat separate from the perceptive functions. Similar observations were made by Wilhelm Preyer in 1888 and 1889 of the development of his son.

W. Ament (1926) found that at three years of age there is no resemblance between the child's drawing and the model. Later the first recognizable drawings were of a man made up of loop units, and then of animals made in the same way. Some of Ament's illustrations of children's drawings of animals are of particular interest. They were made in such a way that there was a long horizontal loop for the body and a small round loop at the left side for the head, but the body loop extending to the right was bent around a little and was terminated by a curling tail that bent with the whole figure in a clock-wise direction. Near the head was the first small loop for a leg and this was perseverated five or six times without regard for the natural number of legs. All were curved with the figure in a clock-wise direction so that the whole gave the marked impression of a whirl or vortical design. In the same way the child made a stork, cow, pig, mouse, dog, and cat. Marie W. Shinn in following the development of her niece, 1893 to 1897, found that the child could recognize "O" in her 12th and 13th month although she then tended to confuse this letter with "C" and "Q," which, however, she learned

---

[3] Baldwin, James M.: *Social and Ethical Implications of Mental Development.*

to distinguish in the next few weeks. In the 109th week she drew circles in imitation of her aunt's arm movements and made many spontaneous scribblings back and forth over each other.

Florence Goodenough from a careful analysis of published studies and from her own material concluded that in young children there is a relationship between concept development as shown in drawings, and general intelligence. Drawing is primarily a language or form of expression for the child. In the beginning he draws what he knows. This is the ideoplastic stage of M. Verworn (1907). Later the child attempts to draw what he sees; this is the physioplastic stage. The features of the ideoplastic stage are seen in the child's tendency to exaggerate items that seem important or interesting, and to minimize or omit the other parts. The child pays little attention to the details of the object before him. Florence Goodenough summarized her psychological interpretation of children's drawings as follows: Association by familiarity; analysis and evaluation of component parts and their spatial relationship and proportions; judgment of the same; abstraction, reduction, and simplification of parts; coordination of eye and hand movements; adaptability.

These conclusions were influenced in part by those of G. Paulsson (1923) that "meaning" is the guide to graphic structure in the child's development from the primitive schematic stage to the highest manifestation of the artistic mind; that association by similarity is an important part in graphic art, and that the first impulse towards graphic expression has its origin in the desire for emotional outlet and in the pleasure derived from objectivation of emotions.

A much earlier analysis by L. S. Cushman (1908) seems to give us more insight into the subject. She said, "All the fine arts have this in common—they interpret the human mind. This mind is so constituted that it seeks organization of the material with which it deals. Therefore logical unity or arrangement is the basic principle of all art. In those parts which appeal through the eye the unity must be spatial. This unity is more important than detail."[4] Coming as early as 1908, this is an interesting anticipation of the gestalt theory of sensory organization. Of course Wolfgang Koehler goes much further, stating that "order and distribution in the sensory field is in each case the result of sensory dynamic interactions," and "that all experienced order in space is a true representation of corresponding order in the underlying dynamic context of the physiological process."[5]

The classical statement that the "child draws what he knows, not what he sees" seems to have had undue influence on the psychological interpretation of children's drawings. It is obviously unfair to the child, who knows

---

[4] Cushman, L. S.: *The Art Impulse, Its Form and Relation to Mental Development.*
[5] Koehler, Wolfgang: *Gestalt Psychology.*

a great deal more than he draws. Thus Florence Goodenough herself points out the fact that the small child can recognize his mother or even a small photograph of his mother, although neither he nor indeed most adults could tell by what details or combination of details this is possible; nor could he or most adults draw a recognizable picture of the mother, either from life or by copying a photograph. Or again, as Goodenough points out, a child of three years can point to his own hair or that in a good picture, but he almost invariably omits the hair when he draws a picture of a man.

It thus becomes apparent that what the child knows is based on perceptual and therefore conceptual recognition of certain constellations or gestalten that have significance for him, and that this capacity is not based upon his recognition or analysis or evaluation of details as such, but of their relationship to each other and to his whole world. On the other hand, his graphic representation of his world is based on his ability to make symbols that represent these relationships of parts, and their total meaning to him. This ability is one that, even in the average adult, falls far below what he knows about his world. The problem, therefore, and one to be discussed fully later,[6] is to discover the mechanisms for the origins of the graphic symbols.

Of course, in such a problem there are both motor and sensory elements so interwoven that they cannot be separated, which form an organized perceptual motor pattern. Kurt Koffka has pointed out that even during development all motor acquisitions have a sensory component, and it is also held that movement is a necessary condition for perception, at least in the primitive stage of development. Thus the organism is an organism-as-a-whole or it is no organism at all.

It is not possible to eliminate particularly the motor side of the problem in children. They do not have the language facility to describe their perceptual experiences and it is better to deal with the visual motor pattern in their drawings. Before he can draw at all the child must first be able to manipulate his own hands and the tool. It appears that the motor activity develops first or at least independently of the optic imagery, that the child's earliest productions are purely motor phenomena or merely hand movements or scribblings without meanings, and that his first satisfaction is derived from the simple rhythmic movement. Later he adds meaning to his own scribblings, and only subsequently starts his drawing with some preconceived concept. This purely motor stage persists even to an age when a child recognizes and reacts to many complicated sensory patterns in his world.

In this chapter, interest is focused on the spontaneous productions of children in chalk drawings on the sidewalks and open pavements of parks. The numerous small parks that dot New York's east side afford a great

---

[6] Katz, Dora: *Der Aufbau der Tastwelt*, 1925.

wealth of material, for during pleasant weather they are so frequently covered with the drawings of the neighborhood children. These drawings present several advantages over the usual paper-pencil or slate-chalk drawings, the main one being their absolute spontaneity. The children draw for the fun of the thing and apparently with no other goal than the immediate joy of activity and production, except in case of sidewalk games such as hopscotch, where the drawings afford the setting for the game.

The sidewalk drawings also afford us an opportunity to study drawings produced under varying motor conditions. The child may be either sitting or kneeling on the ground on which he is drawing, or leaning over from a standing position, or even balancing himself on roller skates and drawing with large arm sweeps. Yet the pictures produced in this way are in many respects quite similar to those described so extensively in the literature, which were obtained by the usual paper-pencil method.

Perhaps one of the important differences is dependent upon the unlimited amount of space. A child with plenty of chalk, with pavement all about him, with plenty of time, and totally unconscious of any observation, rarely draws a complete isolated figure. He draws and draws and scribbles all over the place, delighted when his scribbles display some unexpected form; experimenting with this, he modifies it first this way and then that by some such simple variation as enlarging a loop or extending a line, often leaving some fragment of design incomplete in order to try a new variation. He may for some reason leave this place and at some subsequent time take up the game again in some new location, or other playmates may adopt his idea and play with it in their own way. Thus definite schools of design may prevail throughout a neighborhood for days at a time.

It becomes evident that the satisfaction derived from these sidewalk productions is certainly largely a motor one. This is especially true of the younger children, but it occurs also in the older ones. They may simply make large arm movements with circular swaying lines until they have filled all the nearby space or have used up the chalk (Fig. 1a). At times they whirl themselves around, making large circles, and then they may fill them in, block by block. At other times simple designs or directional features are presented, such as making one block of cement white or colored, leaving the others as background, or lines may be drawn from various fixed points on the pavement, or the child simply moves along, drawing lines in the direction in which he is going. Numbering things is a frequent pastime possibly closely associated with the impulsive trends of children. We have elsewhere reported our studies on impulsions in children[7] among which counting, preoccupation with space, and drawings play a prominent part. Impulsions have their ori-

---

[7] Bender, Lauretta and Schilder, Paul: *Impulsions, a Specific Disorder in the Behavior of Children,* and Chapter 5; Billy—who was one of the children reported in this study.

gins in early infantile situations and desires appropriate to young children. They may be exaggerated into a behavior disorder in some prepubertal children but they do not take on the nature of compulsions and obsessions until after puberty. Blocks of city pavements are numbered consecutively, or simple designs such as oblongs are made and marked off in parts and numbered. As a result, any given area is usually filled with many of these different activities as well as with the better organized pictures of older children. In

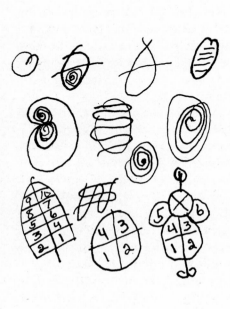

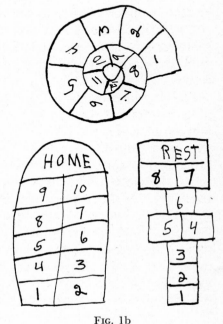

FIG. 1a

FIG. 1a. Sidewalk scribblings (*chalk*).

FIG. 1b

FIG. 1b. Hopscotch drawings (*chalk*).

the latter case loops and circles in many variations are gradually worked into more elaborate designs (Fig. 1a).

Our studies of the genesis and maturation of visual motor gestalten in normal and defective children, as well as of native, "primitive" children, showed that whirls and loops were characteristic of the most primitive levels.

Dora Musold, working with Karl Buehler and H. Vokelt (1926), tested children for their ability to discriminate the size of spheres, surface circles, contour circles, and straight lines. She found that the small children had better discrimination for spheres than the adults or older children, but had much poorer discrimination for straight lines. This is further evidence to show that, in the developing mentality, spheres (in the case of three dimensions) or circles are biologically more primitive as perceptual experience than straight lines. The child is first acquainted with his own and his mother's body, his own feces, her breast, and face. James Sully has made the interesting comment that the earliest pictorial forms have embryonic characteristics. The possibility is impressive that the postural model of the body[8] is the first perceptual experience and helps to determine the organization of the visual field, but as Kurt Koffka says, "It is not the simplest forms but those biologically most important which are the first evident in infantile perception."[9] However the visual field may have underlying physiological features of its own that determine its organization into movement of a whirling, circular, and wave type. Leo Kanner and Paul Schilder[10] have shown that the characteristic properties of optic imagery are movements of a wavy and circular nature, with scintillations and multiplications or fading and diffusing of the image or parts of it, and participation of the background in the same process.

Preliminary to a discussion of the more elaborate pictorial designs of children, some of their sidewalk games may be considered. Hopscotch is a game that has several variations which are dependent upon the different age levels, that is, on the maturational level of the perceptual motor pattern. Of course this is not absolute, as older children often play with a younger group and vice versa; also, older children sometimes revert to simpler forms, and younger children sometimes emulate their elders. But in general small tots just able to hop on one leg make a simple whirl design on the pavement, mark it off in blocks and hop from block to block until they reach the center (Fig. 1b). The aim is always to hop on one foot, without putting the other foot down and without touching any line. The size of the loop depends on the abilities of the members of the group; it is readily enlarged or made smaller at the open end. This is a very simple game but it apparently affords considerable satisfaction for youngsters of four to seven years. One sees in it an almost pure example of a perceptual motor game involving the principles of a *visual* pattern of a primitive whirl and a *motor* pattern involving a rhythmical hopping in a whirling direction. Whirling is an activity that young children enjoy very much which appears to be dependent upon their primitive postural reflexes and vestibular sensations.[11] Wolfgang Koehler's apes played similar whirling games.

The more mature children make a hopscotch design, the general outline

---

[8] Schilder, Paul: *Image and Appearance of the Human Body.*

[9] Koffka, Kurt: *The Growth of the Mind.*

[10] Kanner, Leo, and Schilder, Paul: *Movement in Optic Image.*

[11] Schilder, Paul: *Brain and Personality.*

Joseph D. Teicher in *Preliminary Survey of Motility in Children* investigated the maturation of the whirling postural reflexes and found that the tendency to whirl when the head is turned disappears at about 8 years. It is at this age that various whirling games are so important in children's play. In children with retarded or regressed motility, the whirling pattern persists. See Bender, Lauretta and Schilder, Paul: *Mannerisms as Organic Motility Syndrome.*

of which is more rectangular, although it is rounded at the top where "heaven" or "home" or "rest" is located. The lower part is marked off, by crossed lines, into eight or ten square sections. The aim is also more complex. A block is used and the child hops kicking the block from one square to the next until it reaches the top. The player must not touch a line or put down the elevated foot and the block must each time be kicked into the next space without stepping on a line. This involves several more complicated processes. The primitive circular form used by the younger children has organization only from the periphery to the center and in a clockwise or counterclockwise direction. But in this more advanced form, there is a top and a bottom, and a right and a left side, and there are also straight lines crossing each other. The motor pattern requires a better adaption; it includes the accurate control of an inanimate object and also a back and forth direction.

A still more sophisticated form of this game is played by girls of eight or ten years. They make a cross-shaped design such as is seen in Figure 1b. The pattern includes the alternate position of form, and the motor activity includes an extra step over paired spaces between each hop in the individual spaces, at the same time kicking a block from one space to the next. This represents merely an elaboration of the previous game by the addition of an alternating rhythm in both the sensory and the motor patterns.

It will be noted that there is a close resemblance between the scribblings shown in Figure 1a and the hopscotch designs shown in Figure 1b. These smaller scribblings were often found near an area where girls were playing hopscotch on larger forms of a similar configuration. This shows the tendency for the games to grow out of the primitive scribblings and for drawing designs to be influenced by the motor games, by a reversion back to the simpler forms.

Of great interest are the drawings that were found scattered lavishly on the sidewalks in a spirit of experimentation, such as are reproduced in Figures 2 and 3. In Fig. 2a, is seen a study in whirligigs, sometimes just for their own sake, or, as the tail of a cat, but most often as the central theme in a human figure; here it is featured as the hair. The rest of the body is suppressed in various ways; once the legs and feet are missing but the hands are exaggerated, again the arms are missing but the legs are better represented, but at best any of the limbs are unimportant as compared to the hair. The body is always shown in a similar way, as is also the face, in which the eyes are the only feature to appear. Even in the cat a similar pattern is shown. In different parts of the same park, numerous modifications of this design were seen, and continued to appear for several days. This might be looked upon as a period in which the school whirligigs dominated the art tendencies in this particular locality.

Fig. 2b shows a Halloween study, and was found at Halloween time.

The simple incomplete primitive loop is used with variations to form an apple, a pumpkin, a jack-o'-lantern, a bouquet, and several human forms. The surrounding neighborhood was covered with several more of these in various forms of fragmentation, duplication and evolution.

Fig. 3a represents an experiment in angular creatures. Its similarity to the second form of hopscotch is evident, although no hopscotch was seen in this park at this time.

A well developed girl of about 7 years was seen experimenting with tri-

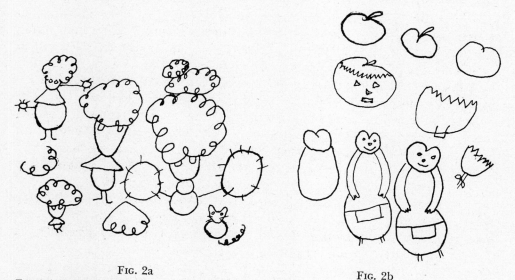

FIG. 2a

FIG. 2b

FIG. 2a. Whirligig sidewalk drawings (*chalk*).   FIG. 2b. Halloween sidewalk drawings (*chalk*).

angles and squares in the study in Fig. 3a. It might be commented along the way that the trend in cubistic art represents about a 7 year level in the maturation of form representation.[12] It is as though the cubist artist said: "Lo and behold, I have outgrown the infantile levels of loops and circles and can now accomplish and appreciate squares, cubes, and crossed lines!"

The more sophisticated drawings of the older children are often isolated figures and do not differ much from the paper and pencil drawings which have been extensively studied by many observers, and standardized by Florence Goodenough. However some pertinent observations may be pointed out: As a rule the child does not draw man in general, with the interest focused on the correctness of details. Neither is it any special man, with the emphasis on the form details. Rather it is a man doing something. As C. Guillet found (1909) the small boy is chiefly interested in drawing what men

---

[12] On the Stanford-Binet and other standardized tests, the child is expected to copy a diamond at 6½ or 7, a triangle at 5, and a square at 4 years.

and animals are doing and he is not interested in their form nor in other details. The young child also defines words in terms of their use. Kurt Koffka says that for the child who is drawing, a man is not made up of his members, but the members belong to the man. Therefore if the drawing is depicting some concept that does not utilize some part of the body, that part is likely to be deleted (Fig. 3b). Thus a man walking does not need arms, and the man urinating needs genitals, and the man wearing a hat does not need legs,

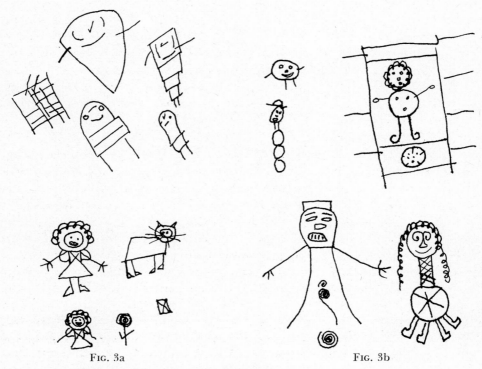

Fig. 3a.   Fig. 3b

Fig. 3a. Sidewalk drawings from geometrical figures (*chalk*).
Fig. 3b. Sidewalk drawings of people doing things (*chalk*).

etc. Nevertheless one is impressed with the pictorial success of the prominent idea, as in the case of the urinating man, with his spread legs and strained facial expression. The walking girl (with braids) gives us an excellent example of the influence of the sensory field on the pictorial forms. We know that she is walking by the multiplicity of her legs.

It has been experimentally shown by Paul Schilder and Leo Kanner, and also by Max Wertheimer that the perception of motion is accomplished in optic imagery by frequently recurring or many static figures.[13] The 27 month

[13] Kanner, Leo and Schilder, Paul: *Movement in Optic Image.*

old Ruth said, when remonstrated by her aunt, Elizabeth E. Brown,[14] for putting so many little dashes about the round loop that she called a mouse, "I give dat mouse many legs so he can wun wight away." That children's drawings are sometimes apparent symbols of unconscious concepts is shown in Fig. 3b. This is only a fragment of a very extensive design made up of many interwoven forms like the simplest circular hopscotch, with the cross lines apparently representing many stairs up which girls were apparently climbing at more or less regular intervals. That they were girls is evident by the breasts and umbilicus (infantile vagina) and the curls. There were about twenty-five such girls, all similar, varying in the absence of different details; some without hair, or arms, or legs, but all showing the sex features. At the top of this intricate stair design (inside of the many loops) was a house. It would appear evident that this was an unconscious sex fantasy.

In psychological terms it may be said that the goal in children's drawings is to establish an equilibrium between the mental symbols as determined by the biological background of the perceptual motor pattern at the different stages of maturation of the organism as a whole, and the reality of the world as it is perceived. The traces that are used must correspond not alone to the stimuli that produce them but also to the organization characteristic of the sensory field. Kurt Koffka and F. Wulf have done some experiments on traces that bear on this matter. They showed a variety of simple geometrical forms to adults and asked them to reproduce them after intervals of from twenty-four hours to a month or more. In many successive productions, there were constant progressive changes towards a simplification or exaggeration of the figure but generally towards a balanced or symmetrical form. It thus appears that the traces that were originally produced by the stimuli were modified by the biological character of the field in favor of closer organization. Kurt Koffka has said, "The development of such configurations cannot be conceived as a simple combination of sensations or an outward manifestation of juxtaposition of repeated sensations but as a result of a process which alters, refines, recenters, enriches the configuration throughout its entire make-up—a procedure in which maturation participates largely,"[15] and it may be added, organization also participates as a function of the sensory field as emphasized by Wolfgang Koehler; probably also the motor pattern, the postural model of the body, and other sensory experiences may participate.

[14] *Notes on Children's Drawings.* University of California Studies, 2:75, 1897.
[15] Koffka, Kurt: *Principles of Gestalt Psychology*, 1928, p. 105.

～ 4 ～

GENESIS AND MATURATION IN VISUAL
MOTOR GESTALTEN[1]

I. INTRODUCTION

GESTALT psychology holds that the whole or total quality of the image is perceived. This is in contrast to association psychology, which states that stimuli are perceived as parts and built into images. According to gestalt psychology, the organization of the stimuli into the image is based upon laws of perception which include proximity, similarity, direction, and inclusiveness of parts of the stimuli. The perceptual experience is a gestalt or configuration or pattern in which the whole is more than the sum of its parts. Organized units or structuralized configurations are the primary form of biological reactions. In the sensory field, these gestalten correspond to the configuration of the stimulating world. This is the static concept of the classical gestalt psychologists Max Wertheimer, Wolfgang Koehler, and Kurt Koffka. It fails to take into account the drives and tendencies of human conduct, growth, retardation in growth, or regression.

It was Paul Schilder who emphasized the importance of dynamic concepts in gestalt psychology. He stated that "there are not only Gestalten but Gestaltung," signifying that the organism in the act of perception always adds something new to the experienced perception. He said that "the organism does not react to single local stimuli by single responses but by a total process which is the response of the whole organism to the total situation."[2]

The organism has a "gestalt function" which is defined as that function of the integrative organism whereby it responds to a given constellation of stimuli as a whole, the response being a constellation or pattern or gestalt which differs from the original stimulus pattern by the process of the integrative mechanism of the individual who experiences the perception. The whole setting of the stimulus and the whole integrative state of the organism determine the pattern of response.

There is an innate tendency to experience gestalten not only as wholes which are greater than their parts, but in a state of becoming (Arthur Ed-

---

[1] This and the following chapter have been partially compiled from data relative to children in: Bender, Lauretta: A Visual Motor Gestalt Test and Its Clinical Use, Research Monograph, #3, *American Orthopsychiatric Association*, 1938. Manual of Instructions and Test Cards for the Use of The Visual Motor Gestalt Test, *American Orthopsychiatric Association*, 1946.

[2] In the Introduction to Bender, Lauretta: *A Visual Motor Gestalt Test and Its Clinical Use.*

dington) which integrates configurations not only in space but in time. Furthermore in the act of perceiving the gestalt the individual contributes to the configuration. The final gestalt is the result of the original pattern in space (visual pattern), the temporal factor of becoming, and the personal-sensory-motor factor. The resulting gestalt is, accordingly, more than the sum of all these factors. There is a tendency not only to perceive gestalten but to complete gestalten and to reorganize them according to principles biologically determined by the sensory motor pattern of action which may be expected to vary in different maturation or growth levels and in pathological states organically or functionally determined.

The factor of becoming is present in the physical world (Arthur Eddington). It accounts for the continuous integrating physical processes and tendencies. In the individual personality it accounts for tendencies to action and drives. In the final analysis the two are the same working towards the necessity for completing gestalten in all the realms of nature.[3]

Working against the tendency of becoming are the destructive forces whereby all gestalten are simplified or destroyed. This is seen when deviate organisms experience the perception of the stimulating pattern. Even in these individuals the drive to experience complete gestalten and to contribute to the integration of gestalten is always present. Even in retarded or regressed children a gestalt is always experienced, but a more primitive form tends to emerge in which the whole is still greater than all its parts including the processes which contribute to it.

II. THE VISUAL MOTOR GESTALT TEST

The visual motor gestalt test is a pencil and paper test in which configurations, originally used by Max Wertheimer for research in visual gestalt psychology, are presented to the individual for copying. The writer's first use of this test was with defective and schizophrenic adults at the Springfield State Hospital of Maryland in 1929 under the auspices of the Phipps Clinic of Johns Hopkins Hospital. Its use was further extended in the Psychiatric Division of Bellevue Hospital, especially for adults with organic psychoses. It was soon found that the test had a wide use for children as well as adults. By applying its use to children we have been able to arrive at an understanding of the genesis of perceptual motor gestalten.

Nine of Max Wertheimer's figures[4] are reproduced on cards and are offered to the child, one at a time, to be copied. Figure A which is readily experienced as a closed figure on a background is made up of a circle horizontally contingent to a diagonally placed square. This is used as an introductory figure.

---

[3] Whyte, Lancelot L.: *The Next Development in Man*. New York, Holt, 1948.

[4] Instructions, for the Use of the Visual Motor Gestalt Test and test cards are published by the American Orthopsychiatric Association.

The figures 1 to 8 are then given in sequence. Sheets of plain white unlined paper 8½ by 11 are used. One sheet is often enough, but more may be necessary especially for individuals of the lower intellectual levels or those who are confused or disturbed. A pencil with an eraser should be used. There should be no mechanical aids such as a rule or coins, etc.

The cards may be presented one at a time by being laid on the table at the top of the sheet of paper correctly oriented and the child to be tested should be told simply "Here are some figures (or designs) for you to copy. Just copy them the way you see them." It may be necessary to discourage the turning of the test card to some new position. If such turning is not easily discouraged, it should be permitted and noted. It is well to encourage the placing of the first figure near the upper left hand corner of the paper although if the suggestion is not really accepted, it too should not be insisted upon. The orientation of the figure on the background and in the series is also a part of the gestalt function. All other instructions should be non-committal. For example, if the question is asked if the dots should be counted, the answer should be, "It is not necessary but do as you like." Several attempts at any one figure may be permitted, and all trials should be left on the record. Erasures to improve lines may be permitted but not encouraged. There is no time limit on the test and the figures should not be removed until they are reproduced. Memory does not play a role in this test. Many individuals prefer to have all of the cards before them in a pile and to look at them all and orient the whole test to the sheet of paper. This can be permitted, but the test should start with figure A and run through the series in order. Many succeed in orienting the whole test situation to its background on the sheet of paper without the initial exploration.

This is a clinical test.[5] It should not be so rigidly formalized as to destroy its function which is to determine the individual's capacity to experience visual motor gestalten in a spatial and temporal relationship. Deviate behavior in the course of the test should be observed and noted. It in no wise represents a test failure. Notes may be made on the test paper of anything unusual in the way the test is organized, in the manner and behavior of the individual being tested and in his reaction to the test situation.

The test has been used as a maturational test in visual motor gestalt function in children, and to explore retardation, regression, loss of function, organic brain defects, as well as personality deviations, especially where there are regressive phenomena.

It may be given at any point in a battery of tests and may also be a restful change between more verbal or emotionally weighted tests. If given when the

---

[5] There have been efforts made by psychologists to standardize this test. See Pascal, Gerald, and Suttel, B. G.: *The Bender Gestalt Test,* 1951.

child is fatigued, this should be noted, as fatigue tends to exaggerate disturbances in the gestalt function, increasing perseverative tendencies, or calling forth other energy-saving processes or regressive tendencies. In the writer's own clinical work with children, an examination includes this gestalt test, the Goodenough drawing of a man, a few minutes of observation with some play material, observation of motor activity or play, a neurological examination, and a psychiatric interview. There is, however, no regular order, each child requiring a different pattern for the total examination depending

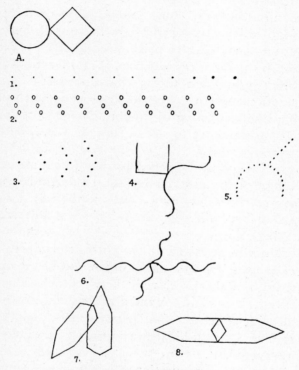

FIG. 4. The visual motor gestalt test figures.

on his clinical state at the time of the examination and on many external circumstances.

Evaluation of the test does not depend solely upon the form of the reproduced figures but on their relationship to each other, to the spatial background, to the temporal patterning and to the clinical setting.

Fig. 4 shows the figures of the test, adapted from Max Wertheimer. As has been noted, they are reproduced individually on test cards and are presented to the child one at a time to be copied with a pencil on a sheet of unlined paper.

Figure A, then, consists of a circle and a square, the linear figure touches the circle in such a way that it is perceived as a diamond. This design was chosen as an introductory figure because: it soon became evident that it was readily experienced as closed figures on a background. According to Wertheimer, "this configuration is recognized as two contingent figures because each represents a 'gute Gestalt.' " (A "gute Gestalt" refers to a complete, consistent and coherent configuration.) "This principle over-rules the principle that parts which are close together are usually seen together. In this instance the contiguous parts of the circle and square are closer to each other than the two sides of the square."[6]

Figure 1, according to Wertheimer, should be so perceived that the dots appear as a series of pairs determined by the shortest distance, or with "remnants" left over at each end. Such a pairing would be more readily perceived if the differences in the distances had been greater. This is an example of a gestalt formed on the principle of the proximity of parts.

Figure 2, again according to Wertheimer, is perceived usually as a series of short, slanting lines consisting of three units (of loops) so arranged that the lines slant from left above to right below. It, too, is determined on the principle of proximity of parts.

This is also true of Figure 3 formed by dots which are arranged in such a way that one, three, five, and seven dots form a design in which the middle dots of all these parts lie on the same level and the added dots are arranged in relationship to this midline like the two sides of a diamond, converging towards the first single dot.

Figure 4 is ordinarily perceived as two units determined by the principle of continuity of geometrical or internal organization; the open square with the bell-shaped form at the lower right hand corner. The same principle holds for the introductory Figure A and also for Figure 5 which is seen as an incomplete circle with an upright slanting strike made in dotted lines.

Figure 6 is seen as two sinusoidal (wavy) lines with different wave length, crossing each other at a slant.

Figures 7 and 8 are two configurations made up of the same units, but they are rarely perceived as such, because in Figure 8 the principle of continuity of geometric form prevails—in this instance it is the straight line at the top and the bottom of the figure.

III. VISUAL MOTOR MATURATION
IN CHILDREN

It is important to see how perception arises genetically in children and what the processes of maturation of perceived experience are. It is quite evident that the infant does not experience perception as the adult does. Never-

---

[6] Wertheimer, Max: *Untersuchungen zur Lehre von der Gestalt.*

theless, the school child who is able to read and write must have visual motor experiences similar to those of the adult. Dorothy (Fig. 5) who was a bright 14 year old girl, copied the test forms as a normal adult would be expected to do. It will be interesting to observe the manner in which the small child must pass through many stages of maturation before it is able to achieve this stage of efficiency.

It is known that the first drawings of children are scribblings representing pure motor play. They are made for the pleasure of the motor expression, the scribbled pictures being a by-product and having no meaning. They are performed by large arm movements in a dextrad, clockwise whirl or pendulum waves if the child uses its right hand, and in sinistrad, counterclockwise whirls if the left hand is used. Soon the child produces such scribblings on command for any suggested picture or in response to any test form offered, and then calls them by some other name if it so pleases him. Such are the scribblings of Eva at age 2-9,[7] when asked to draw a man and to copy the test forms (Fig. 5). She was delighted with the fun of the game and called the resulting scribbles "ropes." Sara at age 2-11 already showed a tendency to inhibit her scribbling to a more continuous form of loop. Furthermore, she could be influenced by watching the examiner perform the motor act of drawing some new figures, rather than by the figures which were offered her to copy. She made arm movements similar to the examiner's, about the sample form of Figure A which represents a well inhibited part of a loop accomplished in one arm stroke. She perseverated this response several times with great joy and tended to emphasize the single stroke aspect of the game. She offered the same response for Figure 1, although it was entirely inappropriate.

Next, she was shown how to make dots. The motor part of the dot-making game pleased her very much. She emphasized the stab of the pencil into the paper. Then she made a loop form out of dots instead of by means of the single arm movement. At this stage she gained a sudden insight into the game as a whole. She discovered that some of the figures were made of single stroke loops and some were made of dotted loops. For the next several figures she responded accordingly without further help. There is certainly some resemblance in Figures 4, 5, and 6, especially in Figure 6 where the long horizontal loop doubled back and crossed itself in the middle. However, the examiner could not resist trying to show her how to make Figure 6. Sara observed the zigzag arm movement. She tried it herself and was pleased with the result. She had also observed that there were two parts to the movement, that one stopped and started again, but she could not properly orient the two zigzag lines so that they would cross. In Figures 7 and 8 we see how well Sara really understood the problem and how well she used the modified form of her loop to express the gestalt principles implied in the test forms, except that

---

[7] Exact age of children will be given as follows: "Age 2-9" meaning 2 years and 9 months.

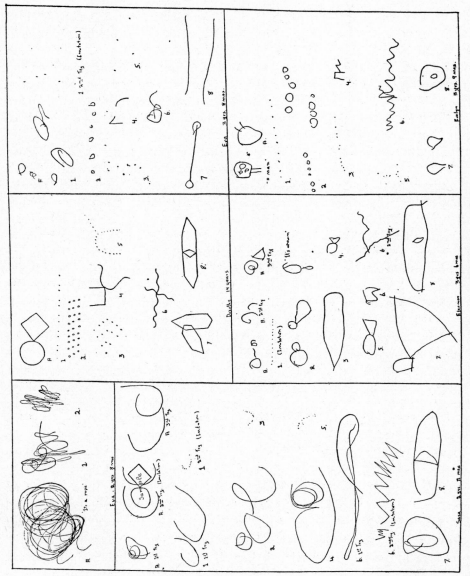

Fig. 5. Gestalt drawings by children 2-8 to 3-9 years of age.

in Figure 7 she showed a concentric relationship of the two loops which is the most primitive form of a relationship of any two parts in a whole. Of course, the very simplest visual motor gestalt relationship is an enclosed loop on a background. As has been seen, the principle of this relationship arises from the motor behavior of the small child which adapts itself to resemble the stimulus perceived in the optic field.

Eleanor, who was age 3-6, understood the use of loops very well. However, she sometimes spoiled her results by an uninhibited tendency to closures. She could make dots in Figure 1 only after she was shown how, but she gave them up and continued to experiment with loops and parts of loops. In Figure A. she made two loops and showed their relationship by a graphic connection. This tendency graphically to depict relationship occurs very often. She was not satisfied with her results and tried to tighten both loops, but that did not work either. The third effort in which she showed a real differentiation in the two parts of the figure is very good. She looped the loop freely in the first part and in the second part constructed a figure with several little parts of loops, the exact number of which did not bother her. Dots were made in Figure 1 in imitation of the examiner. She experimented some with little loops in Figure 2, but was not entirely satisfied and finally called one of them "a man" and then stopped. Figure 3 is a single enclosed loop resembling the whole figure on a background. Figure 4 shows the adjacent relationship of the two parts, one loop less round than the other but both enclosed. Figure 5 shows this overwhelming tendency to closures, which was best observed by watching the child perform the test.

The round loop was made and the upper right hand dash was added so that the figure would have been excellent (even though her arc was a complete circle) if only she had stopped there. She studied it several seconds in doubt and finally completed the right hand side of the figure. The close resemblance to Figure A and parts of Figure 2 will be noted. This is the infantile tendency to utilize a similarly constructed form for different purposes. In Figure 6, the lower wavy line was drawn and an effort was made to cross it with one little line, but after some hesitation she enclosed the whole figure. A second effort was better, due to the inhibition of primitive tendencies, but the crossing was still difficult and as a result occurs at the tip end of the line. Figure 7 resembles A, 2, and 5, but was modified to adapt better to the form offered. Figure 8 is the typical response of the young child, easily done because it represents the concentric relationship of two enclosed figures.

Eva at 3-8, just one year after she made her scribbled "ropes" showed how much she had matured in her ability to control her scribblings. She represents figure A as two adjacent loops; Figure 1 as a series of loops until she is shown how to make dots; Figure 2 as a series of little loops; Figure 3 as a mass of dots; Figure 4 as two loop segments (somewhat disoriented in their

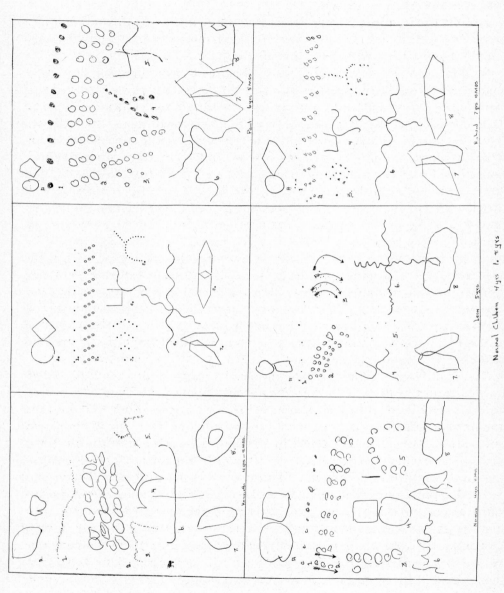

FIG. 6. Gestalt drawings by children 4-8 to 7-10 years of age.

relationship to each other); Figure 5 as a mass of dots; Figure 6 as one loop crossing another; Figure 7 as two related loops, and Figure 8 as possibly a perseveration of the line she drew in Figure 7.

Evelyn at age 3-9 shows considerable motor control and a tendency to differentiate the different forms and gestalt principles. First, we see the kind of man she can draw. This man scores her a mental age of four years on the Goodenough scale. Figure A is a modification of this man. Figure 2 is of special interest as it shows that the child does not experience this figure in accordance with the Wertheimer laws, but as a horizontal series of loops. Eva was satisfied with one series, but Evelyn has discovered that there are three horizontal series, though their exact relationship to each other is not so important. Figure 3 is always the most difficult figure. She sees it only as a series of dots. Figure 4 is somewhat disoriented; Figure 5 is a little sketchy but the principle is all there; Figure 6 was difficult to cross but it was accomplished; in Figures 7 and 8, the proper relationships, the first essential in gestalten, are shown, although the exact sizes, distances, and details of shape are not represented.

In the study of these visual motor patterns in children from age 2-6 to 4-0, the following principles may be deduced: Scribbling is at first a motor activity. It may acquire significance after production. It tends to take on a differentiated form by inhibition into single closed loops or parts of loops. Patterns or gestalten are formed by combinations of those which are adapted to resemble the perceived stimulus or to represent it symbolically. The child finds it difficult to reproduce patterns, but by various motor experimentations pictures are produced which may finally represent the pattern desired.

It is easier for the child to imitate the movements of another person so that scribbling may be limited to single arm movements, to dashes, dots, and zigzags. Once these are learned by motor imitation or experimentation, they may be more freely used to resemble test figures. Thus, any dotted form may call forth the motor behavior that produces dots, but the tendency may still persist to produce them in loop formation, masses, or series. An enclosed loop is the basis of all perceived form. There is also a tendency to perseverate any one learned (even if self-discovered) pattern wherever adaptable to other perceived figures, or, at the most primitive level, to use the first experienced form or behavior pattern in response to any figure that is offered. This merely represents to the child a stimulus that calls forth the pattern. Direction, especially dextrad horizontal direction in the right-handed child, is more important than distance or size. It is more overwhelming than Wertheimer's principles of proximity (as in Figure 2), or similarity of parts. This predominance of the directional factors is probably due in part to motor features, and in part to the principle that the optic field is organized on movement. Such concepts as "series" and "masses" are more readily grasped by children than absolute number or size. Wertheimer's principle of continuity is important to the extent that it involves direction and series; these principles of "gute Gestalt" and natural geometrical figures are important to the extent that they arise out of the primitive loop. In other respects the principles of gesalt given by Wertheimer do not apply to the genesis of gestalt in the maturation of the child's visual motor patterns.

There is a rapid differentiation of form between the ages of 4 and 7 years (Fig. 6). This is the age at which children are sent to school and expected to learn to read and write. Henrietta who was age 4-8, reproduced the test figures in such a way that her figures closely resemble them. Figure A is two closed forms, the right-sided one less round, but the distance between the two is not a matter of importance to her. Figure 1 is a series of little dash-like dots. Figure 2 is three horizontal series of little loops. Figure 3 is only a series of dots to her; Figure 4 consists of two open forms widely separated as in Figure A. Figure 5 is quite well done. Figure 6 expresses the crossed relationship in its simplest form. Figures 7 and 8 show the side to side and concentric relationship of primitive loops. It will be noted that any slanting or oblique relationships are not depicted at this maturation level.

Norman at age 4-11 used some form of the loop or enclosed figure in all his responses. In Figure A he has produced a pretty good square although not obliquely oriented. Figure 1 is a series of tiny loops, but there is no pairing. In Figure 2 for the first time we see the vertical series of three loops, but there is no slanting. Figure 3 is still too difficult for him. Figure 4 is a modification of Figure A. Figure 5 shows an interesting displacement of the dash, perhaps the very effort it required for this child to make a dash when he was still dealing in loops, displaced it. In Figure 6 he got the idea of two wavy lines but he could not cross them. In comparing this with the previous child, it is seen that often a child can get one new principle in a gestalt but is unable to combine two of them in the same gestalt.

Leon at age 5-0 shows several advances in progress. In an effort to slant the vertical series in Figure 2 he has displaced the whole figure. Figure 3 shows the first real effort to produce this pattern. It is a series of concentric dotted curves, the number of series or the number of dots in each series appearing not to matter. Figure 6 is a crossed wavy line but the crossing is not slanted. There is, however, an oblique overlap in Figure 7.

Paul at age 6-5 made a real diamond in Figure A and showed a better accomplishment in details of relationships in Figures 3, 4, 5, 7 and 8 than any of the younger children. He still always uses loops instead of dots, although he sometimes fills in the loops to make them look like dots. He was unable to cross the lines in Figure 6 or angulate those in Figure 3.

Richard at age 7-10 does all these things, except that even yet his dots resemble little loops, some of his slanting relationships are not very accurate, and the pairing does not occur in Figure 1. Degree of perfection in size, shape, distances, and motor control is still not as great as it was in the work, first shown, of Dorothy, aged 14.

It will appear from these experiments that visual motor patterns arise from motor behavior that is modified by the characteristics of the visual field. This motor behavior is organized about the primitive enclosed loop with directional tendencies (usually dextrad and horizontal at first) and perseverative behavior. There is a constant interplay or integration between the motor and sensory features which can never be separated, though either one may advance more rapidly than the other in the maturation process and appear for a time to dominate any given stage in the evolution of the gestalt.

Kurt Koffka pointed out that even during development, all motor acquisitions have a sensory component. It is also held that movement is a necessary condition for perception, at least in the primitive stages of development (Dora Katz). Thus the organism is an organism-as-a-whole or it is no organism at all. Wolfgang Koehler makes the point that behavior is not the response of the organism to the stimulus, but is rather the response of the organism to its own sensory organization of the stimulus. The child, therefore, responds to a much more simply conceived world than does the adult. G. W. Hartmann speaks of the greater dynamic unity of the child making the isolation of a single action more difficult for the child than for the adult. He quotes Koehler's color-box experiment with his three-year-old daughter to show that the native and primitive perceptual responses in children stress totals and wholes. Similar principles may be demonstrated in children's spontaneous drawings.

The genetic significance of verticalization was not properly evaluated until Abraham A. Fabian observed it while he was working with educational disability in the problem children at Bellevue. He used the gestalt test to help in his exploration, and checked it on normal children in one of the city public schools. He stated, "The tendency to rotate horizontally directed configurations to the vertical position is found in the normal child of pre-school and beginning school age. It is a developmental phenomenon which is gradually corrected as the child matures but does not disappear until he is seven or eight years of age. Physiological, psychophysical, and psychological forces contribute to the tendency." Under these headings he has shown that "muscle mechanics of the arm favor movement in the vertical direction."[8] Movement tendencies in the gestalt function also contribute. Finally, body-image factors which are described by Paul Schilder as all of the perceptual experiences integrated into a schema, or which represent one's experiences about one's own body, influence the projected sensory experience of the developing child. Here upright posture is a factor. The close relation with the visual motor gestalt function and with language development is emphasized by A. A.

---

[8] Fabian, Abraham A.: *Vertical Rotation in Visual Motor Performance.*

Fabian. Those children who show reversal tendencies in reading disabilities may be shown on testing with the gestalt test or similar tests to persist in the tendency to verticalization of horizontal figures or to rotation of figures.

The close relationship between the genesis of visual motor gestalten and body imagery has been pointed out by Paul Schilder and Lauretta Bender. The Goodenough drawing of a man is not the man visually perceived, but a projection of one's own body image acquired by lifelong integration of all perceptual experiences. The body image as projected into the drawing of a man is an excellent sensory motor gestalt test. Its maturation runs parallel with the maturation of the visual motor gestalt test. The standardization of the two tests is similar. Deviations occur under similar circumstances in both tests. In our clinical work we usually use the two tests together.

Plasticity, as a feature of the very young child, which is readily recognized in the gestalt test especially when it is viewed as a total gestalt on one sheet of paper, was not sufficiently emphasized in our earlier work. It has been seen most frequently in very gifted children, in schizophrenic children, and in some organic brain disorders in children; also in some of the gestalt test material of native children from the island of Saipan in the Marianas, which will be discussed next fully.

IV. VISUAL MOTOR MATURATION IN THE "PRIMITIVE" CHILD

Some data which appears to give evidence that the evolution of gestalten is a maturation process rather than an educational or imitative one is derived from drawings obtained from native African children. H. W. Nissen of Yale University secured these drawings in Pastoria, a laboratory of the Pasteur Institute (Paris) situated in French Guinea, Africa. In May 1930 while making some nature studies of chimpanzees he administered ten psychometric tests to fifty native Negro children 5 to 13 years of age (the exact age could not be given and had to be estimated). Among these tests were included the drawings of designs (Test 6) from the Army performance tests[9] (see Fig. 7a). Although these designs are not the same as the figures which were used in our study of visual motor gestalten, they lend themselves to the same sort of analysis. (About half these children had never used paper and pencil before.) In the Army test the scoring has been standardized on adults and allows only two to five possible scores on each design. The scoring of these drawings of native Negro children by H. W. Nissen and his co-workers resulted in no score for many of the children, but an analysis of the drawings as maturation of gestalten showed that every child's response was directly related to the stimulus.

---

[9] Yoakum, Clarence S. and Yerkes, Robert M.: *Army Mental Tests.* New York, Holt, 1920.

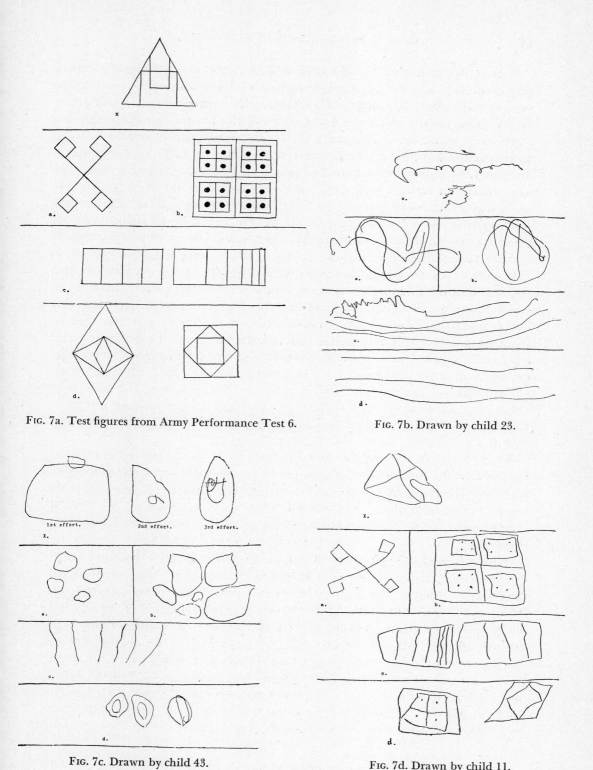

FIG. 7a. Test figures from Army Performance Test 6.

FIG. 7b. Drawn by child 23.

1st effort. 2nd effort. 3rd effort.

FIG. 7c. Drawn by child 43.

FIG. 7d. Drawn by child 11.

FIG. 7. Army Alpha Intelligence Test designs.

The term "primitive" child[10] is here used to mean the näive unsophisticated child who has not been subjected to the educational or cultural regime of the child of our civilization. It assumes no difference in native intelligence. H. W. Nissen, Saul Machover and Elaine Kinder in analyzing the results of these studies[11] maintain that there is no available evidence for any clear-cut racial difference in intelligence. Nor can any conclusions be drawn concerning general ability or adaptability of primitive native potentialities from any known test materials. However, some test materials do show differences in "specific immediate present abilities." In their own battery of tests these investigators found that the best results were obtained in the native children from tests which involve imitative functions, immediate memory, perception and retention of visuo-kinesthetic cues and which were without representative content; the poorest results were obtained from the tests which had pictorially representative content, or symbolic material, or which required combinative activity based on the perception of part-whole relationships. The authors felt that no conclusions as to native endowment could be derived from their data. They emphasized, instead, the influence of cultural sets and group phenomena "in conditioning the development of functions with consequent cumulative differentiation" somewhat in the terms of Charles M. Child's dictum on neuro-anatomical data that "Development is a process of functional construction, that is, beginning with a given structure and function the continuance of the function modifies the structural substratum and this in turn modifies further function and so on."[12]

These drawings were made available to us by H. W. Nissen before the investigators had completed their analyses. The drawings were analyzed and classified by us in accordance with the gestalt principles which have been observed in the drawings of hundreds of children who copied the figures of the visual motor gestalt test. Seven levels or stages of accomplishment were distinguished.

The first or most primitive level showed large whole-arm scribblings which were produced in such a way as to fill the space allotted without much regard to the form which was presented. The drawings of three children were of this type (see Fig. 7b, Child 23 of H. W. Nissen's series). Design X is essentially a meaningless scribble. In Design A there appears to have been some effort to use the scribble to form a cross. Design B is essentially a perseveration or carry-over from Design A. In Design C there is some resemblance to the form given, in that one sees a horizontal figure, but again the child's production may have been influenced as much by the space allotted as by the form pre-

---

[10] See Mead, Margaret: *Research on Primitive Children.*

[11] Nissen, H. W., Machover, Saul, and Kinder, Elaine: *A Study of Performance Tests Given to a Group of Native African Children.*

[12] Child, Charles M.: *The Origin and Development of the Nervous System,* 1921, pp. 114, 115.

sented. However here there is also some suggestion of perseveration of vertical lines on the left-hand side. Design D is essentially a perseveration of Design C. Perseverative tendencies are strong and may well be determined by the motor pattern or by kinesthetic clues. These results represent essentially the simplest form of motor response to the stimuli. There was, nevertheless, some slight evidence of a response in accordance with the sensory pattern, at least to the extent of adapting the response to the background, which is the first principle of gestalten (Kurt Koffka).

In the second level of production there was a good loop formation and the tendency to produce patterns by perseveration of loops in a horizontal plane without regard to the form offered but with the apparent intent to fill the space allotted. Two children formed drawings of this sort. There was also evident some tendency to put loops inside of loops and they were formed both clockwise and counterclockwise, and perseverated in both the dextrad and sinistrad directions.

The first clear evidences of gestalten with an inner structure are seen at the third level. They are produced by the spatially related loops, and by the perseveration on the horizontal plane of vertical, radial wavy lines. Four children are represented in this group (see Fig. 7c, Child 43). In Design X, the child after three trials gives some idea of the original form by means of three inclusive loops. In Design A, four loops are properly related to each other, but show no connecting crossed lines. Similarly, Design B is formed by a grouping of loops. Design C is a simple perseveration of vertical lines. In Design D, we again see loops inside loops.

In the fourth stage of development, the relationship between lines and loops, and of lines to each other was seen. So far, lines have been only segments of loops. Even in Design C by Child 43, the lines are probably only small segments of large arcs perseverated in a wave-like manner. The inclusions of such perseverated segments into other loops, or the connection of such a single segment to a loop, or the crossing or angulated relationship of such segments, is a special stage in the development of gestalten. In these primitive levels of development the child is found to be experimenting with any one of these new combinations, but a higher level of development is required for the utilizing of more than one combination in any design.

Up to this point, H. W. Nissen and his co-workers had not been able to give any score to any of the drawings by the standard method, although our analysis shows a definite gradation in performance.

In the fifth stage are found either a better utilization of the same elements or the capacity to utilize several combinations in the same design. This included the drawings of eight children, all of whom made the lowest possible score on the standard scale.

In the sixth stage, better produced forms and more accurate relationships

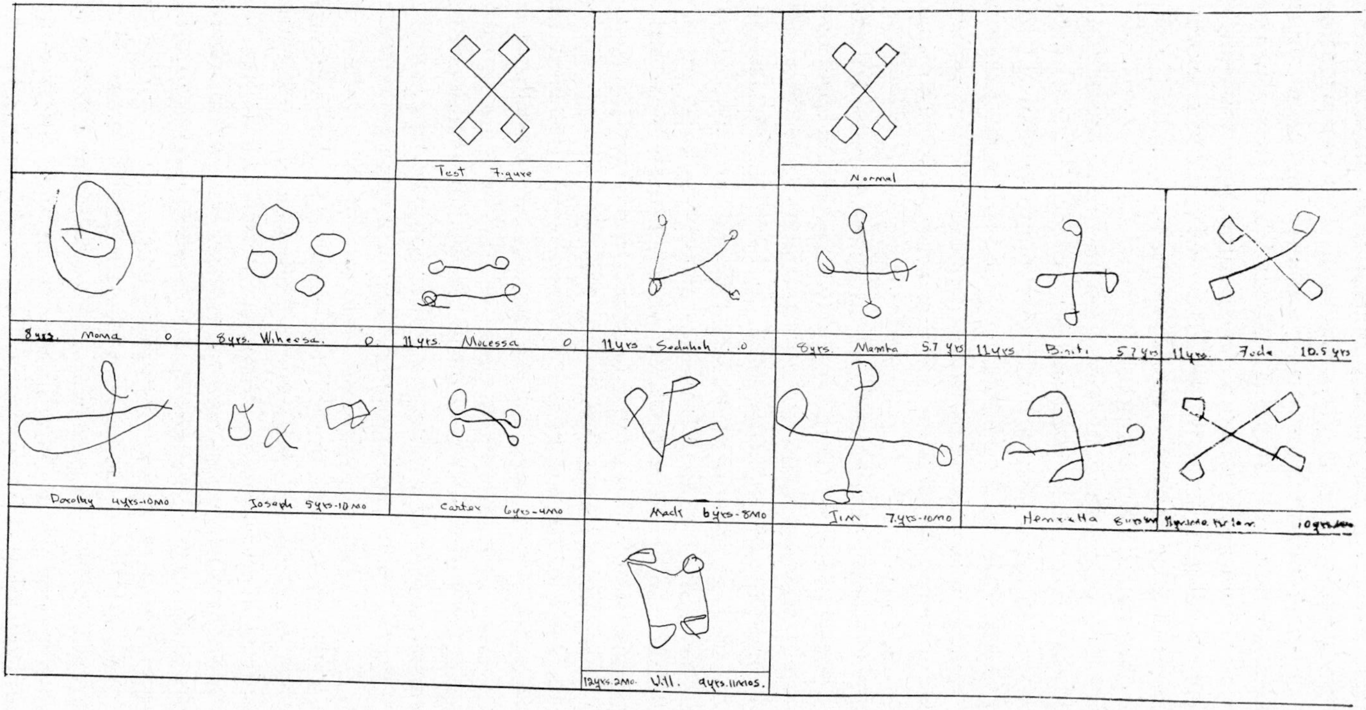

FIG. 8. Army Alpha Design "a" by native African and New York City school children.

occurred. Eleven children produced drawings that fell in this classification.

In the best or seventh group of drawings which was obtained from eleven children, all of which received the highest possible score on the standard scale, a higher grade of perfection is to be seen. There is more accuracy in reproducing details, numbers of parts, and spatial relationships. In these drawings we note for the first time the ability to make diagonal gestalten with acute and obtuse angles (see Fig. 7d, Child 11).

The best of these productions compare favorably with drawings of the same designs by American Negro children of known average intelligence, born in New York City and educated in New York City schools. This was determined by comparing these drawings with those of 50 American Negro children. A number of these drawings of the Design A are shown in Fig. 8. Among the native African children there were found more drawings of the more primitive type, but all levels of maturation are seen in the native African group as well as in the children educated in New York City schools. It will be seen in Fig. 8 that the drawings of an American child of 4 years are compared with those of one of the African children whose age was estimated at 8 years. In the same way the various recognizable levels of maturation may be found at progressively higher mental levels in the American child, as compared with African children of various ages. However, the two best and practically normal drawings were furnished by an American school girl of 11 and by a native boy of 11 who had had no formal schooling. By way of contrast, the drawings of a child of 12 who had been in a state hospital since the age of 8 is shown. He was 12 years old at the time of the test and scored a mental age of 9-11. His drawings show a new relationship of the parts which occurs in schizophrenia and which will be discussed in more detail in Chapter VI.

From this material it appears that a native child who has had no schooling whatsoever and who has had no previous experience with paper and pencil may produce copied forms with the same facility as does an average American born and American educated child. Among the native children there appears to be a greater range of maturation levels even at similar age levels. They show features which are the same as those that are observed in New York City children when they are studied at different age levels. It may be noted that copied form evolves as a motor pattern adapted to a given background. The simplest principles of structure depend upon loops which may be perseverated inclusively or on horizontal planes. Lines occur as horizontally perseverated segments of loops in wave-like relationships. More intricate structures are formed by combining loops and segments of loops, to make angles and crossed forms. Small loops may become dots, segments may represent lines, and angulated forms may represent rectangles. Several of these relationships may be utilized at once. Perfection in forms and spatial

relationships and accuracy in number of parts (by inhibition of perservera-
tion) are accomplished by some children. The best drawings show slanting
forms, angles other than right angles, alternating and diagonal relationships.
The children who produce such sophisticated drawings score the highest on
the group of psychometric tests given by Nissen. The majority of these include the older children.

The analysis of this material by Nissen and his co-workers led them to the
opinion that the variability of this test was somewhat less than that of the
maze test, although the designs seemed to show, to them, a greater discrim-
inative value for the estimated age levels of the group as a whole.

In their analysis of the individual drawings they state:

"As will be noted, Design A is so constituted as to make possible the detec-
tion of a 45 degree rotation appearing in the reproduction. The performance
of nearly 50% of our subjects showed this rotation, the effect being the crossing of a vertical line by a horizontal line instead of the crossing of oblique
lines as in the copy. With respect to this feature the design elicited three
types of performance: 1) Inability to approximate the figure presented;
2) reproduction as a crossing of a horizontal and a vertical line; and 3) reproduction of the diagonal crossing. Performance of the younger group
with one exception, was limited to the first two categories. All three categories
were present in the performance of the older group but only 17% of the
responses of this group came under the first category.

"Design B proved considerably more difficult for our subjects. Whereas in
Design A there were fifteen zero scores and thirty subjects receiving one point
each of a possible three points allowed by the scoring standards, in Design
B we find thirty-three zero scores and only twelve scores above zero.

"On Design C all but two of the younger group scored zero on both parts,
these two each receiving one point, whereas of the older group seven subjects
scored on the first part and nine on the second. For Design D the scores were
zero for all but two of the older group. Like Design A, both C^1 and C^2
showed a certain number of rotations, but here the rotation was through
90°, so that the predominantly horizontal extension appeared as predominantly vertical extension in the reproductions. This rotation appeared less
frequently than in the Design A (9% of the attempts of the younger group
and 21% of the older group). It suggests that for our subjects the extensity
of the designs was the more important feature, the direction being secondary.
The tendencies to rotation exhibited in the reproductions in Design A, C^1
and C^2 are probably expressive of the ontogenetically prior prepotency of
verticality and horizontality over obliqueness, and of verticality over
horizontality, of the perceptual organization of, and motor adjustment to,
spatial extensity. The priority in development of certain directional tendencies in copying design had been recognized by Arnold Gesell and utilized by
him in his normative schedule. Tendencies to rotation in the design tests
like the reversals in the cube imitation test suggest the general problem of

orientation and merit investigation as to whether such phenomena appear as prominently among Negro children of comparable age with American upbringing."

This gestalt study investigates this problem and indicates that spatial orientation cannot be spoken of in terms of ontogenesis but in terms of organization of the perceptual motor patterns; also that it follows a definite pattern in the different maturation levels which are alike in the native and American child. Abraham A. Fabian's studies also give us more understanding of the question of horizontality and verticality, showing that this is also a maturational problem. This might lead us to expect that children, such as these native children, who are less fixed or determined in their patterned responses will show a greater variability in their spatial-motor organization.

Dr. Alice Joseph and Dr. Veronica F. Murray studied 149 native children ranging in ages from 6 to 17 years from the Chamorros and Carolinians of Saipan in the Marianas, subjecting them to a battery of psychological tests, among which was the visual motor gestalt test.[13] The work was done under the Pacific Science Board of the National Research Council.

Dr. Joseph and Dr. Murray were good enough to allow us to analyze the gestalt test and we found that it had been well handled by these children. There was a strong drive to accomplish the task and a high degree of conformity. The organization of the test figures on the paper was good. There was never any doubt as to which figure was represented; each one was discrete and clear. The gross deviations were few. Some of the children were retarded but this was reflected also in the IQ rating of the Grace Arthur and Porteus Maze scores, which were likewise made available to us. A few of the children's drawings were distorted with motor, schizophrenic or impulse disorders. Out of the total of 149 there were four retarded or defective responses and six with other disturbances. The maturation level of the gestalt figures agreed with the IQ rating of the Grace Arthur score; when the Grace Arthur and the Porteus Maze scores differed, the gestalt responses were closer to the Grace Arthur score.

The maturation of the gestalt test progressed smoothly to 8 or 9 years when it tended to fixate at the 7 to 9 year level according to the previous standards for the gestalt test; it lagged behind the gestalt test and the Grace Arthur score. This appears to be a function of the test, but perhaps it lies also in the maturation of these native children. The lag in the chronological ages above 12 years is not significant.

There were many indications of fluidity, plasticity or primitive trends, which we have heretofore considered evidence of regression, schizophrenia, or lack of maturity, but which appear to be the norm for this group. In

---

[13] See report (in press) of Alice Joseph and Veronica F. Murray, National Research Council.

straight-line figures, the corners were rounded in squares and diamonds, even when the motor pattern, i.e., of the square or diamond, was clear. There were many rotated figures from the horizontal to the vertical, or from the vertical to the horizontal. The dotted figures tended to be particularly motile, showing wavy formations in Figure 2, for example, or closing of Figure 5. In general there was increased action. One part of a figure was influenced by another part, or one figure was influenced by the one that preceded it.

At the same time a strong effort was expressed to achieve the test, to conform, and to control primitive perceptual experiences. The children used the framework of the boundaries of the paper as background. They tended to make the whole composition of figures horizontal, vertical, or circular, or in some way closely patterned. They put similar figures together, as, for example, horizontally oriented ones, or dotted ones, etc. Thus they showed a spontaneous tendency to classify the figures or to show abstract rather than concrete responses. They often tied figures together by allowing them to touch each other, especially at pointed ends. They tried to make use of mechanical aids, employed counting and tracing, and made soft, tentative lines. Their erasures showed higher maturation levels, from more primitive to more controlled responses, straighter lines, etc.

V. STANDARDIZATION OF THE GESTALT FUNCTION IN A PERFORMANCE TEST FOR CHILDREN

It has been shown that the copying of these figures by children is a test which shows the maturation level of the child in the visual motor gestalt function. It has been found from the studies in sensory aphasia of adults, that the visual motor gestalt function is associated with language ability and closely associated with various functions of intelligence such as visual perception, manual motor ability, memory, temporal and spatial concepts, and organization or representation.

Raymond Street (1931) standardized a gestalt completion test in which he aimed at helping to fill the need for a test which was "clear cut in structure and well-defined in nature," and to help clarify the confusion that has followed from empirical tests, when it is not clear what functions they are supposed to measure. He believed that his gestalt completion test measured a specific capacity that is probably involved in the perceptual process. He used a type of picture puzzle of familiar objects made up of black figures on a white background, or white figures on a black background: "by deletion, parts of each figure have been made to form the ground, so that in order to perceive the picture, it is necessary to complete the structure; that is, to bring about a 'closure.' "[14] It appears that, in the first place, Raymond Street

---

[14] Street, Raymond: *A Gestalt Completion Test.*

overlooked the motor phase of every perceptual function without which the gestalt function cannot be reckoned; and in the second place the deletions were arbitrary and often artificial, and not a functional part of the gestalt.

The visual motor gestalt test has been standardized on 800 school and nursery school children. The children were tested in a suburban (Pelham) grade school,[15] in two public day nurseries in New York City, and in the hospital wards and out-patient departments of the pediatric and psychiatric services of Bellevue Hospital. Children of 3 to 11 years, inclusive, were used, or children of pre-school age and also those in the first to fifth grades, inclusive. Adult drawings were obtained from school teachers and members of the hospital staff. Children of 3 years and younger usually produced only a scribble, unless the figures were produced in front of them and they were allowed to imitate the motor acts. All of the figures are satisfactorily produced at the age of 11 years. Adults add only a certain motor perfection or perfection in detail in sizes and distances.[16]

The test may therefore be considered of value as a maturation test of performance in the visual motor gestalt function between the ages of 4 and 12 which is the age when language function, including reading and writing, is developing.

Arnold Gesell has standardized the drawing ability of small children and finds that a child of 9 months to 1 year can scribble imitatively; that a child of 1 to 1½ years can scribble spontaneously; that a child of 2 years can imitate a vertical stroke; that at 3 years a child can also draw a recognizable figure of a man. He expressed wonder at the inability of a child to produce an oblique cross as early as it could produce a square cross, or a diamond as early as a square. He tried to explain it on the basis of a motor difficulty. It is quite clear from these studies, however, that the difficulty is related to the problem of visual motor gestalt function. According to the Kuhlman standards, a child can make a mark with a pencil at 1 year, and copy a circle at 2 years.

Other workers are inclined to set the age for copying specific forms somewhat later than these two. In the Merrill-Palmer test for pre-school children, copying a circle is expected at 3½ to 4 years. In the Stanford scale, a child of 4 is expected to reproduce a more complicated design from memory. Charlotte Buehler finds that the 4 year old can reproduce a circle by imitation; that the 5 year old can reproduce schematic pictures such as trees, a man, etc., by imitation and that the 6 year old can reproduce a border made of a series of rings, triangles and crosses, around a paper.

From the standardization of the gestalt drawings (Fig. 9) we found that the

---

[15] With the aid of Miss Anita Ruben.

[16] For charts and graphs of standardization data see: Bender, Lauretta: *The Visual Motor Gestalt Test and Its Clinical Use.*

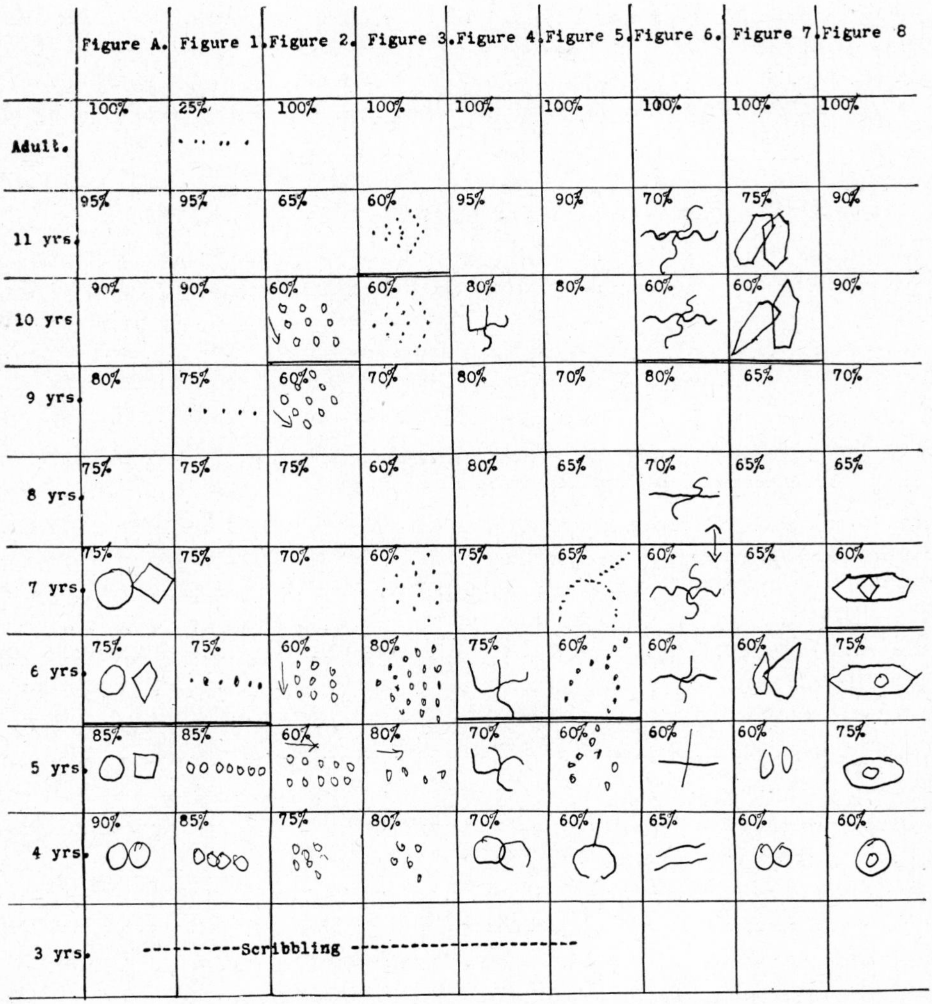

	Figure A	Figure 1	Figure 2	Figure 3	Figure 4	Figure 5	Figure 6	Figure 7	Figure 8
Adult	100%	25%	100%	100%	100%	100%	100%	100%	100%
11 yrs	95%	95%	65%	60%	95%	90%	70%	75%	90%
10 yrs	90%	90%	60%	60%	80%	80%	60%	60%	90%
9 yrs	80%	75%	60%	70%	80%	70%	80%	65%	70%
8 yrs	75%	75%	75%	60%	80%	65%	70%	65%	65%
7 yrs	75%	75%	70%	60%	75%	65%	60%	65%	60%
6 yrs	75%	75%	60%	80%	75%	60%	60%	60%	75%
5 yrs	85%	85%	60%	80%	70%	60%	60%	60%	75%
4 yrs	90%	85%	75%	80%	70%	60%	65%	60%	60%
3 yrs	--------Scribbling ----------------------------								

Fig. 9. A chart of norms for the visual motor gestalt test.

3 year old child usually responds with a scribble which is somewhat controlled; that is, the child stops spontaneously after making a small scribble on the paper before him, and repeats the same or similar response when each new figure is shown to him.

The 4 year old uses circles and closed loops to represent some of the gestalt principles in all of the figures shown to him. Usually, Figure A is two circles in the horizontal plane in the dextrad direction. Figure 1 is a series of larger or smaller circles, or loops, in the dextrad horizontal direction. Figures 2 and 3 are masses of small circles. Figure 4 is two loops in a more or less horizontal direction, with, possibly, some effort to keep either or both circles partly open. Figure 5 is a partially open circle with a dash at the top. Figure 6 may be intertwining circles, or two horizontal unclosed lines, or segments of circles. Figure 7 is two dextrad circles and Figure 8 is two concentric circles. At the age of 4, therefore, the child may use closed circles or loops in horizontal dextrad, concentric, and mass relations. Dextrad horizontal direction may also be represented as a segment of a circle. Partially open circles are attempted. In other words, it may be said that a 4 year old child can express form by loops or circles on a background; direction, by dextrad horizontals; numbers, by mass and perseveration; and to some extent these functions may be combined to produce integration in a pattern. There is a slight tendency to use open loops and segments of circles, but this is not consistent.

A 5 year old child may modify his circles and loops into close square-like figures, into oblong oval figures or into open circles; he may use arcs of circles in various combination, including perseveration of concentric arcs; and he may perseverate horizontal series in vertical direction and cross vertical and horizontal lines.

A 6 year old child may produce closed squares in the oblique direction; and represent oblique relationships by two partially closed loops, and by a segment of one loop in relation to another. He may also make circles so small that they are dots and represent points in space. It is possible, therefore, for him to reproduce correctly Figures A, 1, 4 and 5. He may also produce vertical series alone or by horizontal perseveration; or combine several of these functions in one figure so that he is not only able to cross lines but also to cross wavy lines. Another possible variation is to make Figure 5 an open circle of small dots with an oblique dash at the top, etc.

The ages over 7 add very little more than an improvement of obliquity and an increase in the numbers of combinations. Thus, in Figure 2, the problem of forming an oblique vertical sequence of three small loops is a difficult one. Even after it is accomplished the whole pattern tends to take the oblique direction indicated by this feature. This is often seen at the 9 year level, and it usually requires a 10 year old child to form a horizontal dextrad perseveration of oblique vertical sequences of three circles. An 11 year old child is required to form Figure 3 as a horizontal dextrad series of obtuse angles of increasingly greater spread rather than the concentric arcs used at the younger ages. Only the unusual adult can notice the exact spatial relationships in the pairing of the dots in Figure 1.

Fig. 9 is a summary chart showing type of responses at the different ages. The percentage of children who could do the type of response depicted or better is printed in the upper left-hand corner of each square. This chart may be used as a scale for determining the maturation level of any child or defective adult who may be asked to draw these figures.

VI. EXAMPLES OF THE USE OF VISUAL MOTOR
GESTALT TEST IN CHILDREN

The two following case histories are quoted to show the use of this test in the study of children:

Elizabeth (see Fig. 10) was age 4-5 when she was brought to the Mental Hygiene Clinic because of infantile behavior in the day nursery where she

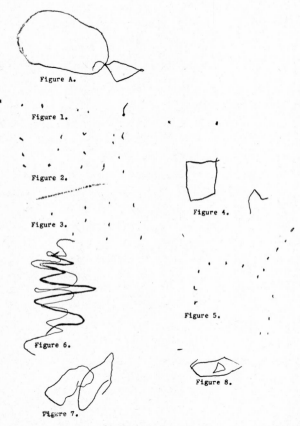

FIG. 10. Visual motor gestalt test, by Elizabeth, a bright, normal child, age 4-5 years.

was daily left by her mother who worked; the father was in jail. She came from a Roumanian home where Roumanian was spoken. Her infantile behavior included poor toilet training, baby talk, restlessness and inattentiveness. On the Stanford-Binet test she scored a mental age of 4-0 with an IQ of 91, but it was noted that her English was limited because of the bilingual home. On the Randall's Island performance test she scored a mental age of 6-3 with an IQ of 142%. She did not do well with the Goodenough test for drawing a man. She blocked on attempting the drawing and became restless and upset. The drawing could not be recognized. She spoke of the devil's eyes and the belly button. The gestalt drawings were performed as shown in Fig. 10. Figure A scores at the 5 year level, being composed of a round closed loop with the second part of the figure modified to resemble a square. Figure 1 scores at the 6 year level; Figure 2, between 7 and 8 years; Figure 6, at 6 years; Figure 4, at 6 years, except that the first part of the figure is

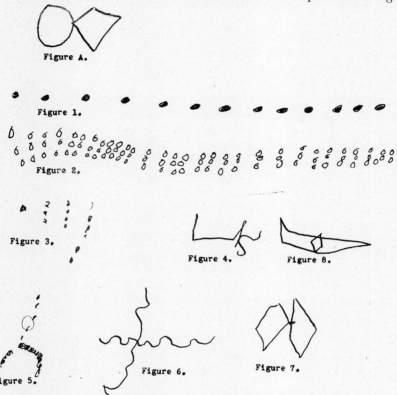

Figure A.

Figure 1.

Figure 2.

Figure 3.

Figure 4.

Figure 8.

Figure 5.

Figure 6.

Figure 7.

FIG. 11. Visual motor gestalt test, by Jesse, a dull child, age 11-6 years.

closed; Figure 5, at 6 years or above; Figure 7 cannot score because her lines are not crossed and both are vertical although both are wavy lines; and Figures 7 and 8 score at 6 years. After a period of treatment on the children's ward for her neurotic problems, she was able to produce a man without fears or inhibitions and scored over 6 years on the Goodenough scale. When this child was 4-6, she had a mental age of 6 years. The gestalt test was in keeping with other performance tests. The Stanford-Binet test seemed to have been performed at a disadvantage because of the bilingual home background and the blocked neurotic state of the child. When she was 8-6 she was returned[17]

[17] The subsequent development of the children discussed will be given whenever it is possible, especially when it is important in confirming data or when it has failed to confirm it. This will prove significant as in many instances the original data was given on children who have since attained maturity.

to the hospital with a severe neurotic anxiety. This followed difficulties in the home during which her mother was hospitalized for depression, anxiety, hypochondriasis. Elizabeth's behavior reflected the condition of the home and the emotional state of the mother. The psychometric examination at that time gave her an IQ of 105 on the Stanford-Binet but it was still recognized that this was a minimal score because of her language inadequacies and her emotional state. Her drawing of a man at this time was superior. At our recommendation she was placed in a cottage-plan institution for normal girls where we have learned that she did well until she was 16 when she was discharged to her mother.

Jesse (see Fig. 11) was a Negro boy, age 11-6. He was accomplishing nothing in school and had not learned to read. He was poorly supervised by a defective mother and beaten so much that he ran away from home. In the Stanford-Binet he scored a mental age of 6-0, with an IQ of 52. On the ward among other children his social adjustment seemed at a somewhat higher level. On the Pintner-Patterson performance scale he scored a mental age of 7-10 with an IQ of 73. On the Goodenough score for drawing a man he scored 7-plus years. With the gestalt drawings seen in Figure 11, all his productions fell between the 7, 8 and 9 year level. The child was a borderline mental defective with a reading disability so that he had gained no educational accomplishments. On the Stanford-Binet test which assumes school and language accomplishments he had scored much lower with a mental age of 6 years. A year later he was returned to the ward from the children's court because of persistent truancy from school and neglect by his mother. It was arranged to send him to a state training school for defective children where his needs would be more adequately met than in his own home or the public school system.

In general it may be said that the visual motor gestalt test agrees rather with performance tests than with language tests and tends to suffer less from emotional disorders than the Goodenough drawing-of-a-man test.

As already discussed in Chapter III, the child's early activities in spontaneous drawings, games and various forms of play represent experiments in form, spatial relationships, rhythms, temporal relationships, and various physical forces such as gravity. This is in accord with Susan Isaacs' teachings that the child has a drive for knowledge as such. It is in contrast to the teachings of Jean Piaget who sees in all the early behavior of the child egocentric tendencies, and to those of Melanie Klein for whom the child's love of knowledge or epistemophilic drives is an instinctual urge for sex knowledge. In their drawings, play, and activities, children show their drive to experience or experiment with physical phenomena. Susan Isaacs has emphasized this early drive for knowledge, but is inclined to look upon it as a drive for the absolute due to fear, insecurity, and incomplete or erroneous knowledge.

Our experience, on the other hand, would lead to the conclusion that the child actually experiments with the different phenomena, getting satisfaction with each new experience which is complete enough for that stage of maturation of the developing organism growing from preceding experience levels. There is, moreover, a continuous reaching out for new experiences in which the child freely gives himself so that his activities become an active part of the knowledge obtained. This becomes a continually expanding "Gestaltung" which is continually reshaping itself in the experience of the growing child, and is both experienced by and produced by the child. It can be particularly well seen in the drawings of these gestalt forms at different maturation levels that the child accepts them not as absolute truths or patterns of the forms which are displayed, but that they represent constellations of stimuli to which different organisms react and which they experience in different ways, and that the reaction or experience of each child is complete and satisfactory for him.

DEVIATIONS IN VISUAL MOTOR GESTALTEN
IN CHILDREN

I. VISUAL MOTOR GESTALT FUNCTION
AND MENTAL DEFICIENCY[1]

MENTAL DEFICIENCY is not an entity; neither is it an isolated deficiency in intelligence. It is a symptom which may be associated with many different conditions. Although the general attitude towards mental deficiency assumes that it is due to an actual quantitative failure in endowment or to loss of function through structural disturbance due to disease processes or injuries to the brain, there are some studies which point to a different evaluation. L. Pierce Clark defines mental deficiency as "the failure in the process of acquiring, absorbing and using knowledge for an adaptive mastery of reality."[2] He points out that even where the deficiency is associated with definite organic injury, there are dynamic or psychological factors that play a part, for "any wound to the physical structure must be reflected in the ego's efficiency and in its sense of power to govern the total organism in its approach to reality." In other words, the reaction of the personality-as-a-whole in terms of the psychobiological unit must be considered. Deficiency must be looked upon as a dynamic response even where there are structural defects. Viewing mental deficiency in this way, impaired intellectual responses may be looked for in association with various conditions. It may, therefore, be expected that a somewhat isolated specific function such as the visual motor gestalt function would show different types of disturbances in different types of conditions which are associated with mental deficiency, and even that they might be more or less specific for different conditions.

A simple retardation in maturation processes with a constitutional or hereditary background will be the most obvious type. Such individuals would be expected to show the responses of a normal child of the same mental age. Specific developmental defects in the field of language might be expected to show disturbances akin to the aphasias resulting from disease processes or injuries to the brain. These conditions have been described and

---

[1] Compiled, with considerable new data added, from Bender, Lauretta: *A Visual Motor Gestalt Test and Its Clinical Use,* 1938, Chapters IX, XII and XIV.

[2] Clark, L. Pierce: *Nature and Treatment of Amentia,* 1933, p. 3.

analyzed by Samuel T. Orton.[3] Congenital word blindness, or congenital alexia, is the best known of this group, and within recent years children with this type of disability are being recognized, studied and given remedial training which helps them to compensate for their specific deficiency. Such children often show directional disturbance in the visual motor gestalt function. Children with congenital aphasia are more difficult to differentiate from the general category of mental deficiency because of the speech retardation and the necessity to utilize special performance tests to show the general intellectual level. Other aphasic disturbances secondary to structural injuries may be present with difficulties in the symbol unit and with perseverative tendencies. Such a case will be discussed below.

Schizophrenia in children with retardation and blocking is not always differentiated from other conditions in which the children are functioning at a mentally defective level. According to Howard W. Potter, institutions for mental defectives probably care for many such schizophrenic children who are not recognized as such. Difficulties in perception or in impulses may also be important factors, either with inhibited impulses or hyperkinesis. Confusional difficulties with disorientation, with essential difficulties in spatial orientation of configuration on the background, may occur with epilepsy or other conditions. Neurotic or emotional blocking of speech and social contacts and infantile reactions are known to be factors in apparent retardation of development where there are no structural or functional disturbances in the realm of perception, memory, ideation, judgment, or reasoning. In other cases the retardation seems to be specific for certain fields, with normal or superior ability in other fields. Some children rated as mentally defective by the standard tests and social criteria are able to handle the visual motor gestalten in a normal or superior fashion.

There is a tendency still expressed by some psychologists to look upon mental deficiency as a simple quantitative problem. Rudolf Pintner recommends the percentage criteria which he believes would divest feeblemindedness of sociological criteria. Thus the lowest X percentage ($1\frac{1}{2}\%$ according to Cyril Burt) of the community should be considered as feebleminded. He also believes that clinical classification has value for the medical profession only. This would be true if the only basis for the classification was the size of the head, anatomical structure of the brain, endocrine features, and body build. But if it is true that classification will also indicate different intellectual and psychic functions with the possibility of different types of training, the classification would seem to be of value to the psychologist, psychiatrist, and educator as well.

Mental deficiency has been studied through the Rorschach test both by its original author and by Samuel J. Beck. It has been observed that the feeble-

---

[3] *Salmon Lectures, New York,* 1936.

minded react to the blot configuration with the fewest number of whole
responses. The number of whole responses is considered by Rorschach to be
an indicator of the energy which is directed towards associational activity
and, also, of a conscious or unconscious will to complex achievement. Thus
it is concluded that whole responses are a function of intelligence. Other
functions of intelligence as measured by the Rorschach test are listed by
Beck as perception of sharp forms, inner creativity, originality, and a low
percentage of stereotyped thought. Alfred Binet has also defined feeble-
minded persons as "stereotyped children." Beck also reports that he found
atypical reactions in 11%—some of which suggested the dissociative phenomena of schizophrenia, and others an unevenness in the maturation processes.

A dynamic theory for feeblemindedness has been offered by Kurt Lewin,
a gestalt psychologist, who directed his studies mostly in the field of personality, will, and social relationships. He has found that the feebleminded
are to be characterized as dynamically more rigid and less mobile. He based
this on studies of feebleminded children's psychical satiation, resumption of
interrupted action, and the values of substitute actions. Thus, when children
are given a task and then interrupted in the middle of it to carry out another
task to completion, 79% of normal children will return to complete the
uncompleted task. It is found in normal children that a high substitute
value (returning to incompleted task reduced from 79% to 33%) may be obtained; on the other hand, in the defective children, the rigidity of the
tension system reveals itself by the low substitute value (94% returned to
incompleted task). Thus the "will" of the feebleminded child is said to be
strong and rigid. Kurt Lewin also quotes W. Eliasberg to the effect that the
feebleminded think more concretely and perceptually. It is said also that
the feebleminded child shows less "stratification," meaning that a feeble-
minded child of a given age shows less differentiation than a normal child
of the same age brought up under similar circumstances. The question still
remains, however, as to whether he really resembles a younger normal child.
On this point the writer would disagree with Kurt Lewin and present evidence indicating that the defective child may be more rigid and less differentiated than the normal younger child of a similar mental level. Similar
problems will be discussed in Chapter 8 in the Goodenough drawing-of-a-
man test in mentally deficient and encephalitic children.

It is interesting to see how mentally defective individuals respond to these
visual motor patterns. It is found that there is not simply a lower level of the
integrated gestalt production commensurate with the mental level determined
by the other standard psychometric tests. There is a much greater variety of
productions among mentally defectives of a given mental age level than
among normal children of the same mental age. There is, of course, retarda-

tion of some one or all of the various maturation processes, but this retardation may be more in one field than in another. Naturally, one sometimes gets results which are commensurate with the mental level. Sometimes one may get results above the mental level indicated by the standard mental tests or by the poor social adjustment that may justify the institutional care. This is partly due to the fact that this is not a test of educational or language accomplishment but of maturation processes and is, in that way, comparable to the so called performance tests. Often the gestalten are produced in a more simple fashion, but with better motor control. There may be more primitive scribbling, but in some way it is better controlled, as the work of Alfred (Fig. 12) will show. In Fig. 12, all of the children were of about the same chronological and mental ages, but it will be seen that the productions vary greatly.

Beside the scribbling of Alfred, one sees how Charles uses the primitive loop almost entirely—but with a greater conservation of energy and with less tendency to experiment than the younger normal children display. Arthur shows a combination of the scribbling and the loops. Often the results are somewhat bizarre and show dissociative and plastic features that are suggestive of schizophrenia, such as is seen in the work of Nicholas. Figures A, 1, and 5 are as they might be done by a bright younger child, while all of the other figures show some mature features with more or less dissociation, scattering, reduplication, etc. In some defective children we find hyperkinetic features. Lillian had suffered from encephalitis and had a defective intelligence quotient. She was hyperkinetic in all her behavior. The hyperkinetic features in her productions are seen: 1) in the tendencies to flight in Figure 2 where the third line is tailed off around in a curved fashion; 2) in Figure 4, where both open figures are closed, and the figure is rotated into the vertical position by a rapid association that she called "doggie"; and, 3) in Figure 7, which is only partially finished when her flight carries her off into much decoration by perseveration, which she called "fishie." Aside from the hyperkinetic features, however, Lillian's productions show the characteristics of retarded mental level, rather than of her chronological age as may be seen in the horizontal series in Figure 2.

A number of mental defective individuals at the Children's Hospital of Randall's Island[4] were tested with the visual motor gestalt test. The cases were unselected except that individuals were chosen whose mental ages ranged from 3 to 6 years. Fifty-six individuals were tested, there being 30 children from age 4-2 to age 10-3, and 26 adults from 16 to 49 years of age. The results of these examinations have been analyzed: 1) to determine if the maturation level could be estimated in the light of the standardized results

[4] Through the courtesy of Dr. Louise E. Poull, Chief Psychologist at Randall's Island at the time this material was obtained.

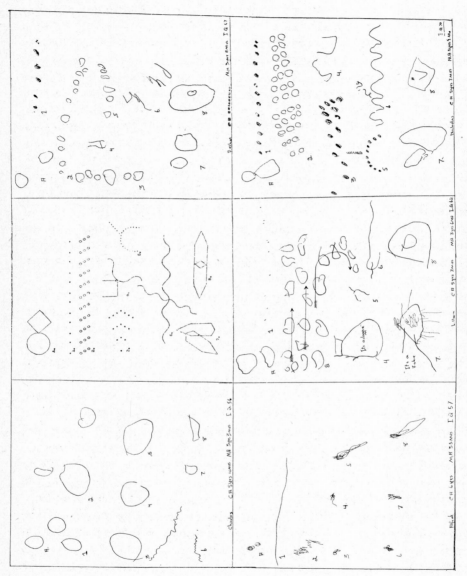

Fig. 12. Visual motor gestalt test of mental defective children:
C.A., 5-7 to 6-0; and, M.A., 3-3 to 4-0.

of the tests on normal children; 2) to determine if the results were comparable to the mental tests obtained by the usual standard tests (Terman, in this group of cases); and, 3) to determine if the test revealed a simple retardation in maturation in the visual motor gestalt in defective individuals, or gave evidence of other types of disturbance.

Ten children had a mental age at the 3 year level. Their chronological ages ranged from 4-2 to 7 years, their IQ's from 48 to 72. In six of these the child responded to each test figure with a simple unformed scribble which could not be analyzed further than to say that there was no evidence of any maturation of the visual motor gestalt function above the 3 year level. One of the children produced drawings decidedly superior to the level indicated by the standard tests and the social criteria. This was a child of age 5-7 with an IQ of 70 (see Nicholas, Fig. 12). The productions were such as would be expected of his actual age or a year better, except that he also showed some tendency to plasticity and to separate parts and split figures in the schizophrenic fashion. Three other children produced drawings which could be recognized as efforts to draw the test figures. In many ways they resembled the drawings of a 4 year old child except that they were more restrained; in two, the unit figure was more rigidly utilized and perseverated; in the third, there were some dissociative phenomena.

Twelve children had a mental age at the 4 year level. Their chronological age was 5-9 to 8-9, and their IQ's ranged from 53 to 80. Two of the children produced drawings normal for their chronological age, one other showed drawings appropriate to his chronological age but with some confusional features due to disorienting the figures on the background. Three children showed a simple retardation in maturation processes so that the drawings were more or less appropriate for the mental age given by the standard tests. Three children showed retardation in the maturation process with preservative or aphasic disturbances. One showed retardation with confusional features, and one showed retardation with dissociative or schizoid phenomena.

Five children had a mental age at the fifth year. Two of these produced drawings at a maturation level that was normal for their chronological age but one showed schizophrenic and the other aphasic phenomena; two children showed a simple retardation of the maturation of the process at the mental level indicated by the standard tests, while one showed retardation with aphasic features.

Three children had a mental age at the 6 year level. One of these made normal drawings, one retarded drawings, and one aphasic drawings. The children examined scored IQ's between 48 and 80 or, in other words, at the moron range. Six of the 30 children were still too young and their drawings too poorly differentiated to be of analytical value; they may possibly have represented a simple retardation. Otherwise, there were six children whose drawings indicated a simple retardation of the maturation process for the visual motor gestalt function, in keeping with other intellectual tests. Six children produced drawings at the maturation level of their physical age, with evidences of disturbances which might be characterized as aphasic due to simplification of the gestalt unit with perseveration; they showed confusional features due to dissociative phenomena.

Of the adults,[5] nine had a mental age at the fifth year level with IQ's ranging from 27 to 31. In none of these did the drawings show the features of a simple retardation to the mental age of 4. Two, however, rather closely resembled the work of a 4 year old child, except for the poverty of the drawings, which may be interpreted as a poverty or blocking of impulses. Three others showed this same poverty of responses which were also distorted and might be considered to be a combination of perceptive and impulse disturbances. Three others showed marked aphasic disturbances; the remaining one showed schizophrenic disturbances. Fifteen adults had a mental age of 5 with IQ's ranging from 33 to 39. One drawing was that of a normal child. Four showed retardation to the mental age of 5 years but with the usual defective features of restricted activity, rigidity of response, and some slight but recognizable disturbances in the way of disorientation of perseveration; seven showed marked aphasic disturbances and three showed marked schizophrenic features. Two adults, with mental ages of 6 and with IQ's of 40 and 41, showed aphasic phenomena.

This group of adults showed a range of intelligence quotient from 27 to 41, thus representing the imbecile group. It is interesting that one individual produced a normal adult drawing. Of the others, only six at the most produced drawings which could be interpreted as a simple retardation in maturation to the mental age as estimated by the other standard tests. Even in these, there were features which are considered typical of the mental defective intelligence. All of the others showed more or less severe disturbances which have been found as characteristic in known cases of aphasia, schizophrenia or confusional states, or disturbances due to blocking of impulses and severe perceptive defects. It would appear, therefore, that in the lower-grade defectives a considerable number of the individuals show some specific type of disturbance which might be comparable to the specific disorders in the speech centers of the brain, or to specific impulse or perceptive disorders, or to confusional features, which may accompany a number of different organic conditions.

It will be of considerable interest to analyze more carefully certain indi-

---

[5] Occasionally data from adults will be included because of the comparable mental level or states, as occurs here, or because we are able to follow the course of the child into adulthood, or because the original writing of a contribution included studies of adults referring to the childhood period or making comparisons which are a significant part of the contribution.

vidual cases where the differential diagnosis of intelligence quotient represents a challenging problem:

Jack (Fig. 13) was a child who suffered speech disturbances in connection with convulsions. He was age 8 when last examined. He was apparently born a normal child in a gifted family. At age 2 he began to show precocious ability in piano playing, and was considered a prodigy by the family. However, following a severe attack of whooping cough, he developed epileptic convulsions of the Jacksonian type. The treatment was neglected as the mother was unwilling to recognize the condition. His mental development was retarded with the frequent severe convulsions. Following a particularly

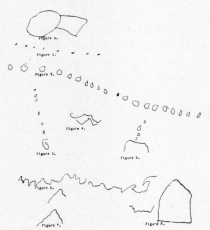

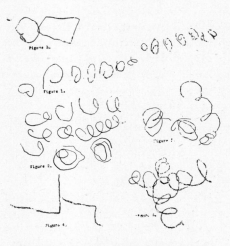

FIG. 13. Visual motor gestalt test, by Jack, an epileptic child.

FIG. 14. Visual motor gestalt test, by Walter, a congenitally aphasic child.

severe series of convulsions he became paralytic on the right side, and aphasic. The mother then consented to treatment. Phenobarbital and ketogenic diet controlled the convulsions, and the child recovered from the aphasia and paralysis, except for some weakness in the right hand. His behavior improved. However, his mental condition remained retarded at 50 on the Stanford-Binet scale. He had lost considerable of his ability at the piano. His gestalt drawings (Fig. 13) show many of the features of a child of 5 to 6 years of age with the tendency to rigidity in response and poverty in impulse often seen in the defective. There is some preseveration seen in Figures 4 and 7 and a poor attention to detail. There are no marked disturbances which may be characterized as aphasic at this time, however. Jack was subsequently committed to the state epileptic colony.

Walter (Fig. 14) was another child who was brought to us with speech difficulties. He reported to the Mental Hygiene Clinic at intervals between the ages of 4 and 6 because of retardation in speech and dull, inadequate social behavior. He was an illegitimate child of an illiterate Negro mother.

A marked discrepancy between the Stanford-Binet and the performance tests was noted at the time of the first examination. When his age was 4-5, his IQ on the Stanford-Binet was 68; it was 83 on the Randall's Island performance test. When he was age 5-11 his IQ was 79 on the Stanford-Binet and 110 on the Pintner-Patterson performance test. The history showed that he had not learned to speak until he was nearly 4 and that then his speech was hesitant and meagre, and could be understood only by his mother. He was shy, quiet, and unresponsive to strangers. His mother assumed an over-protective attitude toward him. Even when he was nearly 6, he would not speak to strangers. The mother claimed that he played and talked with children, but usually only repeated what they said. She asserted that his speech was adequate for her to understand his wants. While he was under observation, it gradually became possible for his teachers to adapt him to situations so that he would speak. His speech was always normal, but very limited. He seemed to have to learn new items of speech either as words, phrases, or sentences, with considerable conscious effort. Some observers felt that his speech was inhibited on a neurotic basis. There was however some evidence against this. The mother gave the history that he had preferred the left hand but she had taught him to use the right. At the time he was under observation, it was very difficult to determine either his dominant hand or eye. He seemed to shift from one side to the other. It was noted, however, that when he used his right hand in writing numbers or copying, he was inclined to produce reversals or mirror images. His gestalt drawings are very significant (Fig. 14). They are not the drawings of a normal child, age 6, who might be neurotically inhibited. They show striking features similar to the adult aphasic.[6] The looped unit symbol is used with many variations and with perseverative tendencies. Difficulties in interpreting the figures are also seen. These features are combined with others which suggest normal mentality. Figure A, for example, shows the diamond formation of a child, age 6. Figure 6 represents a similar level of attainment. It was thus our opinion that this child was suffering from a congenital aphasia, associated with disturbances in cortical dominance together with perceptual difficulties. The unit symbol of loops is used in most figures.

The study of the visual motor gestalt function shows that the problem of mental deficiency is not a simple problem. If one were to assume a slow-up or simplification of the maturation process in a unified way, one would expect less differentiation, a more unified system, a stronger and simpler gestalt, such as is found in the younger normal child. This does occur in some individuals, especially among the higher-grade defectives. Such individuals usually seem to represent the hereditary constitutional defective. Even in these cases, a simple retardation is not found in all of the principles of the integrated visual motor gestalt function. Motor control is usually better than in normal children of a younger age. Small, energy-conserving figures are the

---

[6] See Bender, Lauretta: *A Visual Motor Gestalt Test and Its Clinical Use,* Chapter VII.

rule. The primitive loop is freely used with less motor play or experimentation. The patterns are more rigid. In the majority of the responses of all the mental defectives investigated other features are also seen.

It must be realized that many individuals who function as mental defectives do so not because of a hereditary retardation in maturation, but because they are constitutional deviates of some other sort; or because of some subsequent brain pathology. It is, therefore, possible to get every sort of deviation in the personality reaction and in the gestalt function. Detailed analysis reveals that many individuals who are functioning as mental defectives show evidence in their gestalt drawings of more or less severe aphasic disturbances which are characterized by the use of a perseverated primitive symbolic unit. Some others show the dissociative phenomena characteristics of schizophrenia; others show disturbances in impulses with a poverty of response or hyperkinetic features. Finally, still others show perceptual difficulties, confusional features, with disorientation of whole figures or parts of the figures, on the background. Such analysis leads to the opinion that there are multiple causes of mental defectiveness, which may be classified as simple retardation in maturation; specific disabilities in the language field; dissociative phenomena which distort the whole personality, or schizophrenia; impulse disturbances; perceptual disturbances; confusional disturbances. Such analysis leads also to the hope for a better understanding of mental defectiveness and the hope of classifying some groups and treating them specifically. Furthermore, the gestalt test aids in the analysis, differential diagnosis, and prognosis of specific cases.

The impulse, perceptual, and confusional disturbances are symptoms of organic brain damage. This type of disorder in visual motor patterning in the gestalt drawings of children serves as diagnostic aid for the kind of organic brain damage associated with these features. It is true that all brain-damaged children are not mentally defective, but to the extent that the gestalt function is impaired there is a disorder in intellectual functioning. The visual motor gestalt test is useful as a diagnostic tool in organic brain damages in children.[7]

II. VISUAL MOTOR GESTALT FUNCTION IN
CHILDHOOD SCHIZOPHRENIA

The earliest work done by us with the visual motor gestalt test was with schizophrenic adults at the Springfield State Hospital in Maryland in 1929-30.[8] Since then our knowledge has been extended by the opportunity

---

[7] See Wechsler, David: chapter on Psychological Diagnosis in Israel Wechsler's *Clinical Neurology*, 6th Edition, 1947. Pp. 90-104.

[8] See Bender, Lauretta: Principles of Gestalt in . . . Schizophrenic Persons. *Arch Neur. & Psych.*, March 1932.

to study the schizophrenic children at Bellevue Hospital.[9] Our definition of childhood schizophrenia is a clinical entity occurring in childhood before puberty which reveals pathology in behavior at every level and in every area of integration or patterning within the functioning of the central nervous system, including vegetative, motor, perceptual, intellectual, emotional, and social functioning. This behavior pathology disturbs the pattern of every functioning field characteristically by plasticity in pattern formation.

The motility of the schizophrenic child is especially important and in turn influences the perceptual motor patterns and psychological problems. This motility is characterized by a plastic regressive reflex motor activity including a tendency to whirl about and rotate rhythmically and to engage in a great deal of reflex motor play. There is also a tendency for motor dependency and cohesiveness.

In the schizophrenic child the visual motor gestalt functioning shows a similar disturbance. There is a tendency to use old primitive responses interlocked with the more mature capacities which are to be expected from the maturational level of the child. In the drawing of the gestalt test figures there is therefore an excessive use of the vortical movement even with good diamond forms. A series of figures on a horizontal plane may be pulled around into a vortical figure. The boundaries of circles are uncertain and may have been gone over several times. The centers of circles are uncertain; there are no points but many little circles, and for the same reason angular and crossed forms are fragmented. Action cannot be readily controlled and figures are elaborated, enlarged, repeated. The total product makes a pattern itself with a great deal of fluidity based upon vortical movement. The perceptual patterns lose their boundaries and therefore their relationship to the background. One may speak, too, of a motor compliance and cohesiveness between the boundaries of two objects. Similar reactions are observed in the motor behavior or in the way the schizophrenic child relates its body to that of others. There is also an effort to explore and fixate depth or third and fourth dimensions. In a well-patterned fluid matrix there are areas in which the pattern is broken; a part of a figure is separated from the whole and made to rotate faster; for example, a group of small circles may be separated from the whole mass. It is as though a pebble were thrown into a stream of rippling water, causing a new wave movement. One's best understanding of these phenomena is to think in terms of a disturbance in the time factor in patterned behavior characteristic for each field of behavior, such a time factor being of biological origin and specific for the schizophrenic disease process. Other forms of behavior such as regressive, projective and introjective, elaborative, inhibitive, distractive and concretistic, appear to be efforts on the

---

[9] See Bender, Lauretta: Childhood Schizophrenia. *Am. Jour. Orthopsych.,* 1947.

part of the personality to orient itself to this pathology and to control it, if possible.

When the child draws the human form, it is essentially a projection of his body image and its problems; it is a self-portrait. It is not surprising that the schizophrenic child with his body-image problems, motility, and perceptual disturbances, uncertainty as to his identity and his drive for action, finds ready expression for his problems in drawing the human form.[10] The techniques that are used have a wide range even in the same child. The most primitive use of vortical movement with graduated variations may be the sole form used to draw a human figure, but it expresses just that whirling motility, impulse to action, fluid ego boundary, and uncertain center of gravity which represents the schizophrenic child and his problems. He is by no means limited to this technical device.

The studies we made of visual motor gestalten of schizophrenic children confirmed previously made observations on schizophrenic adults. The visual motor patterns can be understood if we realize that all form arises from motion, which is vortical, and that the schizophrenic disturbance in function is such a fundamental one that there tends to be disturbance in this motion which distorts the form of the units and the relationship of the gestalt configuration. Gestalt drawings of typical schizophrenic patients are easily recognized by the plastic distortions of the configurations produced, by the frequent splitting in figures (not in such a way as to make a "gute Gestalt"), and especially by their showing an unusual cohesion between all the figures and an increase in movement in the figures on the background. Attempts to use these figures as matrices for delusional or confabulatory ideation by ornamenting them with connecting lines, destroying the original gestalt, and creating new figures, are usually noticeable.

Schizophrenic children show similar tendencies in their drawings of gestalten (see Willy, Fig. 8, lower part; Nicholas, Fig. 12, lower right-hand; and Marty, Fig. 15).

Marty was brought to Bellevue in December 1934 at the age of 6 years because of retarded and withdrawn behavior, which had been getting worse since he was age 4 years. He seemed to live in his own fantasy world; it was not possible to make satisfactory contact with him; his speech was scanty consisting of inappropriate ejaculations which were not related to the situation. He had a dreamy far-away look, took no interest in the play of the other children, nor in the routine. He had to be dressed and then would not keep his clothes on. He had to be fed, did not sleep at night, and was disturbed by bad dreams and severe anxiety reactions. The diagnosis of schizophrenia

---

[10] Montague, Allison: "Spontaneous Drawings of the Human Form in Childhood Schizophrenia" in Anderson, Howard H. and Anderson, Gladys L. (Editors): *Projective Techniques*, New York, Prentice-Hall, Inc., 1951.

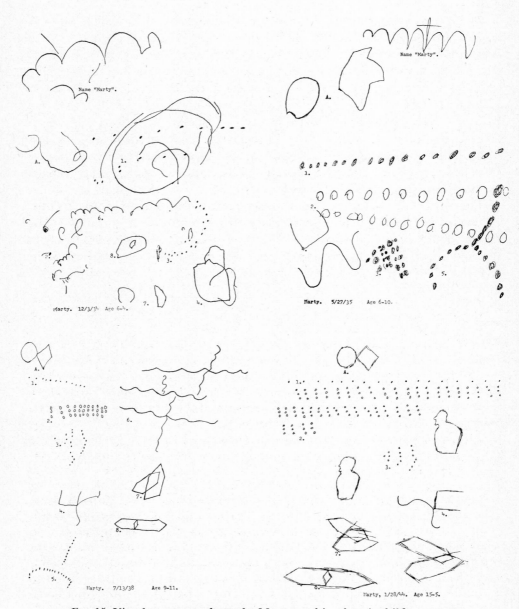

FIG. 15. Visual motor gestalt test by Marty, a schizophrenic child, at ages 6-4, **6-10**, 9-11 and 15-5.

was suggested from the beginning although some of the staff thought that he was a mentally defective child suffering from emotional shock. After a period of hospitalization and therapy there was considerable improvement but the subsequent course confirmed the diagnosis of schizophrenia.[11]

The first successful psychometric examination gave him an IQ of 74 with a marked scattering of responses and many atypical ones. His first gestalt drawings, December 1934 (Fig. 15) were characteristically plastic. They were scattered over several sheets of paper. Nevertheless one can see the gestalt principles in the figures. His own name was an abbreviated distortion and tended to influence some of the other figures. There was a good deal of vortical movement as in Figure A and Figure 1. Figure 4 was closed. There was a tendency for regressive or primitive phenomena, with movement and plasticity and also a tendency for the figures to be influenced by each other. Movement besides being circular seemed to direct the figures upward towards the right. Six months later, after a period of group and individual psychotherapy in the hospital, another psychometric test gave him an IQ of 98. His gestalt drawings were much more compact, each one was readily recognized for what it was intended to be. There were still immature features in the inability to draw a diamond, although the diagonal on Figure 5 was fairly well done even though it tended to be arc-shaped. Horizontal planes were dominant as in Figure 2. Dots were much worked over in a compulsive way. This was the remainder of the strong drive to vortical movement. These plastic features were seen in the rounded corners, the spreading of the two horizontal lines in Figure 2, the movement in Figure 5, and the separation in Figures A and 4, as well as in the vertical activity in all dotted forms.

After this Marty went home and started to school. He was accepted in the class room where he was thought to be dull, if not defective, and where he was inactive and relatively unresponsive. He was not very conspicuous, however, except as a day dreamer and because he was protected by his sister, two years older. Three years later, in the summer of 1938, he returned for metrazol shock treatment which had then become available on our service. On a psychometric examination he scored an IQ of 92. His gestalt drawings were rigid and highly controlled. They were small and carefully done but showed schizophrenic features. The most conspicuous of the latter was the separation of one part of Figure 3, but still showing the definite form of this figure. It appears as though this separated part has been duplicated and projected. Also Figure 6 had been repeated three times and in the middle one the difficulty in crossing was expressed. There was still some tendency for spreading in Figure 2 but now it is in the vertical plane. There was also some rounding of corners. But the figures displayed maturity. Apparently the same defense mechanism which made it possible for Marty to control his anxiety and fantasy life sufficiently to attend school rather inconspicuously, showed in his gestalt work in the closely controlled precise configurations.

After the metrazol shock he seemed a little more active, responsive and

[11] See Chap. XIII for more case history, therapy and drawings.

realistic. He continued in school and entered high school where his work was also fair. In January 1944 at the age of 15-6 he was re-examined. The psychometric examination on the Bellevue-Wechsler test gave him an IQ score of 79, with uneven functioning and unpredictability and unreliability of responses. The Rorschach showed anxiety and compulsive features. His motility was still cataleptic. His gestalt drawings showed good configurations, compulsive precision and repetition. He repeated the small circles in Figure 2 excessively, but controlled the movement of the dots. Straight lines and large circles are gone over excessively as though they could not be defined or controlled. Twice he stopped to attempt the human figure which appears to be merely a variation of Figure A verticalized. This in itself represents a struggle with a maturation problem in identification, appropriate for the ages of 3-4-5 years, and a point at which the schizophrenic child often becomes fixated.

These gestalt drawings of Marty have been analyzed in considerable detail in order to show the nature of the schizophrenic process in the gestalt function and the effect of strong efforts on the part of the individual to control the disorganizing process. It is possible that Marty's ability to control the plastic features in visual motor patterns is significant in relation to the relatively good clinical prognosis.

Marty is now 21 years of age. He has graduated from high school and earns his living while living at home with his mother. He still demonstrates schizophrenic features in that he is cataleptic and shows the whirling motility characteristic of the schizophrenic child. He has the "schizoid" introverted personality. His sister at 17 became acutely schizophrenic and now at 23 is in a hospital.

Francine, a 10 year old girl, was recognized as an obvious schizophrenic child when she came to our children's ward in 1935. At that time the diagnosis of schizophrenia in childhood was not commonly made. Her subsequent course confirmed the diagnosis. After several months she left our wards for a state hospital and has remained there ever since. In 1948 at the age of 23 years, she was a typical chronic delapidated schizophrenic.

As a 10 year old child her motility showed catatonic features with constrained postures and bizarre activities such as twirling her saliva out of her mouth and onto her dress with quick automatic movements. She showed an imbalance of the vegetative function with cold extremities, mottled skin, and episodes of cyanosis and syncope, when she seemed quite ill without evident cause. Her social behavior was inappropriate; her association with other children was impersonal; her emotional reaction was inadequate and lacked spontaneity. Her thought processes were distorted, she could not attend to her lessons, she experimented with words and concepts in a way that gave a philosophical turn to all her utterances. She was preoccupied with delusional ideas especially in regard to the structure and function of her body, sexual problems, her relationship to her mother.

Psychotherapy was attempted in 1935 with all the techniques then available.

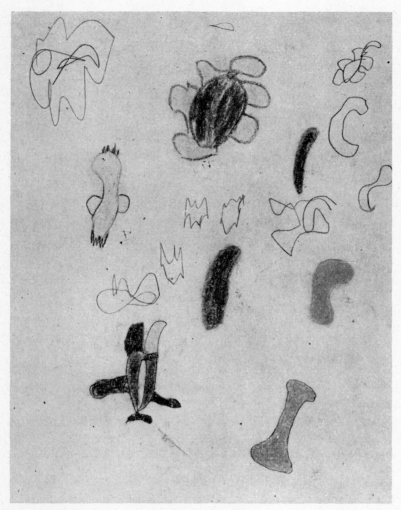

FIG. 16. Brain Bodies, fantasied introjected objects by Francine (*pencil and crayon*).

When she was clay modeling she once said, "There is a mummy. A mummy she is a mummer, I suspect. She gives you ovaltine. Kindly, gentle, animals that your confidence may buy, who will be good and loving to you if you will only be kind. She also gives you lies. She tells aplenty—she is a big frame-up, my mother. This is a mummy I tell you and a mummy is a dead person. A cruel and heartless thing. Yessir, I killed her, I wouldn't live with her." Thus she expressed her ever-present ambivalent attitude towards her mother, the one person in the world that she had every reason to love and feel dependent upon.

She often spoke of a "brain body" and drew pictures of it (Fig. 16). At first she said: "There is a brain body inside me. I found it out from my mother that I had it inside of my body. She happened to mention it. It harms my body. It does a lot of harm I hear. I heard about a brain body doing harm. It comes from my mother." It is probably difficult for anyone not accustomed to the primitive, symbolic thought of the schizophrenic fully to understand what this child meant. It seems probable, however, that in part she was

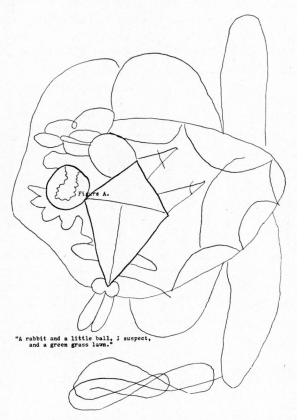

"A rabbit and a little ball, I suspect, and a green grass lawn."

FIG. 17. Gestalt drawing A. A Rabbit and a Little Ball,
I Suspect, and a Green Grass Lawn,
by Francine (*pencil*).

referring to her own bad self inside of herself, for which she blamed her mother for giving birth to her. It also was determined by one of the doctors who worked intimately with her that this represented a girl-child's delusion of pregnancy, the result of her badness. One must not accept any of these concepts too literally, but allow for a good deal of poetic license. We soon learned that in schizophrenic children such "introjected fantasied bodies"[12] were to be found in place of projections or hallucinations.

[12] See Rapoport, Jack: Phantasy Objects in Children. *Psychoanalytic Rev.*, 1944.

Francine was asked to draw the "brain body" which she drew in the form of a bone in yellow, blue, and red. But such comparatively simple forms did not satisfy her (Fig. 16). She soon started to draw complicated indented lines and added irregular little waves in a different color to the simple oval which was her original form. There was never complete symmetry. When symmetry seemed almost achieved, she destroyed it by adding some slight irregularity. In these first schematic drawings long ovals prevailed. Very often they were drawn out in the form of fantastic sausages. This represents primitive play with a form which is not completely symmetrical, contrasting the smooth line with the curves and indentations.

Francine was asked to draw the gestalt figures and her play with symmetry could be directly observed. Figure A was at first copied correctly except that the diamond was lengthened downwards (see Fig. 17). Then she began to distort it until she had destroyed the original gestalt; she experimented with new forms that only slightly resembled the original stimulus. She began by subdividing the diamond and adding new excrescences to the basic line. The excrescences were irregular, sinusoidal waves, half circles, oblong sausage-like figures in which symmetry was sometimes approached but never reached. It is as if the simple form was immediately overshadowed by form principles of a very primitive wavy and oblong type. She gave it the title "A Rabbit and a Little Ball, I Suspect, and a Green Grass Lawn." One can see the motif of the rabbit's ears appearing again and again in the drawing, though often distorted. Of course the ball belongs to the original figure, the green grass lawn is the background which is fundamental to every gestalt, the rabbit probably represents the schizophrenic tendency to action which is seen in every configuration.

III. VISUAL MOTOR GESTALT TEST AND PSYCHONEUROSIS

In the psychoneuroses are found disturbances in the normal emotional development through the infantile stages. The child who is frustrated or traumatized in his demands for satisfaction arising from his relationship to his mother or father or from his own instinctual needs will tend to show a persistent demand for a more satisfying type of relationship or experience. Since the frustration or trauma may occur in the infantile stage when consciousness is not fully developed, it usually happens that the individual remains unconscious of this reason—unless it can be brought into consciousness by some special technique such as psychoanalysis. The unrewarded infantile demand for satisfaction is usually represented by some other activity which stands as a symbol for the real desires and drives of the personality. Since the stage of dawning consciousness is also the stage of maturation of perception or perceptual motor patterns, it would not be surprising to find that some of

these patterns might become the symbol of the individual's unsatisfied infantile drives. In other words they might represent the individual's preoccupations, obsessions, or compulsions.

In 1941, Paul Schilder and Lauretta Bender described a specific neurotic
disorder in the behavior of children which they called impulsions. Impulsions give to the objective observer the impression of compulsions and obsessions, but have a different value for the child who experiences them. This
condition was observed in children between the ages of 4 and 12 years. The
symptomatology consists of continuous looking at and handling of a specific
object, drawing of the object, preoccupation with the object in fantasies or in
thoughts, excessive walking, counting, and preoccupation with numbers and
space. The subjects insist on immediate satisfaction of their wishes. They
cannot stand any interference in the fulfillment of their desires. There may
be greed concerning food and money or a tendency to collect and hoard.
Such children are stubborn, aggressive, show hypochondriacal preoccupations, and may use asocial means to satisfy their strong desires.

The impulsions take their origin from early infantile situations and desires
and can be compared with the preoccupation of children before they are 2
years old. They are never direct expressions of sexual, motor, or aggressive,
drives, but are always related to the family situation and are, therefore, in
many respects the results of transformation, i.e., of sexual motor or aggressive
drives. However, owing to the inefficiency of the ego-superego structure at
this age, the transformation is not as far-reaching as it is in patients with
obsessional character trends which otherwise have a similar genesis.

Billy was one of the boys discussed in our contribution on impulsions. He
had been under psychiatric observation and treatment at the Bellevue
Hospital and Mental Hygiene Clinic since 1935 when he was age 5-6. He was
a child of superior intelligence, the only child of parents of college training.
His home life was not always satisfactory as his parents were not always
compatible; several times his mother had gone to her parents' home with
Billy because of sexual incompatibility, jealousy on the father's part and
nervousness on the mother's. The birth was difficult because the mother had
a narrow pelvis and instruments were needed. It is probable that Billy had
heard this discussed. There was no evidence that his head was injured at the
time of birth, however. He was born with an imperforate anus which was
operated on the second day after birth. The function of his anus was impaired and he had to have frequent manual dilations performed by his
mother until the age of 2, as well as occasional instrumental ones by the
family physician thereafter.

The normal course of his oedipus complex was interfered with because
of the unsatisfactory relationship between the parents and the frequent
visits of the mother and Billy away from home. He openly expressed a hatred
for his father, the desire for the father's death or removal from the home,

and the wish to have his mother to himself. He also identified himself strongly with his mother and expressed a strong dislike for his penis. He wished to be like his mother, wanted to sit on the toilet to urinate and frequently denied his penis.[13]

At age 2-6 while visiting his grandparents, he enjoyed automobile rides as many children do. He was fascinated with the "Stop" and "Go" traffic lights and seemed to think that they made the car stop and go. At home he played in a cupboard where he could sit on a shelf and close himself in with the cupboard door, which was like the door on the automobile. He would play at taking imaginary rides with imaginary "Stop" and "Go" lights that made the car stop and go. He then became interested in doors as such, then with their knobs, key holes and hinges, and finally with door checks. Door checks became an obsession with him that occupied him from this time up to the period when he came to the hospital for treatment. He was preoccupied all day with doors and door checks. He had been rejected from kindergarten because he smashed the fingers of the other children in the doors. He could not play on the streets because he could not be stopped from playing with the neighbors' doors all up and down the street. He was much concerned with the shape of the doors, the door knobs, the casements, and hinges.

All his questions were concerned with how doors open and close. He believed that the door check made the door open and close. When he was told that babies were made inside of the mother, he believed that they got out by door checks. He would also occupy himself by the hour by drawing doors and door checks. He valued these drawings very highly and became very aggressive when an effort was made to remove them from him or to destroy them. It was important in the drawing of these doors that they maintain certain proportions and that the shape of the plate for the key hole and the door knob, the hinges, and the hinge plates bear a definite relationship to the shape of the door. Thus they must all be square or rectangular so that the axis was vertical.[14] If they were drawn for him so that the long axis was horizontal it disturbed him to the point of his having a rage. Furthermore the color of the crayons that were used was important. Green doors and door checks were especially valuable as they represented "Go," while red ones represented "Stop." Thus he was very much concerned with movement and the impetus for movement; for openings and the mechanisms for openings, and he was preoccupied with symbols for these things. When he dealt with them as visual motor patterns, he treasured them very highly and he demanded that they conform to his concepts of such patterns.

After he had been in the hospital for a period of a month he developed some new obsessions. He resented his placement in the hospital away from

---

[13] For more details on the dynamics of the psychosexual development and the development of the impulsion state in this boy, see the original article: Bender, Lauretta and Schilder, Paul: *Impulsions: a Specific Disorder of the Behavior of Children.*

[14] See Wolff, Werner: *Personality of the Pre-school Child,* for the significance of the patterned rhythmic relationship of parts to each other and to the whole in children's drawings.

his mother and was very much preoccupied with the reasons for sending him there, and with his new experiences and associates. An effort had been made to direct his good intelligence into lines which usually interest a child of his mental age. He was taught his numbers and how to read. He was greatly preoccupied with the numbers and especially "6." The children's ward is located on the 6th floor. Much of the day was spent in the school rooms and play rooms of the 8th floor and on the 8th floor open roof. On returning to the 6th floor ward, it was Billy's habit to watch the mechanisms of the elevator and especially a window slit in the door of the elevator whereby the elevator mechanic could determine the number of the floor he was approaching. The "6" which showed through this window slit was a large open faced figure. It was this "6" which fascinated Billy for months, as formerly he had been preoccupied with door checks. He made "6's" out of clay, paper and crayon all day long. He experimented with all kinds of "6's" and noted all their characteristics. He compared other numbers to "6." Thus he said that he liked "6" best of all because it was an open or smiling number. He liked "8" least of all because it was all closed up and sad. Next to "6" he liked "2" and "5." He also liked "6" because it had an edge on only one side of it, but he hated "1" because it was all edge. He didn't like "7" because it was almost like "1." He said that "9" was a "6" upside down, but was not much interested in it.

Due to his increasing aggressiveness under treatment (which cannot be discussed in this limited presentation) he was returned to the ward about eight months after his first admission. On this occasion he became obsessed with the indicators over the elevator doors which indicate the location of the elevators and the direction in which they are moving. These indicators are round in form with a clock-like face with nine numbers for the nine floors in the hospital and, as it happens, with "6" at the top. At the time he had first learned his numbers he had shown some passing interest in the clock with its numbers and moving hands. The elevator indicator, however, fascinated him completely. He believed that the indicator made the elevator come and go. He believed that the numbers on the indicator regulated the numbers on the floor and, since "6" was at the top he had reason to believe that all the floors in the hospital centered about this important floor. He was occupied all day long with the spatial problems of the series of floors from 1 to 9 and the circular series of numbers on the indicator with "6" at the top. To complete these preoccupations he was obsessed with the doors on the elevators. These are sliding doors with little windows in each of two partitions, so that when the doors are wide open by sliding past each other the little windows are parallel. He thus was soon able to preoccupy himself with the nine pairs of sliding doors with the nine indicators each with the complete series of numbers on their faces and always with "6" at the top.

Actually he was preoccupied with the philosophy of space, of sequence, and therefore of time, of movements, and finally of the mechanisms of movements, of doors and the meaning of openings, and of symbols for all these things. By this time "6" probably represented himself. It is also a feminine number not being penis-shaped like "1." At home he made "6's" out of clay or paper and crayon and gave them to his mother as a precious gift. He could not be induced to give them to his father although by this time he was on fairly good terms with his father. It is not possible for us to say what were all the mechanisms which relate these preoccupations with his personal experiences, with the difficulties of his anal sphincter, his hatred of his father and his own masculinity. It is of interest however to note how all of his optic imagery and visual motor patterns which constituted his favorite playthings conform to the principles of gestalten which are discussed here. It is obvious how much he was concerned with the primitive closed figures and with closures in the more active sense. His preoccupation with the different numbers concerns itself with their gestalt. Often in playing with the figure "6" he would state that one must close the lower part tight in drawing it on paper as that made it whiter in the inside. It is a well-known phenomena to gestalt psychologists that the figure on the background determined by an outline has internal organization and really is experienced as whiter or more solid.

It was very difficult to concentrate Billy's attention on anything except his obsessions. Therefore it was difficult to get him to draw the gestalt figures. On one occasion he drew them and they were as well done as a 7-year old child could do them. At other times he became distracted by some detail that reminded him of his favorite preoccupations. Figure A, for example, would remind him of indicators, and he would continue to draw indicators rather than complete the test. Figure 1 would remind him of sequences and he would write the numbers that indicated the floors of the hospital. Figure 7 was joined together by door checks; Figure 8 was turned into a door, and door checks added; at another time this figure was used to indicate the sliding doors of the elevator. Fig. 18 shows a few of Billy's drawings.

This boy may be considered from the point of view of Kurt Lewin,[15] who claims that the structure of the mind is composed of psychical systems, stratums and spheres in different degrees of tensions, striving for equilibrium. It is possible artificially to create an experiment with a psychical tension system by requesting a child to start a task and continue it to the point of satiation. It was found by Koepke[16] that 79% of 7 to 8 year old children would resume the uncompleted task.

Thus Anitra Karsten[17] ordered children of 8 to 9 years to draw moon faces until they had had enough of it. The normal child of this age drew moon faces for 55 minutes and then drew figures of his own choice for 3 minutes more. It is hard to compare Billy with these experiments since he was younger, was excessively restless, had poor attention and a strong resistance

---

[15] Lewin, Kurt: *Principles of Topological Psychology*, 1936.
[16] Koepke is quoted by Lewin, Kurt: *Ibid.*
[17] Karsten, Anitra: *Psychische Saettigung*, 1927, pp. 142-254.

to complying with requests. It must be considered that he was in a constant psychic tension state in regard to his obsessional interests. It was thought that it would be of interest to try to determine his satiation point and to utilize this mechanism as a possible therapeutic measure.

At the time when his interest in "6's" seemed to be at its height, he was given a roll of wrapping paper and to his delight, requested to draw as many

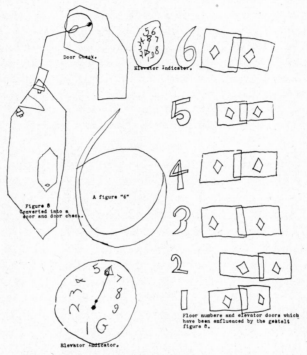

FIG. 18. Billy's drawings: Showing the influence of his psychoneurotic preoccupations and the gestalt test figures.

"6's" as he could. He drew "6's" with apparent satisfaction for 50 minutes. Once he stopped to draw an indicator which was half completed before the observer noticed it and asked him to set it aside and draw more "6's." He continued as requested and during the next 5 minutes became very restless and began to draw large "6's" to fill the paper more rapidly. He finally begged to stop. When offered the elevator indicator to finish, he did not wish to do so. The next day on entering the office and seeing the roll of paper and pencils, he asked if he could draw some other number. He was told he could choose to draw whatever he liked provided he continued with the same thing for the whole period. He drew elevator indicators but drew very large ones in order to fill the large roll of paper that was given him. This continued for some time but although he got very restless during the period and found many excuses to stop and had to be watched to keep him at the task, he resumed it again the next day with satisfaction. It appeared, however, that during this time he had many more interests than usual, and he kept at the usual routine of the other children, showing more interest in puppet shows. In art classes when given paper and pencil he drew other subjects and on one occasion drew a car going to a festival, driven by his psychiatrist, this being the first expression of his positive transference to the psychiatrist.

Billy's reactions to puppet shows[18] allowed a still deeper insight into his problems. Primitive oral and anal trends and an enormous aggression came into the foreground. He was particularly preoccupied with a play called *Casper and the Devil.* Day after day he would play in an impulsive manner with the puppet characters, the Devil and Casper. He played the following scene:

> The Devil appeared with a pitchfork with which he stuck Casper. Casper whimpered and cried. The devil laughed, "I am going to take you down to hell; ha-ha-ha." The Devil took Casper down to Hell. After that both characters were held up again and the whole scene re-enacted. Billy was observed to repeat this scene as many as twenty times in the course of one afternoon. During the play Billy let the Devil threaten Casper by saying: "I'll cut your eyes out. I'll chop your head off. I'll cut your stomach out." On a few occasions the Devil also took Billy's mother to Hell. Frequently Billy kept Casper down in Hell and let the Devil attack him with a pitchfork. When Billy was told that the devil was a bad character, he denied it. He said, "He is Billy's Devil. I tell him to do these things."

There is not much doubt that one is here dealing with an extreme sadistic aggressiveness and anality. This discussion does not attempt to exhaust the psychogenic problem. Billy's hate of his father was outspoken. For this reason he denied the existence of his own penis as well as his father's penis. One might be tempted to connect the whole problem with his congenital defect, the specific anal difficulty, the infantile period of manipulation, his mother's necessary preoccupation with his anal function, and Billy's resulting psychological problems. However, in our opinion, the marital problems of the parents were important as well as the local organ inferiority and the sensations connected with it. It is tempting to bring Billy's primary impulsions with the "Stop" and "Go" signals and the door checks in relation to the obstruction of his anus. However in this interpretation one must not forget that the preoccupations of young children with the opening and closing of doors may also be present without any difficulty with anal functioning. Billy was fascinated with his impulsions and could hardly be induced to give up acting in his customary impulsive manner. As long as he performed the impulsion he

---

[18] See Chapter 15 for puppet shows and more details about Casper and the Devil.

was satisfied, although he sometimes remarked that he had to do so. The distress started when he was hindered by outward circumstances from following his impulses. In other respects Billy was a difficult child, full of sudden and destructive impulses. It is remarkable that the impulses changed from time to time. All of them seemed to have symbolic character, although they were based on real interests, such as doors, numbers, and watches.

In 1949, it is possible to write the last chapter in Billy's case history. He left the children's ward in 1936 when he was 6 years old, but we had a continuing psychotherapeutic relationship with him afterwards, sometimes at long intervals and sometimes intensively. During latency he was preoccupied with his father's car which he called a jalopy, and which he fantasied would break down. He then for a while fantasied and dreamed that his mother was in a plane crash in which she was killed. He would draw pictures of these preoccupations and play them out with miniature toys. At the same time he desired to have knives in his possession which he polished and sharpened compulsively. He fantasied that he attacked his father with these knives. He slept with them under his pillow. On one occasion his mother found his knife blade buried in the kitchen floor.

As he passed puberty he became distressed by the obsessive compulsive force of these activities and their symbolic meaning. He never found it difficult to discuss them with whichever one of the three psychiatrists was treating him at the time.[19]

In early adolescence he became interested in the subway cars, the intricacy of the light signal systems, the schedule for the many subway trains and the possibility of crashes. He would ride the subways for hours and get off at various major transfer stations and watch the systems in action. He rapidly developed an interest in motors and how they were made from magnets and electric batteries or other sources of electric currents. He would make his own basic motor and bought stronger and stronger magnets, carrying them about with him in his trouser pocket, sleeping with them under his pillow and always fingering one. He became concerned with the idea that this was a masturbation substitute and a fetish, and developed absorbing sexual preoccupations.

He thought a great deal about the functions and sensations of the woman and the various female organs, especially the breasts. He asked the woman psychiatrist many questions in regard to this. He then became interested in ether, chloroform, and other volatile anesthetic drugs which would produce, unconsciousness and began carrying about with him bottles of these substances which he inhaled. He was concerned with death and various states of consciousness, and as he felt unable to solve his problems, and was driven by his obsessive compulsive tendencies he frequently thought of suicide as an easy solution. Once he had to be revived by a physician from a state of coma.

Meanwhile he had done quite well in his grammar school and high school,

---

[19] Schilder, Paul; Bender, Lauretta; and Montague, Allison.

with camps in the summer, and had graduated from high school. His parents moved to a distant state where he entered college. His problems apparently became overwhelming and after two more instances when a physician had to revive him he was sent to a sanitarium where the frustration arising from isolation and lack of any opportunity to exercise his compulsions led to serious anxiety outbursts and open expressions of hostility. This in turn led to further isolation. A transorbital lobectomy was performed when he was 18 years old. For some time after this he felt some relief from his tension states and compulsive obsessional activities. However when they returned, he ended his problems by a self-administered overdose of a soporific drug.

～ 6 ～

THEORIES OF ART AND ITS RELATION TO THE PSYCHOLOGY AND PSYCHOPATHOLOGY OF CHILDHOOD[1]

CHILDREN and animals play, but they also take their activities very seriously. For instance, when you watch a kitten it seems to be in continual movement, but there also appears to be an element of playfulness in its motion. Karl Groos developed a theory that the play of animals serves as a preparation for later biological functions, but he was merely expressing the point of view of the observer who already knows what the later development of the animal will be. From the point of view of the kitten its play does not represent preparation for the future. The kitten takes life and the world seriously. Its actions bring it into contact with the world, and with every new action new qualities of the world merge into the kitten's experience. The emergence of new qualities of the object is, obviously, but one of its immediate psychological aims, but the animal also wants an inner relation to the object. It wants to get hold of it and sooner or later to incorporate it into itself. In addition, it gets pleasure from its muscular activity and not only learns about the object but also learns about itself when acting. Parallel with this development, control over its own movements increases. External world, body and muscular control merge in this active process, guided by the urge towards the world and towards satisfaction of biological needs. It may be said that there is no immediate evidence for the assumption of certain psychological processes in the kitten. In the development of the child, more evidences for psychological processes can be offered. In its play the child learns something about the world, satisfies its needs and gains control over the mechanics of its actions.

This play is, of course, primarily a process of maturation and development.[2] However, the psychological adaptations connected with motility give final shape to the developmental process. The aim of every activity is mastery of the object. This can be attained only by continuous experimentation which does not stop even when the object is removed, because it remains in the child's mind. Objects and situations are revived in the memory, either

---

[1] This chapter was written by Paul Schilder in 1939, a part of a manuscript on *Art and the Problem Child,* not heretofore published. See also Chapters 9 and 19, and the section on schizophrenia in Chapter 7.

[2] See the studies of Arnold Gesell, Helen Thompson, and Mary M. Shirley.

wholly or in part. With this revival of the actual world, processes of experimentation continue. Parts of experiences of the past are put together in new sequences until finally a satisfactory unit of imagination and memory is reached which furnishes a suitable basis for new action and experimentation. Such units may be called gestalten or configurations.[3]

These configurations are parts of the world and emerge during action, but they may also be reached by the processes of imagination and memory. They are "good" configurations, or "gute Gestalten" as they have been called by Max Wertheimer, only when they fit into and are part of the world. The process of imagination and remembering contains elements of action as well. There is no picture in the mind which is not connected with a set of motor attitudes and small movements, carrying on the process of experimentation which took place in the perception and action. There has been a controversy as to whether the process of thinking can go on without optic imagery pictures. It is known however that thinking can proceed when mental images are indistinct and incomplete. It is, further, of importance that the path from thought to action should be a very direct one. Thinking is an efficient preparation for action, and Freud has justly called it trial action performed with small amounts of energy. Human beings, especially children, are continually experimenting with perception, imagination, memory, and thinking, all of which are based on and interrelated with motor attitudes and actions. Human experience cannot be separated from activity which builds itself up in a sequence of levels by a continuous process of trial and error. It is a continuous construction.

Where does art fit into this scheme?[4] Art does not lead to immediate action. Even when art is used for propaganda it is different from an immediate call for action. A Soviet novel or drama is more than a mere call to direct political action and propaganda. Even when a Diego Rivera or a Jose Clemente Orozco creates revolutionary murals, the message of such murals can hardly be adequately expressed by a political program.

The misfortunes of friends and of those whom we love may be called tragedies; still, the emotions experienced on such occasions are different from those we may experience when we see a performance of Eugene O'Neill's *Mourning Becomes Electra,* in spite of the fact that it would be difficult to imagine that human beings could be harder hit by fate. A storm is an esthetic object only so long as human beings are not threatened with disaster. The emotions experienced in a love affair are obviously more direct than those aroused by any piece of art. One is doubtful about persons who experience their strongest emotions in relation to art and is inclined to object to their estheticism. The conclusion may be drawn that art provokes emotions of a

[3] See Koffka, Kurt: *The Growth of the Mind,* 1928.
[4] See Johnson, Martin: *Art and Scientific Thought.*

quality which is not equal in fullness to those experienced in everyday life. The world of art, music, and fiction is not one of direct emotion and action.

Some objects of art and esthetic enjoyment seem to be present in nature without man's activity. They are not created by man. It almost seems as though they were received as a gift. If the active character of human perception is considered, it is realized that the person enjoying a landscape creates this landscape and has something of the artist in him. It is interesting from this point of view that almost every century, nay almost every generation, has a landscape of its own. The ruins of Nicolas Poussin, the color orgies of Joseph M. W. Turner and the landscapes of Claude Monet are different worlds. It is well to keep in mind that the creator of a piece of art and the person who is in a state of esthetic enjoyment have much in common with each other.

However, the artist seems to change reality in a much higher degree than does the person who merely enjoys the beauty of a landscape or picture. Leonardo da Vinci has often been quoted advising his disciples to get their inspiration from the chance forms of a crumbling wall. This shows that the objects of art are not merely created from eerie imagination, but portray features of the objective world. Great sculptors have often spoken of the pattern coming from the material, as if the statue was contained in the marble before it was hewn out. The creative artist does not invent something outside of reality but helps reality to its own creation.

Actions have aims. They are directed by the desires and needs of the individual. The artist obviously wants to show that he has discovered something which nobody else was able to discover before him. He promises enjoyment and a new approach to action. He wants to be praised for it and to gain something in everyday life by discovering esthetic realities. Whether the art manifests itself as music, painting, sculpture, poetry, or drama, the fundamental principle remains the same. Since the world of art does not lead to ultimate emotions and actions, the esthetic enjoyment must of necessity have something to do with the preparation to action, and is related to play. The question remains, why should it be valued in spite of the fact that no direct satisfaction of biological needs comes out of it.

Sigmund Freud has shown that one of the central experiences in human life is the so-called oedipus complex,[5] by which he means the wish of the child (especially between the ages of 3 and 5) to have sexual relations with the parent of the opposite sex, and to remove and kill the parent of the same sex. The name for this fundamental desire is taken from a tragedy of Sophocles. The classical tragedy leads man back to one of the essential biological and psychological conflicts of human existence, to the solution of which it

---

[5] See Mullahy, Patrick: *Oedipus: Myth and Complex.*

contributes but vaguely. The great tragedy was created for the community and was the concern of the community. The origin of tragedies lies in religion. The first tragedy was obviously a ritual ceremony which promised the individual an actual solution of his conflicts. In so far as this conflict was psychological the primitive rites fulfilled a part of their aims.

For primitive man, religion was beyond doubt a serious business. It was an attempt to act by magic. We owe to K. Th. Preuss the insight that primitive art and religion had as their core magic wishes and ceremonies.

Magic is based upon strong wishes and urges which demand fulfillment in reality, even when the actual tools are insufficient or when the nature of the wish makes fulfillment impossible. With this insight into the close relation between magic and art, a further step is taken in the understanding of the fundamental functions of art. Whereas the original Dionysian cult, and for that matter also the Holy Mass of Catholicism, promise immediate psychological satisfaction to the community, the art production and the artist do not attempt such direct satisfaction but imply that it might be finally derived from art.

In the child, experimentation and play, although serious in intent, are further away from final completion and final mastery of the world. On the other hand, for the child, play is reality and is in some way comparable to the magic intentions of the ritual. The esthetic character of the behavior and actions of the child and the great esthetic enjoyment which can be derived from observation of the child are closely connected with the preliminary character of the activities of children. It might furthermore be expected that the child when untrammeled by conventional education may produce objects of art with comparative ease. It is very doubtful whether for the child its art production actually means mere play in the adult sense. Its drawing and painting may be expected to denote a serious attempt to do something with reality, perhaps in a magical way.

In studying the art of children it must be realized that the child has only limited technical capacities. Its motility prescribes comparatively simple forms. As has already been outlined in previous chapters, this motility is so arranged that primitive loops and whirling movements are dominant at first. In the drawings of small children these primitive units are repeated again and again, and are the units prescribed by the child's motility. There is reason to believe, however, that this primitive unit is also of paramount importance in perception. Knowledge and activity of the child develop step by step until more complicated configurations can be mastered.

The human figure is drawn by the young child in primitive loops more or less round or oblong. This is not the perceived world of the child, but the child's motility in response to his perceptions. The child is satisfied with its product and recognizes it as a part of the world. Perhaps though, it means even more to the child, who probably has discovered that some geometrical patterns are also present in the human figure, and has learned that by its own movements it can reproduce forms which have at least some relation to what it perceives. The child has thereby conquered a part of the world in its drawing. There is no reason to believe that the child at this stage of development interprets its attempt as a magical act. However, sooner or later the picture drawn becomes more than a mere picture; it may contain a promise of that reality which the child desires. Magic procedures in the strict sense is obviously a great step beyond this.

The art of the child leads us back to the primitive forms which mankind has almost forgotten. The fascinating impression of children's drawing is based on the fact that they reopen to adults a reality which has long since been obliterated. At the same time it inspires the hope that man may be able to start this process of experimentation all over again. It is possible that in this way deeper insight can be gained into what art in general means to man. At any rate, the play of children and their creative art are not so different from each other—both are serious endeavors.

In the art of children two fundamental principles can be differentiated—the tendency to draw what is seen, and the tendency to draw what is known about the object. Both tendencies are decidedly realistic although the technical capacity to express them is often incomplete. In the first few years of life the child struggles with elementary forms, and therefore simple form principles dominate its efforts. Even the human figure is drawn as merely a configuration of simple loops. Arms and legs appear as simple lines, and hands and feet are hardly emphasized as distinct entities. For the child, however, such a drawing signifies the human figure, and the objective incompleteness of the drawing does not hinder him from seeing in the figure a complete representation of what he wants to draw. At this stage of development the child is not aware which part of his image of the object is given to him by visual perception and which part comes from memory and previous knowledge. Both are used indiscriminately in the drawing. Full face productions prevail; profiles appear only later on. Perspective is in general a late achievement and is attained early by only partially gifted children. In no phase of this early development does the child attempt to symbolize. He may find pleasure in simple geometrical form principles and ornamental designs. However, his chief desire is to draw reality as it is. Even if the result of his striving has little similarity to the object from the adult point of view, the young artist offers his production as a full presentation of the object.

It is interesting in this respect that the oldest documents of prehistoric art are decidedly realistic in intent. In the caves of Southern France and Spain there is a monumental and realistic art of animal portraiture. These paintings, termed Franco-Cantabrian art, are polychrome and of considerable size.

The Eastern Spanish or Levantine style shows shadow silhouettes in monochrome in which men and animals are usually depicted in active movement. In general the figures are smaller than in the Franco-Cantabrian style. However by the time of the Bronze Age art ceased to be realistic and sought its ultimate goal in static geometrical patterns.[6]

There is reason to believe that for the child as well as for primitive peoples the picture does not always merely represent the object but *is* the object. The individual is so intent on attaining the object, that everything which can be used as its symbol, though in completely differentiated form, actually becomes the object itself. The relation between primitive art and magic and ceremony thus becomes obvious. One understands also that primitive art is often part of a ceremonial, although this is not invariably true. At any rate, the child has not given up experimentation. In the long run the child cannot be deceived. He differentiates the object very decisively from the drawn or painted picture of the object, when the experimentation is not prematurely interrupted. The primitive individual also will not be forever satisfied with pictures which represent the object. Bound by his customs and institutions, he may remain in the sphere of magic and refrain from differentiating between magical causality and sequences in reality. The art of primitives and of children opens the way to reality, but one cannot always be certain that they will follow all the way through to this end.

The fascination of the attempts of both the primitive artist and the child is due partially to the fact that they represent an effort which has not yet led to definite results. In many respects modern art has gone back to the perception of the essentials of form. In the art of Pablo Picasso, Fernand Leger, and Georges Braque, form patterns are rediscovered which the adult has tended to forget. The principle of seeing simple geometrical forms at first appeared in the so-called analytical cubism in which the abstract form is seen merely as a part of the fully developed form. In abstract cubism and in synthetic cubism, the interest in form of primitive type again dominates. The relation to some of the drawings of children in which the child struggles with form principles is obvious.

Primitive form principles have in no way disappeared from man's perception, but he has turned to a reality which is more or less finished and crystallized. Levels of human existence may come into the foreground which belong to more primitive stages of development. Psychoanalysis emphasizes the tendency to regression in the diverse neuroses and psychoses. Experiences emerge which belong to the different levels of childhood. Primitive form principles which appear in the drawings of children and in some ways also in the art of primitives may be expected to reappear in the art of psychotic

---

[6] See von Wiegand, Charmion: *Prehistoric Rock Pictures,* an article based upon the exhibition of prehistoric rock paintings at the Museum of Modern Art.

individuals. This expectation is indeed fulfilled in the drawings of schizo-phrenic individuals, which have been collected by Hans Prinzhorn, R. A. Pfeifer and others.[7] It seems that the schizophrenic person has access in his art to primitive form principles which so-called normal persons have lost.

Prinzhorn's material contains the work of many schizophrenic artists who had no training before they started to draw or to sculpture. They drew orna-mental designs in which more lively structures which suggest organic forms suddenly appear. Primitive drawings of the human figure occur but they are combined with rhythmical principles which give artistic qualities to the whole picture.[8]

For example, in the drawings and paintings of a psychotic house painter (reproduced by Prinzhorn) dots or flowers in the garden are repeated in a rhythmical way like the faces in a group of saints. It may be said, accord-ingly, that rhythmical principles are used by the schizophrenic in a much freer way than by other untrained artists. In these pictures one also notices that even artists who are in better command of the techniques and would seem to be capable of drawing the human figure in correct proportions, handle the problem with great independence and freely change the propor-tions. They experiment with organic forms in general, much more fully than most normal persons would dare. This may be called the principle of free experimentation with the organic form and especially with the human form. The average artist feels rather closely bound to the forms of space as he per-ceives them.

Primitive artists do not appear to recognize perspective, and add figures to each other without attempting to indicate a perspective relationship. It is well known that the knowledge of perspective is an achievement which comes late in the development of art and is incomplete even in Japanese woodcuts which in other respects reach such a high degree of perfection. Obviously, perspective is a convention, and drawings and paintings which do not use the principle of perspective may yet be of very great value. The schizophrenic artist does not feel bound by this convention and achieves effects which the more conventional individual does not attempt. At the same time the schizo-phrenic artist is not impressed by the ordinary laws of gravitation, and lib-erates the individual from its bonds. The figures may be placed anywhere, without close relation to the earth. They may float lightly in space, no longer bound to the earth. One of the most astonishing effects in art is accomplished when the artist attempts to experiment with spatial relations. Often the lib-eration from the rigidities of space and gravitation also gives a greater free-

---

[7] See Anastasi, Anna and Foley, John P., in their several studies on the artistic behavior of the abnormal.

Werner Wolff speaks of a "rhythmical index" in young children's drawings.

[8] See Chapter 5, Figures 15, 16, 17.

dom concerning the problem of numbers. Objects are multiplied and various faces may be united into one composite figure.

Schizophrenic art might be characterized by the following principles:

1. Primitive form principles make their reappearance. They are used to characterize the forms of the inanimate as well as of the animate world.

2. Geometrical and organic principles are often used in an indiscriminate way.

3. There is a naïve pleasure in rhythmicity and multiplicity. Rhythm and multiplication are applied to the organic as well as to the inanimate world.

4. The proportions of the human figure are changed in an experimental way.

5. The problems of space, size, number, and perspective are dealt with in an experimental way.

6. The laws of gravitation are disregarded.

It is undeniable that freedom from convention helps the schizophrenic artist to the possibility of almost unlimited experimentation. This is a condition which may lead even the untrained person to achieve artistic creations. It is obvious that such a release from the conventions of everyday life will have an effect on the content as well as the form of the artistic creation. The schizophrenic often will choose his subject matter from the sphere of the cruel, or the weird, and especially from the field of frank sexuality. He will over-emphasize the lower part of the body at the expense of the upper part, as for example in the drawings of Joseph Sell in Prinzhorn's book. The motif of the face may be transferred to the genitals or to the kneecaps. Freedom from conventional form principles creates a mythical world in which the human body blends with the animal body and with the limbs or other parts of other human bodies. On the whole it cannot be denied that the artistic capacities of the individual are increased by the psychosis. This idea may be formulated by stating that the artistic process consists partially of reversal to a stage of free experimentation with the body and the world.

However, neither the schizophrenic patient nor the child are artists simply because they use primitive principles. Obviously something else is required. When one examines the artistic productions of a number of schizophrenic patients, one sees immediately that the severity of the schizophrenic process and the artistic value of their productions do not parallel each other. It is clear that a production is artistic only if it shows primitive form and in addition uses experimentation in order to approach the mastery of reality. Modern psychiatry is of the opinion that the schizophrenic is an individual who cannot master the intricate situations of a complicated world and under stress and danger reverts to more primitive modes of experience. Such a world within may offer security and enjoyment when the differentiated external world has become a threat against which defense is not possible. However, the schizophrenic is not satisfied with a limited world. As a living human being, he is fascinated by the world and wants to go back to the more complicated external forms again. He may cling to those parts of reality which he is still able to master. Primitive form principles and modes of experience which make their appearance in the schizophrenic may represent stages in his retreat from reality, or they may represent stages in his new attempt to return to reality or to try to recover it. The schizophrenic artist reveals problems which are important for art in general. Ernst Kris surmised that in this process of recovery and in his efforts to regain the world, the schizophrenic's earliest concern is with the human face. The human face is one of the first objects with which the child comes into close personal relation. Paradoxically enough relations between human beings are to a great extent interfacial ones. One is perhaps justified in drawing the conclusion that the artist has not merely the task of bringing to light the experimental stages of human existence, but also the possibility of advancing beyond this experimental stage to a fuller experience of the world. Schizophrenic art is often lacking in this respect, and even when the first step is taken, the variability of such endeavors is limited. Ernst Kris has further noted that the schizophrenic artist frequently remains monotonous in his themes and patterns. However, it is better not to be too severe in setting of this criterion, since the successful artist, too, often becomes rigid, using again and again the same pattern which once had a meaning. Of course, the successful normal artist who has become rigid has not necessarily also become a schizophrenic. However, he shares with the schizophrenic artist the impossibility of varying his experimentation in his approach to the world.

So far schizophrenic art has been referred to as one instance of the art of persons who are mentally ill. There are many types of mental disease. The mentally ill person has an approach to reality which is different from that of the normal person. Also, the severe psychopathic personality, in his art productions, may use specific form principles in connection with emotional disturbances. The change which has taken place in the world of the depressive or elated (manic) patient will also be reflected in his artistic endeavors. An underdevelopment of the brain which expresses itself clinically in mental deficiency or an organic lesion of the brain which has caused deterioration may give the individual access to primitive form principles which are unavailable to the normal individual. The emergence of such forms of expression is by no means without artistic significance.

Artistic talents are obviously much more widespread than has thus far been surmised, but by most human beings they are never developed. Human beings show great differences in their artistic ability. It is probable that almost anyone has some capacity to express himself in music, poetry, painting, or building, but the degree of ability varies widely. In the art of singing physiological differences can be the basis for the variation in expressive ability. The fate of the individual in early childhood is another factor to be considered; in the schizophrenic artist endowment is naturally also a factor determining artistic capacity.

From this point of view it is interesting to study the life history of artists who have been psychotic. The psychiatric diagnosis of Vincent van Gogh is still a matter of controversy. Some believe that he suffered from a certain form of epilepsy, others, that he was a schizophrenic. However, the problem of diagnosis is of no special importance here. In all his letters he appears as an individual who wanted reality and nothing but reality. He was interested in forms and colors and wanted to get hold of them. Such a thirst for reality can be found in individuals who have been insecure and are full of fear that they may lose their access to reality. In the first phase of his artistic career, van Gogh painted realistically but without much imagination. However, the "Potato Eaters" shows decided distortions in the faces. The caricaturist clings to one trait of the human face when he is not capable of approaching the subject as a whole.

In his most fertile painting period van Gogh painted objects with a direct approach that was almost uncanny. The "Chair" is a characteristic masterpiece of this period, in which the reality of color and form is striking. The chair is almost more than real. Its colors have become more glowing. There are many pictures of a similar type. On the other hand, the arrangement of the chair in his picture shows a decided tendency to rigidity of form. When an individual clings very fast to reality it becomes overdistinct, and form principles which are almost geometrical immediately appear. In the landscapes which van Gogh painted during this time, formal principles become more and more paramount. Clouds are drawn in more or less primitive vortices which repeat themselves. The principle of parallelism of lines is often used to the neglect of other structural qualities of reality. The colors of his sunflowers are so intense that they look more like suns than flowers, and their forms come nearer to geometrical than organic patterns. Towards the end of this period, formalistic principles are overwhelming and the rhythm of lines based on primitive principles almost destroys the pattern of the object. There are pictures of haystacks and gorges in which vortices and curves, partially in parallel arrangements, extend over the whole picture and destroy the "object."

Van Gogh's portraits, too, are of interest from this point of view. It is worth noting that in the majority of landscapes which he painted, human figures are absent. Parallel lines are predominant, although they are often waved. In the picture "Doctor Gachet," the composition is dominated by inclined planes. Other pictures are strongly symmetrical. "L'Arlesienne" is dominated by triangular form principles; the colors are schematic. It is worth while comparing the copies he made of Jean François Millet and Eugene Delacroix with the originals. The great fascination of the work of van Gogh lies partially in its striving for reality and partially in its renewed attempt to experience reality in primitive geometrical and color principles. It is a valuable human document of an individual who strove with great power toward optic reality. It would be difficult to explain van Gogh's achievement without recourse to the specific gifts for optic perception which developed in his emotional battle for optic reality.

Thus far children's efforts to use drawing as an attempt to approach reality more closely by experimentation and repetition have been considered. As in children's play in general, there has been seen in this a preparation for action which is based upon an insight into structure. It has been found that in their search for reality children use primitive form principles such as the loop, the vortex, the wave, and the simple geometrical forms. It has also been found that the simple geometrical forms and primitive patterns are used in children's approach to both the animate and inanimate world, especially to the human figure.

In the most primitive documents of art in prehistoric times has been found the urge to reality which approached specifically the animate form, either at rest or in motion. In these primitive stages of development space is not seen as a distinct problem but more or less in terms of the sum of objects to be included. Since the effort to attain reality is incomplete it has to be repeated over and over again. Repetition and rhythm are closely connected with the basic organization of human motility. In schizophrenic art there was found regression to primitive form principles, rhythm and formal patterns extending into the animate forms, as well as condensations of the various parts of reality into one, and free experimentation with the principles of space.

In all these various experiences an unquenchable thirst for experimentation was noted, and the wish to master parts of reality and reality as a whole; however, the experimentation of the schizophrenic, the child and the artist is incomplete. The child needs its growth to complete it. The schizophrenic artist reverts to primitive forms under the onslaught of a reality which he cannot master, but he does not completely give up the struggle for the richer world which he finds threatening him. The so-called normal artist points again and again toward new structures of reality although he never reaches a definite end or takes a definite action. The less he is bound to convention the freer he is in his experimentation and the greater is his chance for new discoveries. A psychosis may help him to get rid of banal everyday attitudes and open up the way to new experiences. He may be a real artist, with or without a psychosis, if his descent to the primitive layers of experience contains at least a hope for a new adaptation to a world which can be shared by the community. The art of prehistoric times may in part have had magical and ceremonial implications. The moment art becomes ceremonial it sets itself definite aims and becomes a tool, and a not reliable one, at that. This definiteness of purpose implies an irreversibility and a loss of freedom which transgresses the realm of art as it is today understood. Religious and magic ceremonies are indeed devious methods of conquering the world.

Human beings have to live with other human beings. Their emotions and actions take place in a community. Even the lonely thinker is not isolated from his social group. In this sense all experiences are social ones. The imagination of the dreamer becomes meaningless unless he can experience his imaginary thoughts and ideas in the life of the community. Charles Hartshorne has called attention to the social character of every perception.

Even when man turns to the inanimate world he does so with the unformulated but definite knowledge that it is also the world of other human beings. Art is a highly social phenomenon. The child who draws does not do so merely for himself but he also draws for the adult who encourages him. The social attitudes of the child, his individual history and the history of his experiences of love and hate will be reflected in every line.

The schizophrenic has sometimes been called autistic and narcissistic, meaning that he withdraws his interest (libido) from the world and diverts it to his own personality. However, this conception is not entirely valid. The schizophrenic merely gives up his interest or relationship with objects outside of himself which have become too dangerous and too complicated for him to master. For the complicated human relations he substitutes simpler ones by which he can better protect himself. It is obvious that the artist directs his art to his fellow human beings. Through his art he wants to excite in another individual the same attitude which he has experienced in himself. He communicates his vision so that the other individual may know what is going on in him and also to excite the same vision in his fellow human beings. Whatever his gains may be, they are for the benefit of the community and he expects praise and compensation from the community. The communal character of art was more obvious in previous stages of history; it is however never absent although it may be veiled in the most sterile periods of art. Art is, therefore, not only an experiment of a single person but one by which the community tries to reach through art to higher forms of life.

In our study of the art of abnormal children it may be expected that form principles will appear which are enlightening because they represent the early phases of development and also because they emphasize certain aspects in relation to the psychopathology. From the newer developments of psychology it has been learned that the so-called "pathological" is merely a particular aspect of the so-called "normal." In psychopathology, new facets of fundamental problems of the psyche make their appearance. However, nothing extraneous is ever added to the psyche and the variation allows a deeper insight into the fundamental problem.

It has been emphasized that the problems of personality form the fundamental basis for every product of human endeavor, and especially for art productions. In order to understand the art of abnormal children the life history of the child and its emotional problems must be studied. After an insight has been gained into the psychological problems of the child, the basic form principles appearing in his drawings must be examined. The question must be asked whether the primitive perceptual units such as the loop and vortex, or curved lines and geometrical forms which belong to a later development are more prominent. Attention must be paid to how often the same motif is repeated and whether it is repeated in the same form or is varied. It must also be considered whether the forms are geometrical in the narrower sense or whether they approximate the forms which one finds in nature, as in the formation of a river or a hill, which may be regarded as organic forms. It will be particularly interesting to note whether attention is given to the specific form of animate objects, i.e., of animals and human beings. In modern art human and animal forms often have been approached under the impact of geometry, and cubism has emphasized particularly the geometrical principle in the human figure. When an attempt is made to analyze the drawings of children, the question to be asked again and again is whether they are more interested in geometrical or in organic forms. It must also be noted whether they use geometrical form principles in the drawings of human figures.

The human figure has always been the outstanding subject of the arts. In every art production it is of fundamental importance to analyze the way in which the problem of the human form is handled. In primitive experience the human body has no definite form. Even the concept human beings have about their own bodies, the body image, is not fully differentiated.[9] Primitive perception and the dream, change the relations of the different parts of the body freely, and qualities which belong to one part of the body image may be transposed to other parts. Children like to hear stories about dwarfs and giants.[10] It is important to know whether greater attention is given to the face or to the other parts of the body. What attitude toward the genitals is reflected in the pictures? When distortions in the body image take place they are bound to have a close relation to the specific human problems of the child. When the body is seen merely from a geometric viewpoint, there is justification for believing that such an attitude shows either a particular primitivity and form perception or a particular aversion of the full perception of the human body.

Many drawings have more than one object, and even when there is only one it often has several parts. These parts may retain their natural arrange-

---

[9] Schilder, Paul: *Image and Appearance of the Human Body.*

[10] In the *Carnival of Nice* enormous heads are attached to the disproportionately small bodies of real human beings. The images of Indian gods are endowed with a multiplicity of limbs or heads; breasts are multiplied.

ment or may be handled more or less arbitrarily. One may want to show one's power by changing and transposing parts of an object or the relation of different objects to each other. One may attempt to organize the parts or the different objects into a unit, or may be satisfied merely to juxtapose one object on another without any attempt to organize them. The question will also arise as to how well the parts of an object are organized into the whole, essentially a spatial problem, and there may be a question as to the degree of insight into spatial relations displayed in the picture. Some artists, whether they are children or adults, psychotic or not psychotic, respect the relations of the three dimensions of space. Others arbitrarily contract or expand one dimension at the expense of the others. In the drawings of Du Maurier, for instance, human figures are not only elongated beyond their measure but the lower parts of their bodies are too large in proportion to the upper parts. Some sculptors see their figures almost flat, others exaggerate the dimensions of depth.

Human beings, whatever they may be otherwise, are bodies with heavy masses subject to the laws of gravitation. Although psychologists have often neglected the question, human psychology cannot be understood unless problems are considered in relation to gravitation. German poets speak of Erdenschwere (literally, the heaviness of the earth) pointing to the subjection of human beings to gravitation, which immediately becomes the symbol of libidinous constellations. The wish to fly is one of the oldest wishes of humanity.[11] In art, gravitation and firm relation of objects to the earth may be taken for granted, or one may prefer to experiment with gravitation, have things standing on their heads, and have objects floating in the air although they do not usually do so because of their physical quality. It is interesting to note how freely an artist experiments with gravitation, and it is equally interesting to inquire into the significance of such experimentation. An artist may experiment with spatial relations and gravitation. He may also experiment with the number of objects. He may like to draw hundreds or thousands of people or apples or chairs or houses. He may attempt to draw realistically thousands of houses in New York, or he may use the picture of one object and its repetition as merely a form principle.

In general, one might ask whether an art production reveals more interest in form principles, or in objects seen as real objects. Conclusions concerning personal and emotional problems can be made from art productions, but it is more significant to recognize that the understanding of the form of a picture will be possible only on the basis of knowledge of the personal and emotional problem of the individual and especially of the emotionally disturbed child. It is obvious that not only the form principles have to be understood in this connection, but also the more or less realistic choice of

---

[11] This is the motif in many modern comic books for children, such as Superman.

colors. However, one should not forget that an individual may use well developed form principles and may attempt to draw a fully differentiated reality, but still may choose scenes and colors with specific personal value as an object for his endeavors. When an individual prefers to draw scenes of cruelty in which the red of the blood or the red of fire become paramount, some inference may be made in regard to his emotional life. Whatever the form principles may be, the choice of subject matter has to be studied carefully; and it is a problem of no mean importance whether an individual prefers to draw landscapes or circus people. The content, the chosen color and form principles can only artificially be isolated from the life problems of the individual. Every art production has to be studied from the point of view of whether it expresses the desire for a fully developed reality, whether it is an attempt to escape from reality, whether it is an overcompensation, or a magic gesture.

Finally, the social significance of these art productions must be evaluated. Does the child want to gain the love and admiration of adults or does he merely reluctantly obey the request from a teacher for an art production? Is the art product a token of good will, or an attempt to bribe? In what way does it express the competition between this child and other children? Does the child suspect that the adult seeks his art production for specific reasons? The problems of the adult artist who is not psychotic do not differ fundamentally in this respect from the problems of our neurotic and psychotic children.

The various questions posed in the above paragraphs represent an ambitious program. We cannot hope to answer them completely. However, we may arrive at some understanding of the art of the abnormal child and may open the way for a deeper understanding of art in relation to human life and its problems.

❧ 7 ❧

ABSTRACT ART AS AN EXPRESSION OF
HUMAN PROBLEMS[1]

I. ABSTRACT PAINTINGS BY PSYCHONEUROTIC ADULTS

ABSTRACT ART has repeatedly attracted the interest of psychiatrists. Hans Prinzhorn, for example, reproduced an abstract picture called "motivated presentation of God"[2] to which the patient-artist remarked, "This is God who looks like a monkey with a purple cap. . . . On the right side is his crystal eye with which he looks into world space, below is his anal eye with which he looks to the earth." It will be shown that mentally deficient children have a great interest in abstract problems of form and color. In schizophrenic and severely neurotic children, the interest in abstract form problems may become paramount, as we have seen in the gestalt drawings of Francine (Fig. 17) and Billy (Fig. 18). It is almost as if the patient has to begin by experimenting with primitive forms, and especially geometric forms.

In the sidewalk drawings of children, it was seen that abstract form problems are basic to the games which acquire significant social emotional value. It seems interesting to ask, what is the meaning of abstract art from a psychoanalytic point of view. According to our studies, and those of Frank Curran in adolescents, art production helps in many respects to a deeper understanding of psychological problems. It was therefore decided to have an artist[3] assist in the group psychoanalysis of neurotic adults.[4] The patients were encouraged to draw freely whatever they wanted to draw, and were assisted only slightly in the use of the medium. The artist was not supposed to suggest or ask questions concerning the meaning of the pictures. This task was reserved for the analytic sessions.

Fig. 19a comes from a 24-year-old patient of high average intelligence, whose chief complaint was that "I don't understand anything, and I don't know anything, and I am continually bewildered." The picture which is

---

[1] Partially reprinted from: Schilder, Paul and Levine, E. L.: Abstract Art as an Expression of Human Problems, *Journal of Nervous and Mental Disease, 95*:1-10, 1942; and Bender, Lauretta and Schilder, Paul: *Art and the Abnormal Child,* Chapter I, The Use of Color in American Negro and Puerto Rican Children with Emotional and Social Problems, and Chapter V, Graphic Art as an Approach to the Psychology of the Schizophrenic Child (unpublished).

[2] Prinzhorn, Hans: *Bildnerei des Geisteskranken.*

[3] Levine, Esther L.

[4] Schilder, Paul: *Results and Problems of Group Psychotherapy in Severe Neuroses,* 1939.

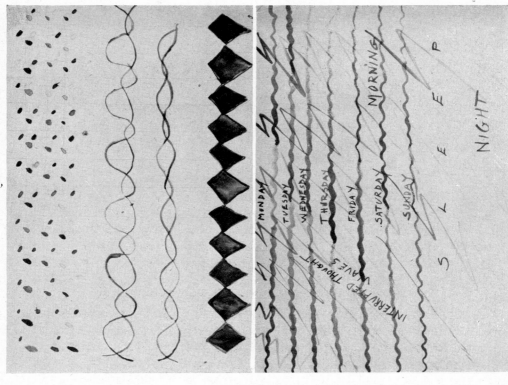

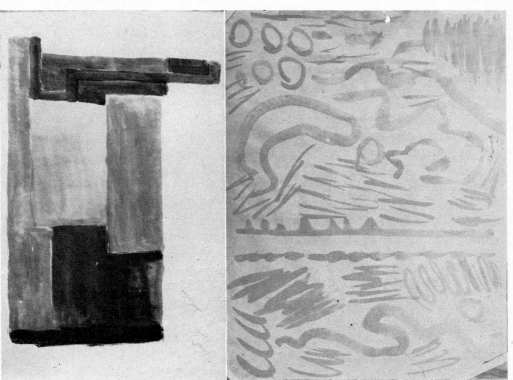

Fig. 19. Four abstractions, by adults (*water color*).

reproduced was done in yellow, orange, brown and red with the exception of one small blue vertical stripe at the right side. The patient says: "Don't ask me what it is. I have always something of such a picture in my mind. I always like to look at the sun. The sun has a lot of power, it keeps everything alive, something to sustain life. It pours it through the rays all over the earth. I see everything and myself in golden and brown color. Sometimes in the morning the sun gives everything the golden glow. . . . The angles are too weak and too dead. I cannot draw it any other way. I used the blue only for contrast."

These associations of the patient have a close relation to his fundamental problems. He says that he was already "confused" at the age of 3 years. At that age he asked, "Why does the sun shine?" However, the patient was proud that he could ask such questions at that age.

His father was for him the embodiment of strength and intelligence. He would like to be like his father. The yellow and brown colors, etc., express his wish. He is, however, afraid that he is too weak to do so. The angles are, paradoxically for him, symbols of weakness. It is very probable that he does not believe in this weakness, and that the paradox expresses his own deeper conviction of his intellectual and physical capacities.

There is some creative effort shown in the way in which he distributes colors and masses although the artistic value may be doubtful. It is remarkable that he did not use any curves but sticks to the straight lines. "The straight line stands for lucidity, mastery and affirmation." André L'Hote has said, "One can hazard the opinion that the curve, the unique element of our spontaneous instinctive expression, is the sign of the relaxation of reason, the symbol of some vital and profound urge."

The patient had drawn only one other abstract picture consisting of red and black parallel stripes. Of this he said: "The red is more living than the brown, and the black is emptiness and coldness." This picture evidently also expresses his fundamental conflict.

Fig. 19b is the drawing of a 37-year-old patient with an obsession neurosis. In the foreground of his obsessions stood the fear that he would make awkward movements and these awkward and unnatural movements would cause disaster and destruction, for which he would be punished and might lose his arms.

The associations to the drawing, which was done in light yellow, were as follows: "I drew a border—a border is a fortress. I always believed in keeping things to myself. I like a border that is sharp on the outside and the inside not pointed. Sharp is clearness-definite. Before you make a remark that according to law my brother is not a criminal. I want something sharp to hold on to. I like singing and dancing. I always like a pencil or a tool. It has unlimited prospect. That came to my mind with the brush. You can make unlimited things by moving your hands. I used to be enchanted by standardization in this country. I also like the movement of armies; I like filling in things—simple production—yet plenty of it. I like to break down foolish laws. You annoyed me by your remarks about my brother not breaking the law. In my line first you make the design and then you fill it in. In the factories the women would just feed the machinery with cloth."

This is an abstraction which has no parallel in visual experience. Because of definite opposing movements the picture is dynamic. For instance, the open and closed forms build up from the lower right-hand side in an upward direction as opposed to the downward movement indicated by the direction of the banana-shaped form, from the center top. The left side of the drawing was constructed in a similar manner. The snake-like lines build upward in opposition to the downward movement of the right side lines. The technique which the patient used also carries out this phenomenon—the jagged, scratchy lines oppose the smooth, wavy lines.

The forms and lines resemble the patterns in cloth and textiles the patient may have seen in his father's factory.

In this drawing one sees primitive space perceptions like the spiral and the vortex. The rhythmical arrangement of lines and forms are caleographic in character. This drawing is different from an ornament as it is a freer evaluation, and is therefore in closer relation to the patient's vital problems.

Prior to this drawing the patient had drawn cherries with very sharp outlines. He liked sharp borders; he wanted to have everything decisive and distinct. In fact, he thought that he knew everything better than others did and he could not stand it if other persons did not see how right he was. Indistinct forms or indistinct contours in the wood meant that something was rotten—cancer or syphilis. The patient usually drew rather stiff houses and trees. The chief problem in this case centered about his aggressive impulses which come out in his motility. His movements became unnatural because they expressed his destructive wish. He had continually to restrict his movements. His history showed that this was in connection with early experiences concerning pogroms, and with attitudes of a severe father whose hands were often hurt while repairing textile machinery. The patient was very much afraid of attack from the outside or of being destroyed by infection, dirt, or cancer. In order to avoid walking on spots on the floor he made the unnatural movements which were destructive. Thoughts concerning dangers which were inflicted on him or which he inflicted, made every object present at this time a weapon of destruction. The object had to be torn and discarded by throwing it in the toilet.

It is of fundamental importance that the abstract forms have a definite meaning in connection with central problems of the personality.

The next case (Fig. 19c) was also one of obsession neurosis in which the motor problems were of fundamental importance. The patient, a girl of 19, was afraid that she might throw things like knives and ice picks at other people, killing them in this way. Furthermore, she thought that she gave cockroach powder to them. She was also afraid that she might set a street car or an elevated car on fire. She was very active and talkative. Her drawings showed a rather outspoken symmetry. To the drawing she made the following remarks: "The rhythm—I always wanted to lead an orchestra. I like the motion of the arm." (*What is in the lower line?*) Diamonds. I always hated jewelry. At one time I believed in free love. A woman could sell her body for jewelry. I once wanted to have a string of pearls around my neck. He'd insult me. I would rip the pearls off and throw them in his face. The man would go out beaten. He would try to pick the pearls up and I'd kick him."

The same patient liked to draw wavy lines as illustrated in the drawing (Fig. 19d). The lines are parallel to each other and have the names of the week days written over them. In this drawing one sees regularity and order which is disrupted by freer movements. Again this disruption saves the picture from being merely an ornament. The patient also liked the opposition of morning and night. She drew a quadrant—the one half in red and the other half in black. She made out of it, "rain or shine, reconciliation or fight." Then she drew blocks with which she had played before. Other drawings also represent night and morning. Her figure drawing and drawings of objects show a very strong urge toward symmetry.

Analytically, the hate against the father who was crippled plays the outstanding part. This hate was based partially on early observations of parental intercourse in which she felt that her father behaved like a beast. In the drawings the motor impulses and the tendency toward opposition again play the outstanding part. In a previous study,[5] it was shown that simple drawings may represent the culmination of a schizophrenic episode and the lines of such a drawing may represent for the patient deep thoughts which are in close connection with his fundamental problems. There is no question that for this patient a very sketchy and oddly drawn head represented the power and energy of her father and similar simple lines meant for her the energy of the universe, the fertilizing power in nature, etc. This patient certainly was not playful concerning the contents of her drawings which represented for her important archaic thoughts. However, her drawings like those of the two preceding patients did not have any deeper connections with any form principles.

---

[5] Schilder, Paul: *Wahn und Erkenntnis*, 1918.

ABSTRACT PRODUCTION AS A WAY OF IDENTIFICATION FOR SCHIZOPHRENIC CHILDREN

The gestalt drawings of Francine, the 10 year old schizophrenic girl who also drew for us her introjected "brain bodies," have already been discussed.[6] In these drawings, which were done on request, her play with symmetry was directly observed. Even when she followed a simple block design, also on request, she soon added colors and conglomerations of her primitive shapes. A series of dots became the basis for long finger-like shapes.

In the art class, Francine's impulse for drawing forms showed more and more freedom of expression with the result that she produced many interesting and often beautiful abstractions. Oblong, circular, and ellipsoid forms which deformed each other in an irregular way were used to make many new patterns, just as the same principles distorted her gestalt drawings. She never had straight lines but always designs. The edges were often scalloped. She sometimes filled large spaces with one color. The borderlines were either wavy or crenated, there was a tendency to strong color contrasts, and irregular lines were sometimes drawn in between, in different colors.

Primitive colored forms were used such as the circle, the ellipse, the round and oblong shape, the sinusoidal wave, crenations. Irregular transformations of these basic forms made by compressing them are arbitrary pieces of these forms. At this phase, the child experimented continually with primitive experience, with the help of motility. In primitive space perceptions, the spiral and the vortex prevail. This child sank back to a more primitive attitude toward the spatial problems, she retreated from objects, from definite configurations, and was satisfied with a more primitive configuration which might perhaps lead to a new interest in space, such as is shown in some of her best drawings.

Generally, one is inclined to think that symmetry is one of the most primitive gestalt principles. It is very probable however that the impulses are never completely symmetrical and regular, but merely approach symmetry and regularity, and that a specific effort is necessary to make them completely symmetrical. Francine did not make this effort.

Werner Wolff believes that abstract drawings of children which he calls schematisms, especially when they display lack of symmetry indicate an inadequate security in the child's emotional life. Lack of security certainly existed in Francine's life, but the form problems expressed in her art work seem to point to many other factors as well.

In a "Still Life" (not reproduced) circular and elliptic forms prevail in lively colored designs of great beauty. Although this picture started as a

---

[6] See Chapter 5, Figures 16 and 17.

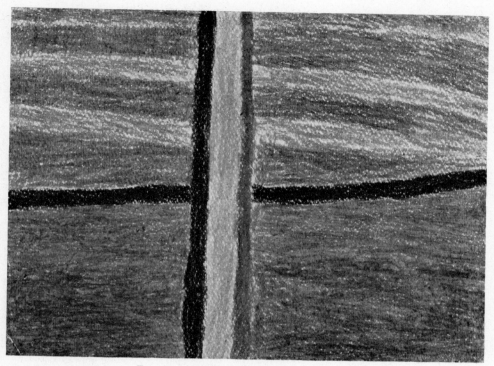

FIG. 20a. A Flag, by Francine (*crayon*).

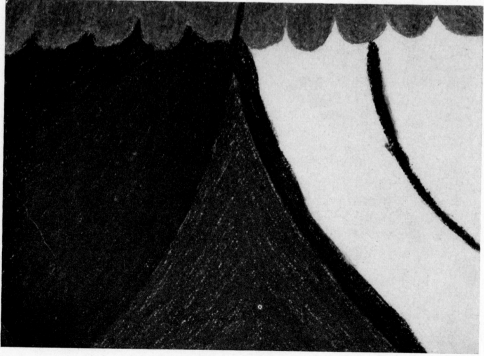

FIG. 20b. A Bulka, by Francine (*crayon*).

play with form and color, it conveyed a meaning to the artist which came during the process of creation. The circle of orange became a "canteloupe," the yellow a "honey dew melon," but the blue half-circle which broke up the irregularity of the design in an interesting way, was called a "roni which is not macaroni." The arbitrary breaking up of words parallels the breaking up of regular forms.

Flower-like designs (Frontispiece) result from the combination of ovals and creations, but it is called "An Aeroplane." Straight lines appear only once in a more elaborate picture which she called "A Flag." It is remarkable for the vivid color sense and the fascinating way in which the planes are broken up by vertical and horizontal stripes (Fig. 20a). A picture which she called "A Bulka" uses experimentation with the same forms and their breaking up in a more complicated way (Fig. 20b).

In order to perceive space, primitive experiences have to be crystallized

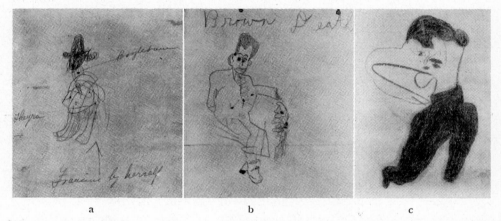

a   b   c

FIG. 21a. Francine by Herself (*pencil*). b. Brown Death Puppeteer, by Francine (*brown crayon*). c. Bender, by Francine (*brown crayon*).

with the help of motility. Since it is known that waves, circles, ellipses, together with the spiral and vortex are the primitive visual motor experiences, it can be said that this child was continuously experimenting with primitive visual motor experiences which easily combine with colors. This experimentation was so important for the artist that she tried to dissolve every other form principle into this primitive one. Her work may be compared with the products of the Orphic school; but this girl had a greater freedom in handling the primitive forms. In both artistic endeavors, the primitive form is victorious over the more crystallized configurations.

Francine was asked to draw the human form. She drew a picture of herself (Fig. 21a) which is so fluid and the boundary lines of which are so uncertain that one can hardly tell where the body boundaries are. This is due not to technical inabilities, as may be seen from her other drawings, but expresses her great uncertainty about her body, its images, and its functions. She uses neologistic terms to refer to her genitals (thegra) and her throat (boglebum) about which she had some special feelings and manneristic behavior, refusing to swallow her saliva, but spitting it about, and constantly clearing her throat.

Shortly after she had reached the peak in her Orphic drawings she burst forth into a series of portraits which showed a rather high degree of technical ability. It is true that her puppet teacher's portrait (Fig. 21b) does not show a photographic likeness to the original, and she unrealistically calls it "Brown Death," but the characteristic posture is caught and the features of the faces are merely emphasized in a caricature way. One is inclined to believe that she could see distinguishing features in faces and wished to overemphasize them in order to keep herself interested. These pictures were drawn very quickly as an immediate reaction to a situation, and she immediately lost interest and wanted to destroy them as she did all of her work.

Later, more primitive features and distortions occurred, as in the figure, especially the mouth, of "Bender" (Fig. 21c). Pictures with distortions characterized the end of this period, after which she gave up drawing altogether.

These pictures represent a last attempt to grasp something of the reality which otherwise was slipping away from her. The real organic form substitutes for the pseudo-organic bone-sausage-flower, and the caricature was merely a redoubled effort to see what reality looked like.

Similar problems were found in other schizophrenic children. However, in this particular case, the experimentation with primitive forms was successful and more beautiful. In such cases it may be surmised what the basic psychological attitude is one which leads to experimentation with primitive forms. However, the patients themselves do not offer any specific explanation nor do they offer associations which open a direct avenue to the understanding of such forms.

Joan, another schizophrenic child, was 4 years old when she was first referred to us because of her overactivity, choreiform motility, running about on her toes, anxiety, temper tantrums, and aggression against other children. Her habit of scratching the faces of babies in baby carriages was especially distressing. The diagnosis of schizophrenia was not made at that time, but was made when she was returned to us at 8 years because of her inability to attend to her school work, or to play with other children, her continued activity, anxiety and aggression. At this age she was very prolific with art work of two types. In the art class she made abstractions with water colors as in Fig. 22a. These were all made in a similar way, yet no two of them were alike. They were divided into square forms with dark paint, the boxes washed over with variegated or almost rainbow or sunset colors, and into the total pattern was woven Joan's name. It seemed that Joan's abstrac-

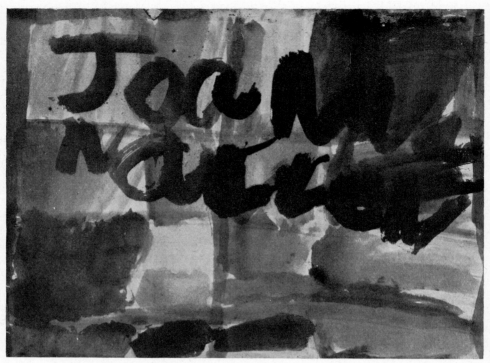

FIG. 22a. Abstraction, by Joan (*water color*).

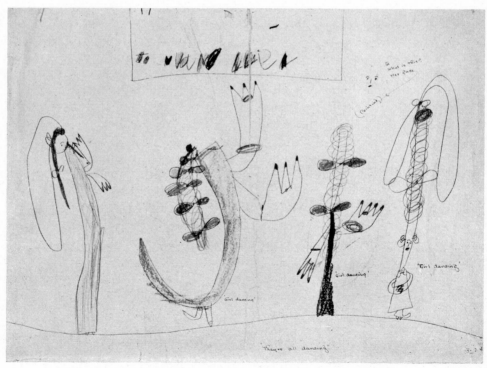

FIG. 22b. They're All Dancing, by Joan (*pencil and crayon*).

tions which were made of simple geometrical forms and primitive colors represented her effort to identify herself in time and space. Similar efforts to express this have been seen in other schizophrenic children.

In the school room, Joan drew pencil sketches of human figures in various dramatic but usually aggressive behavior (Fig. 22b). The human figures were grotesque; they showed exaggeration of all the peripheral features such as arms, fingers, fingernails, hair, breast—even the coccyx. Sometimes the features are further exaggerated by ornaments such as bows in the hair, rings on the finger, ear rings. They always showed some form of vortical circling, indicating that they were sometimes whirling so fast that the facial features could not be made out; furthermore the figures are elongated upwards in relation to the whirling. A face is also detached and in some of her drawings, eyes and limbs would become detached from the bodies, and appear to be flying off into space. Joan used her drawings of human figures to deal with problems of movement, action, aggression, and relationship in somewhat the same way that she used her colorful abstractions to deal with form, space, identity, and individuation.[7]

After a course of shock treatment Joan seemed to improve to the extent that she was less anxious, disorganized, and preoccupied. She was better controlled and freer in her behavior and relationships with people. However she was also freed of inhibitions and her impulses for aggression against children such as scratching their faces with sharpened pencils were too often carried out. She was sent to a grandmother out in the country where there were no children. Later she was able to return home and attend school until she was 12. At this time she became disturbed by hallucinations of the devil underground and by attacks of anxiety. She entered the hospital for another course of shock treatment but episodes of disturbance continued that necessitated a longer period of hospital care. At 12 years her art work did not include abstractions. On request she drew some rather banal human figures which did not interest either her or the psychiatrists very much.

III. THE USE OF COLOR IN ABSTRACTIONS AND ABSTRACT-LIKE PAINTINGS BY AMERICAN NEGRO AND PUERTO RICAN CHILDREN WITH EMOTIONAL AND SOCIAL PROBLEMS

Some American Negro and Puerto Rican children have had to deal with social and emotional problems which have caused them to remain immature and naïve. The inherent primitive features in their art work have been made articulate in their use of color in form abstractions.

Pauline was an 11 year old Negro girl, born in the South, who came to

_____

[7] Montague, Allison: The Art of Schizophrenic Children in *Projective Techniques*. ibid. This paper deals with the psychological problems of the human-form drawings of schizophrenic children. One of Joan's drawings is included.

New York when she was 5 or 6 years old. Her father was reported to have been an infantile, abusive self-centered individual; her mother inadequate but devoted to the child. Pauline boasted that she had chased her father out of the house when she was 7 years old. She dominated the mother and was completely uninhibited and self-willed. As one might expect, troubles arose in school because she refused to recognize authority or to accept routine. All of her teachers complained about her. She did poor school work, and showed no capacity to apply herself to a task or to concentrate. She craved attention, annoyed the other children at their work, defied the teachers, and would completely lose control of herself under any form of discipline. It was known that she could do good work in the handicrafts. Our examination showed that she was of average intelligence. She had the mentality to do good sixth-grade work and was placed in that grade, but actual tests showed that she had mastered work only to the third grade. This was due to poor motivation, interest, and work habits.

She was found to be a child with poorly directed adolescent drives and infantile behavior patterns. She was uninhibited, overactive, constantly seeking immediate satisfaction for her impulses, and had no sense of responsibility for the social situation.

Her drive for self-determined action made it possible for her to find pleasure in the directed activity of drawing and painting. Since her activity was undeniably greater than her capacity to grasp the full structure of the world, it often expressed itself in simple geometrical designs such as stripes and rhomboids which would have been monotonous if they had not been brightened by simple and glowing colors of bright yellow, red, green, and blue (Fig. 23a). This pleasure in geometrical figures and lively colors was evident in her use of water colors and in drawings made with crayons. The painting became more varied when she substituted for the simple geometrical designs, snake-like and worm-like designs in bright color contrasts to the background. There was green on red, brown on green, violet on white and brown. The mosaics of brilliant colored spots of irregular shape remind one of the simple beauty of some of the pictures of Pieter Mondrian; although this Negro child artist did not attempt Mondrian's severity of form; she lived in an orgy of color which is foreign to the more sober Dutchman. She succeeded in one composition of great beauty, in which the irregular geometrical forms were elaborated in brightly colored hills bordering on a stream (Fig. 23b). The house in the foreground, and the tree offer formal problems which the young artist did not completely master, although the construction of the house uses the mosaic pattern not without success. The organic form of the tree entirely defied the undeveloped technique of this child.

Clarence was a 10 year old Negro boy with similar problems. He was the older of two children. His parents were devoted to the child but they were immature and easy-going. They had no control over him and he ran about the streets, truanted from school, and stole anything he wanted. In school he would not attend to his work and interfered with that of the other children. In our examination he was found to have adequate intelligence but was sullen and defiant and said he would be as bad as he wanted because he had more fun that way and his parents didn't care. In our schoolrooms he would not apply himself to the usual school work but found satisfaction of a type new to him in the art work.

His productions have many similarities to those of Pauline, but he preferred more sombre colors, and the soft-flowing line was of much greater importance than the angle and irregular patterns. It is of interest that in the execution of curves he produced patterns which are similar to letters. Two of his pictures are reproduced to give an idea of his work (Figs. 24a and 24b). From the work of this boy we may draw the conclusion that the great urge for action may express itself in curves as well as in angular forms such as are seen in the work of Pauline. But it is also seen more clearly here that the abstraction is used in an effort to identify the child in a confusing world, with the child's name appearing in every painting as do other efforts at symbol formations. There also seems to be an effort to divide space into meaningful parts.

These two children were difficult problems for the community due to their restlessness and aggressiveness, but they had a good conception of what they themselves wanted. Their pictures of their respective worlds were rather unified ones. They displayed a pleasure in color which appears to be part of their racial characteristics which often find exuberant expression in dancing and spirituals.

Pleasure in bright and glowing colors is obviously a primitive trend. According to Ruth Staples children react first to the color red. In our own experience, pleasure in bright colors is already noted in the four month old infant. In the course of development this primitive delight in colors becomes subordinated to many other attitudes. More of it may be expected to be preserved in races which are under less cultural pressure, such as Negroes, Puerto Ricans, Indians, etc. Furthermore, it may be expected that such overemphasis of color might become dominant when low intelligence (cf. Chapter 9) releases other cultural barriers; and that every breaking through of strong emotions due to whatever cause may carry with it something of the naïve pleasure in color which is otherwise obliterated.

Joseph was another 13 year old Puerto Rican white boy who came to the United States when he was 4 or 5 years old. He was the second oldest of the six children in the family. The family had never made a good social adjustment in the United States and were constantly being cared for by social agencies. As a result Joseph and his siblings had spent many years in institutions, and Joseph had been in an orphan home from the age of 6 years until he was 11 years old. He had not been happy there and had made no friends. As an infant he had learned Spanish and although in the course of the years he had lost that language he had not gained much English. This of course handicapped his schoolwork, and in all of his social contacts he gave the impression of being a very dull boy. At best he was not very bright.

After the institution had returned the children to their home, the family began to seek other means of having them cared for. Previously, Joseph's younger brother Ignacia had been on our wards for aggressive, asocial and mischievous behavior. Born in this country, he had a better command of English and appeared brighter than Joseph. The latter reacted to a world which seemed not to welcome him, with aggressive, antagonistic, clowning behavior. Since Joseph had been home his parents had complained of silly as well as dangerous actions, such as starting fires on the roof. They tried to encourage the school to complain that the boy was troublesome, but the school reported that if the boy had been left alone he would have managed fairly well. With the advent of puberty and its problems, and the child's increasing feelings of rejection, inferiority, and hopelessness, his behavior became more inappropriate, asocial, and withdrawn, and he appeared duller than before.

On our wards in an interview with adults he appeared very dull, unresponsive, emotionally flat, and silly. He responded to standard intelligence tests like a mental defective. Among the children he showed fluctuating behavior: for days at a time he was apathetic, unresponsive, and disinterested in the play and other activities of the other children. He made a hebephrenic impression. At other times he became spontaneously restless, aggressive, and even destructive, especially of his own work. At these times he would be silly and clownish. Then for very short periods he would show interest in some activity and become almost gay and appealing. But in the art class he often applied himself with concentrated zeal and produced works of interest, which seemed to give him pleasure. It is probable that only at these times was the boy really himself.

Almost all of the features of the artistic work so far mentioned in this section are represented in the pictures by this boy. It may be pointed out that his intelligence was not high and that in addition he was blocked by his emotions. In the one of the house (Fig. 25b) this rejected and unhappy boy uses colors which have something uncanny about them. The yellowish-green of the windows and the bluish-green of the background have a maliciousness in their content. The tree at the right (Fig. 25a) in a greenish-brown and black, might almost be a ghost. Even when this child used reds, they are subdued. In all of the drawings at our disposal, the whole paper space available is covered with darkish colors from which the dark reds, yellows, and blues emerge. In his drawings Joseph uses primitive forms, such

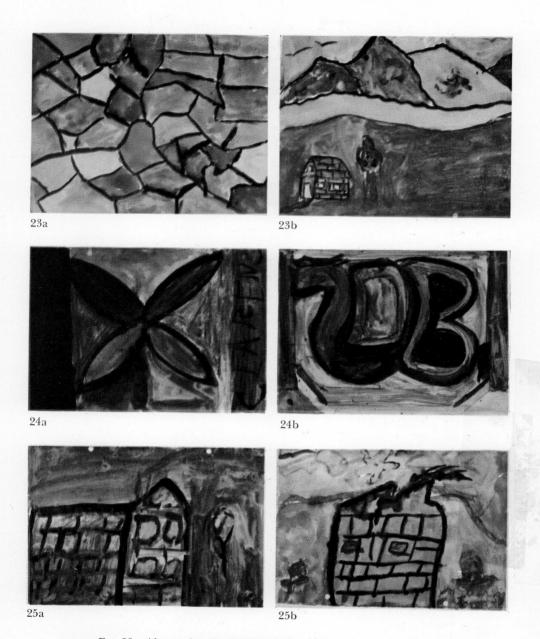

FIG. 23a. Abstraction, by Pauline (*water color*).
FIG. 23b. Landscape, by Pauline (*water color*).
FIG. 24a, b. Abstractions with Symbols, by Clarence (*water color*).
FIG. 25a, b. Houses, by Joseph (*water color*).

as the loop, to represent flowers. The houses are drawn in a rather awkward fashion. Very often the roof shows strange indentations. It is realized that this child—rejected, helpless, unprepared to take his place in the world— expresses his primitive fear of the world by depicting it as a somber place. However, it is not the somberness of black and gray but of colors in which the blue end of the spectrum prevails.

The color red and aggression obviously have close relation to each other. Charles Hartshorne in his *Philosophy of Sensation* writes, "Red is precisely the most dramatic and stirring of colors and there is no other color that it is so necessary to take seriously. Nearly all of the great instinctive emotions, social solidarity, everything save sex are represented in red which is the color of blood."[8]

Abstract art relies upon form, space, and color values which are all deeply related to general human experiences. This differentiates abstract art from mere ornament, in which the general form principles are more stylized and have less relation to action.

Its decorative and ornamental aspects may form an essential part of an art work, but they may also serve merely as the milieu for its more vital functions. When our patients use abstract forms one may be in doubt about the artistic value of their productions, yet the foregoing material makes it clear that abstract forms have specific connections with life experiences.

Abstract art is a form of art dealing with forms and colors as objects and is interested in content only in so far as they are in close relation to form problems.

In obsessional neurotic cases the abstract principles in drawing have a deep connection with the basic motor drives of the individual. The problems of curves, of straight lines, of angles, of borders, of crenations, of sharp or blurred contour have a deep meaning from the point of view of fundamental problems of aggression and of being attacked. Very often the drawings satisfy the wish for unimpeded movements which are not as dangerous as the movements otherwise performed by the patient. Specific topics which illustrate opposition, such as day and night, rain and shine, dark and light are represented by specific choice of form and color.

Even in schizophrenics the form problem may be incidental to the deeper-lying schizophrenic meaning expressed in comparatively simple lines. However, a deep regression to the essentials of form principles can occur in schizophrenics. In such cases, the patients experiment with the fundamental forms and figures of primitive visual motor experience. They also experiment with time and space and try to orient themselves in these verities. Such an experimentation may lead to form productions which are very satisfactory from the point of view of aesthetics.

---

[8] Hartshorne, Charles: *The Philosophy and Psychology of Sensation.* 1935, pp. 255-256.

In the naïve and immature Negro and Puerto Rican child, abstractions are a means of dealing with the insecurity of the world and of identifying himself in time, space, and by some type of symbol formation.

Drawings which are offered during psychoanalysis or therapy can be used in the same way as dream material, irrespective of whether they have contents in the common sense or whether they are to be classified as abstract art. The drawing corresponds to the manifest content of a dream, and abstract forms also are basically the expression of human problems and conflicts. The material at hand permits the conclusion that in abstract forms particularly primitive and important drives make their appearance. Study of such forms is therefore revealing, not only from the point of view of art, but also from the point of view of therapy.

8

THE DRAWING OF A MAN BY CHILDREN WITH CHRONIC ENCEPHALITIS[1]

THE Goodenough test, or the drawing of a man, has been established as a reliable intelligence test for normally developing children. In 1926 Florence Goodenough published her standardization of this test. It is essentially a maturation or performance test independent of verbal function, language ability, or educational attainment.

It has been found by workers preceding Goodenough and quoted by her, that when children are allowed to draw whatever they choose, they most commonly draw the human form. This is probably due to the child's preoccupation with the image of his own body first, and secondarily of others about him. The scoring of the test is based on the number of individual body details, their relationship to each other, and the motor coordination. This suggests that the drawing of the child is an experiment in the visual motor interpretation of the integrated pattern of the kinesthetic, motor, cutaneous, and visual impressions. This is in part Paul Schilder's concept of the body image. It is of considerable interest that this proves to be a maturation test for general intelligence. The impression that it represents the visual image of the child's own body is further borne out by the fact that some children with severe defect in the body often depict this defect in their drawing of "a man." A child who had a short leg from earliest infancy always drew her "man" with one short leg. Several children with congenital anomalies in the skull have depicted the anomaly in their drawings. A child with a disabling neurological condition of the feet drew one-legged men or men riding in carts.[2] The younger children often drew the genitals, breasts, umbilicus, etc. Older children suppress these details or draw their figures with clothes. It is not uncommon, especially among the younger children, that their drawings will throw light on the child's preoccupations which have emotional value, and consequently aid the psychiatrist in the interpretation of psychological mechanisms.[3]

Goodenough summarizes the work of previous authors who had analyzed

---

[1] Reprinted in part from: Bender, Lauretta: The Drawing of a Man (Goodenough test) in Chronic Encephalitis in Children, from the *Journal of Nervous & Mental Disease, 41*:277-286, 1940.

[2] See discussion of Morris, Chapter 13, Fig. 42.

[3] See Machover, Karen: *Personality Projection in the Drawing of the Human Figure.* 1949.

the differences in the drawings of normal children and those of retarded or sub-normal children. The drawings of the sub-normal children resembled those of younger normal children in lack of detail and defective sense of proportion and sometimes also in qualitative deficiencies such as in the relationship of parts to each other, but primitive and mature features might be combined. E. Neumann (1907) stated that the factors that make for defective drawings are lack of analytical observation, defective visual imagery, defective eye-hand coordination, interference with memory images due to imperfections in the actual work as the drawing progresses, lack of related drawing schemes, difficulties with three-dimensional space, and defective manual skill.

However, in the specific task of drawing a man, a special disability may be more important. This is in the form of a specific imperception of the body image. The body image is built up as a maturation process by a gestalt integration of all sensory, motor, and social experiences of the child. It probably has a center of localization in the brain. Paul Schilder states that experiences of pain in the body and motor control of the limbs are important factors in its development. It runs parallel with sensory-motor development. In the same way the child's drawing of a man develops and Schilder points out that since the child is satisfied with his drawing, it probably represents his knowledge and sensory experience of the human body.

The drawing of a man or the Goodenough test was used by J. C. Earl (1933) in studying feebleminded adults with mental ages of 5 to 9 years. He found that the feebleminded adult did not draw the human form in the same way that a normal child of the same mental age does. There is a different handling of details and in general the adult feebleminded person has a greater wealth of detail than the child who is more concerned with the body as a whole. However, the defective adult shows many discrepancies in his use of details. He is unduly concerned with unimportant details. There is a special concern with sex symbolization and a tendency to be meticulous, to perseverate. Dissociative phenomena also occur and generally there is a wide scatter in the test performance. That is to say, primitive and more mature capacities often occur in the same drawing.

The following characteristics for deviate functioning in the drawing of a man in psychopathic children were suggested by Florence Goodenough: The "verbalist" type of product with a large number of details but few ideas; the "individual responses," incomprehensible to anyone but the subject; "flight of ideas" as for example a drawing with only one ear, or hair on only one side of the head; and scattered or uneven mental development shown by the unusual combination of primitive and mature characteristics appearing in a single drawing. In a group of 450 school children, nine were found who produced drawings with one or more of these characteristics. These children rated by their teachers showed more psychopathology than the other children in terms of over-sensitivity, proneness to worry, muscle twitches, poor concentration, absentmindedness, timidity, instability, and flightiness.

Florence Goodenough also discussed drawings produced by fourteen children referred to a child guidance clinic. These children showed the combination of mature and primitive features or "scatter," but showed none of the other features. It was noted that a large number of the drawings showed the characteristics of those drawn by the opposite sex and that there was evidence of relatively poor motor coordination. F. K. Berrien (1935) followed Goodenough's suggestions and obtained drawings of a man from fifty-two children and adolescents from a state mental hospital which included postencephalitic, psychopathic personalities and borderline mental defective children. He found evidence of sex reversal characteristics in the postencephalitic children and "scatter" in all groups, but few of the other criteria in any of these children's drawings.

W. E. Hinrichs (1935) obtained drawings of a man from delinquent and non-delinquent boys and feebleminded children with and without behavior disorders. He found that the delinquent boys were on the whole inferior in Goodenough score as compared to the non-delinquent. The qualitative differences were in terms of incongruity or internal inconsistency in the drawings which included the "scattering" referred to by Goodenough or a mixture of immature and mature features, as well as stereotyping and a relatively immature choice of subjects, such as soldiers and cowboys.

L. N. Yepsen (1929) gave the Goodenough test to feebleminded children from 9 to 18 years of age, correlated it with the Stanford-Binet and found that although the Goodenough test had been standardized for children from 4 to 12 years, it was reliable for older defectives.

E. W. McElwee (1934) found that the total score of defective children was lower than that of normal children with the same mental age due to immature elements such as the absence of a trunk, attachment of legs to neck, and clothing represented by only a row of buttons. Judith Israelite (1936) also found that the scoring of the average mental age was slightly lower on the Goodenough than on the Stanford-Binet. The feebleminded were deficient in proportions and coordination.

Dorothy T. Spoerl (1940), using the Goodenough drawing of a man, studied the developmental tendencies in the drawings of retarded children. She concluded that the feebleminded child showed a marked tendency to draw above the level expected for his mental age.[4]

It has been noticed that children who have been known to be suffering

---

[4] In 1941 Anne Annastasi and John Foley, while surveying the literature on experimental investigations of the artistic behavior of the abnormal, reviewed the use of the Goodenough Scale and reported eleven investigations in addition to Florence Goodenough's original suggestions of deviate findings in her test. Eight of these referred to abnormal children. There have been several additional studies since 1941.

from chronic encephalitis are not able to draw the human form at the level which would be expected of them. In other words, there is a discrepancy between the Goodenough test and the Stanford-Binet test. The Goodenough test is now looked upon as a further diagnostic measure in doubtful cases of encephalitis or similar organic brain disturbances in children. However, the test is not always reliable in the non-specific types of encephalitis or traumatic conditions of the brain, due probably to localization problems. Apparently, damage of certain kinds to the brain, or of certain parts of the brain, are more prone than others to interfere with the child's capacity to draw the human form. If one can look upon this drawing as a test in perception of the body image, one may say that an imperception of the body image occurs as a result of some organic disease processes of the brain, especially in chronic encephalitis in childhood.

The psychometric patterning in post-encephalitic children has been discussed by Lauretta Bender and Florence Halpern in a survey on post-encephalitic behavior disorders in children.[5] This includes case reports on several of the children whose drawings of a man are analyzed here. It was found that tests dependent on spatial orientation, visual or auditory memory, and baragnostic sense are generally failed. Specifically failure was found in copying a diamond (or in a very young child, inability to copy a square), poor memory for digits, inability to reproduce designs from memory, and often also failure to distinguish weights (Yr. IX, Stanford-Binet, 1916 Rev.). The visual motor gestalt test[6] is also of diagnostic value as it reveals disorders in spatial relationships in the visual motor function.

It was concluded that one of the problems of the post-encephalitic child is the specific intellectual defect which is based on difficulties in gaining patterned behavior through perceptual experience; the others are motility and impulse disturbances and the personality disturbance related mainly to the hyperkinesis and deficiency in social orientation. The significance of the perceptual motor disorder is realized when it is pointed out that the inability to draw a man is an imperception of the body image or an inability to integrate all the perceptual experiences of the body; that the hyperkinesis may be understood as an effort continually to contact the physical and social environment and re-experience and re-integrate the perceptual experiences which always fail specifically to satisfy such children. There is thus a continuous effort to gain some sense of orientation in the world. The asocial behavior may be understood as the result of the lack of capacity to live out certain infantile drives and to build up some understanding of one's place in the world in a temporal pattern, to learn from past experiences and to build a concept of aims for future satisfactions.

---

[5] Chapter VIII in Neal, Josephine (Editor): *Postencephalitic Behavior Disorders in Encephalitis, A Clinical Study,* 1942.

[6] See Chapters 4 and 5.

Case 1: Beatrice[7] was born 2/28/24, and had normal development until age 3 years (1927), when she had an obscure febrile illness, the details of which are uncertain. Within the following year she became overactive and difficult to manage by her mother. She came to Bellevue mental hygiene clinic in 1932, at 8 years. The complaint was asocial behavior including running about on the street until 10 P.M., inability to sit still in school, aggressive acts against other children, and temper tantrums. Her school work was good when she attended to it. On a battery of intelligence tests she scored IQ's from 92 to 100. At that time no neurological deviations were noted. She returned to the clinic the next year and was admitted to the children's ward. The mother reported her behavior was worse and beyond control. She was found to be overactive, unable to restrain her impulsive behavior, aggressive and inattentive. She was constantly seeking to get into contact with adults by clinging and affectionate behavior and with children by aggressive behavior. Neurological examination showed poor convergence of the eyes. She was partially exhausted from her overactivity. She quieted down somewhat with ward routine and was discharged. She had two admissions during 1934 at the age of 10. Complaints against her then were running away from home, stealing, sex activities, fighting with other children, and temper tantrums. Neurological examination showed poor convergence of eyes, poor reaction of the pupils to light, and absence of knee jerks. She spent three months in a state mental hospital, was discharged somewhat improved, returned to Bellevue again in 1935.

At this time her IQ tested 92 with a mental age of 10-3 on the Stanford-Binet test. But the Goodenough drawing test of a man scored 5-9 (Fig. 27a). She was sent to another state hospital but removed in a few months by her parents and returned to Bellevue in 1936 at the age of 12. At this time her neurological deviations had increased in the direction of a Parkinsonian syndrome. Her facial expression was flattened, her speech was monotonous, associated movements of the arms during walking were poor, convergence of the eyes was absent and pupillary reaction to light was deficient. Her behavior at home was uncontrollable; she had long since been refused for further school adjustment.

She was sent back to the state hospital where she still was at 16 years when we last heard of her.

Her drawing of a man would not have been recognized as such if it were not that we could compare it with her previous drawing, which it resembled in general contour (Fig. 27a). Her scoring on standard intelligence tests varied between 80 and 90, the drop being due to poor attention and to inadequate handling of school material. Her score on the Goodenough test was 3-6. Her last drawing can be considered little more than a sign of a man. She was dissatisfied with it: she said, "It is the best I can do." This is in sharp contrast to the younger normal children who are always contented with their primitive drawings.

---

[7] *Case 8—Beatrice—*in Neal, Josephine (Editor): *Encephalitis a Clinical Study.* See Fn. 5, p. 374.

Case 2: Lewis,[8] born 4/23/24. Development was normal until 3 years (1927) when he had a severe illness complicated with mastoiditis which left him with "chorea." At the ages of 6 and 7 years he was refused for school admission because of his inability to settle himself to any routine and because of his constant talking. He was admitted to the children's ward of the New York Psychiatric Institute with the complaint of being quarrelsome, fussy, distractible, and always talkative. At that time the endocrine features were emphasized and treated. He showed a Froehlich type of body build and

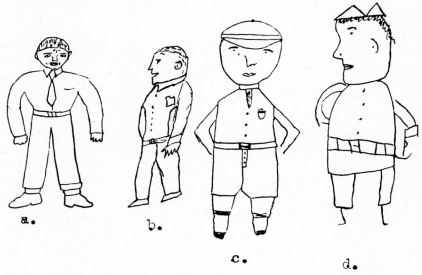

FIG. 26. Drawings of a man by four children, 11 years of age.
a. Superior child with M.A. of 13-6 years.
b. Average child with M.A. of 11 years.
c. Dull child with M.A. of 9-6 years.
d. Defective child with M.A. of 7-6 years.

undescended testicles. With the controlled ward environment, his behavior improved and special school placement was arranged for two years. He was again rejected from school, mainly due to his constant and unrestrained talking. He was referred to the Bellevue mental hygiene clinic and admitted to the children's observation ward.

His unrestrained impulse to talk and to keep in contact with people about him made it impossible to carry on any other activity when he was present. He also presented the picture of a Froehlich syndrome with the additional features of strabismus, nystagmus, oral tics, dyskinesis, excessive appetite, and irritability. Advised institutional care was refused by the parents. He was returned in 1936, showing some evidence of improvement. He was 12 years old. He was less obese and the testicles were descended, though small. He had received a long course of antuitrin S. He was somewhat quieter but was

---

[8] *Ibid.,* Lewis—*Case 7*, p. 374.

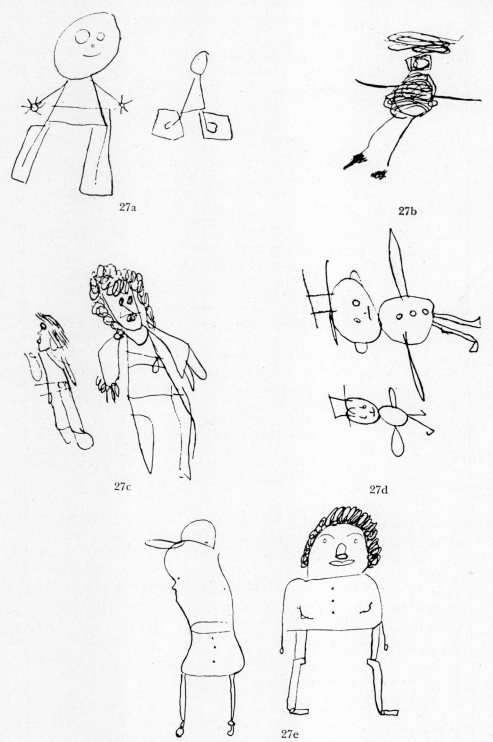

FIG. 27. Drawing of a man, by five encephalitic children.
FIG. 27a. Beatrice. FIG. 27b. Lewis. FIG. 27c. Nan. FIG. 27d. Audrey. FIG. 27e. Leo.

still distractible, meddlesome, and talkative. The ocular signs were still present and in addition there was some facial flattening and asymmetry.

His Goodenough man-drawing test is shown in Fig. 27b. This was made in 1935 when he was 11 years old and was able to score an IQ of 81 on the Stanford-Binet test with a mental age of 8-9. On the Goodenough test he scored a mental age of 4-6. Only in general contour does it resemble the usual child's drawing of a man. It is not the way a normal 4½ year old child would draw the human figure. Facial features do not appear, detail is poor and lines show poor motor control. On the other hand, shading is a more mature accomplishment.

Case 3: Nan, born 3/29/25. She had measles at 1 year and chicken pox at 2 years, but neither sickness was considered severe. At 4 years it was first noted that she was very overactive and showed some choreiform motility. At 6 years when she was ready for school, she was referred for admission to the neurological service of a hospital. Polyglandular disturbances were associated with her condition. She was obese. She was admitted to the children's ward of the New York State Psychiatric Institute at 7 years, and to the children's ward of Bellevue at 9 years. She then displayed a Froehlich body build, athetoid motility, a speech defect, reading disability, and left-handedness. The complaints against her were repeated running away, inability to get along with other children, inability to sit still in school or attend to her work, aggressiveness, destructiveness, temper tantrums, and sex play. She was admitted to a state mental hospital, but was soon removed by her parents, when she ran away through three states and exposed herself to sex experiences. She was returned to the children's division of a state hospital where she has remained for two years. It is reported that new neurological signs have developed which make the diagnosis of a chronic encephalitis beyond doubt.

Her pictures of a man (Fig. 27c) were drawn in 1935 at the age of 10-2. Her IQ on the Stanford-Binet at that time was 80 with a mental age of 7-4. Her Goodenough score was 6-9. Although this is not a marked discrepancy, one must also realize that her Stanford-Binet score was not satisfactory, due to inattention and no schooling. Her drawing of a man showed many mature features in her efforts at detail, but poor motor control. She expressed uncertainty and dissatisfaction in the execution.

Case 4: Audrey[9] was born 2/10/24. In her fourth year she had a severe and prolonged sequence of illnesses with measles, whooping cough, and pneumonia. When she entered school it was complained that she was impossibly restless, domineering with other children, and demanding of adults. She was referred to the Bellevue mental hygiene clinic. The neurological examination was reported to be negative. During the next year she was admitted to

---

[9] *Ibid.,* Audrey—*Case 5,* pp. 372-373.

another hospital for the treatment of "chorea." At the age of 8 she was expelled from school and returned to the Bellevue mental hygiene clinic. She was then found to be fidgety, inclined to drop things, unable to write. She showed poor motor control often falling down. She could not sit still or attend to her work at school and would not stay home but wandered the streets. She was admitted to the children's observation ward where she was found to be athetoid in her motility, and persistently hyperkinetic. She was constantly seeking contact with persons and things, which led her to be overaffectionate or overaggressive and destructive. Convergence of the eyes was poor and the facial expression was flat. She was admitted to an institution for normal children but soon ran away. She was again admitted to Bellevue children's ward and sent to a state hospital where she has remained two years, after one short trial period at home. She was seen there and was noted to have an awkward athetoid motility, defective associated movements, immobile facies, defective convergence of the eyes, hyperkinesis and distractibility.

Her drawing of a man (Fig. 27d) was made in 1933 at the age of 11 years, when she was able to score an IQ of 110 on the Stanford-Binet test with a mental age of 12-1. The Goodenough scores on the two drawings are 5-6 and 6-0, which is less than half the expected scores. The drawings are very immature and primitive. Furthermore, they are disoriented in space. This problem obviously puzzled the child but she could not solve it. It is undoubtedly significant that these children so often draw two or even more figures when asked to make a drawing, thus expressing their dissatisfaction. She was subsequently paroled to her home but ran away to a distant state and had to be returned to the hospital.

Case 5: Leo,[10] born 2/10/24, was normal until 9 years when he suffered an attack of spinal meningitis, diagnosed in a hospital on the basis of the spinal fluid findings. Following this there was a personality change with overactivity and asocial behavior. He became uncontrollable in the home, school, and community and was five times before the children's court. He was sent by the children's court to the children's observation ward of Bellevue in 1935 at the age of 12. He escaped once and had to be returned four times by order of the children's court before the parents could be convinced of the necessity of institutional care. He was found to be diffusely overactive, aggressive, destructive, asocial, and uninhibited. Neurological examination showed poor ocular convergence, uneven facial innervation, and some loss in associated movements in the arms while walking.

He was able to score an IQ of 104 on the Stanford-Binet test with a mental age of 13-9. But his Goodenough score was 4-9 (Fig. 27e).

After several months in the state hospital he became very much subdued.

---

[10] *Case 5*, in Bender, Lauretta: *Cerebral Sequelae and Behavior Disorders in Children Following Pyogenic Meningo-encephalitis in Children*, 1942, p. 774.

He was discharged home and the next year returned to Bellevue for approval for school placement. He was definitely better in his behavior, being quiet, and self-controlled and very anxious to make a satisfactory record. His neurological deviations remained the same. Puberty brought some suggestion of endocrine disturbance with obesity and sluggishness. His Goodenough drawing test was somewhat improved, scoring 7-3, still being almost half of his mental age. Furthermore, at this time he was able to do good art work in landscapes and any subject that did not include the human form. We last heard from him in 1942 when he was 18 years of age and was found fit for military service which he entered.

These five cases offer examples of encephalitis lethargica and other types of encephalitis in childhood. In all, the condition was of long standing and apparently progressive with the exception of Leo, Case 5. There were more or less definite neurological deviations and serious personality defects. The outstanding features were overactivity, inability to inhibit impulses, limited span of attention, tendencies to come in contact with persons and things by clinging to adults, over affectionate or aggressive behavior with other children, touching, handling, destroying things. The secondary symptom disturbance was the diffuse asocial behavior and inability to adjust to school demands. There was no evidence of general intellectual impairment, although there was some tendency for the IQ to drop on tests where school accomplishments were important. Neurological deviations were mostly related to oculomotor control, associated movements, and extrapyramidal motility and endocrine functions. In some cases Parkinsonian-like pictures were suggested as the condition progressed. Institutional care was imperative in all cases.

When these children were asked to draw a man (Goodenough man-drawing test) they all performed the test poorly. They could not score on this test as well as they did on other standardized intelligence tests. Four of them were 11 years old, one 9; none of them could be classified as mentally defective but they performed this test in a way most comparable to a mentally defective child. Their inadequate drawings would not compare with a child of lower mental age. In general, detail was badly handled, motor execution was poor and the drawings expressed their uncertainty as to how to accomplish the tests, while they often verbally expressed their dissatisfaction with the results.

This may be looked upon as a specific disability. It does not represent any difficulty in their technical ability to draw as they can draw other subjects adequately. It represents an imperception of the postural model and probably arises from perceptual integration difficulties in relation to their own body image rather than from optic perceptual difficulties. It is probable that the capacity to draw the human form is not related to a simple visual gestalt but a more complicated gestalt which is based upon sensory impressions of all types coming from the surface as well as from the inside of the body. Besides the sensory impressions of the present, the sensory consciousness of the past are integrated into the present concept. However, it is a most important fact that motor impulses give the final shape to the body image. Only in motility do the various impressions of the senses approach the world of perception. In these cases the motility disrupts the body image as it is represented in the Goodenough drawing. The child, aware of the shortcomings, tries again and again to consociate the picture of the body by renewed contacts. Here we may find a hint as to the importance of motility in the perception of one's own body or the body image.

❧ 9 ❧

THE ART OF HIGH GRADE MENTAL DEFECTIVE CHILDREN DEPICTING THEIR STRUGGLE WITH EMOTIONAL DISORGANIZATION AND THEIR PRIMITIVE PERCEPTUAL EXPERIENCES[1]

THERE ARE many different aspects of the world. In the earlier stages of development, human beings perceive optically a world which is full of color and motion. A person who is born blind and later is enabled to see by an operation, is able first to perceive color before he can recognize form. His perception of spatial relationships is at first imperfect. Persons suffering from carbon monoxide poisoning sometimes sustain damage to that part of the brain which subserves optic impressions. In such cases color perception may remain, whereas the form perception is more or less completely destroyed. As the investigations of visual motor gestalten show there is a gradual development of form perception through maturation. The unit of optic perception in children is the loop, the whirl, and the circle. Angles appear only in later development. The horizontal line belongs to the primitive sphere of experience, and the vertical line appears soon after. The slanted line assumes importance only much later. Before the ages of 6 or 7, children cannot correctly copy a diamond. Nature does not consist of geometrical forms alone; on the contrary, they are rare. On the other hand one finds that in their various creations, human beings tend to produce geometrical forms of more or less simple type. It is as if there are two different worlds: first, the world in which geometrical forms prevail; and second, the world of nature, in which organic forms are dominant. The former is a world created chiefly by human beings, although some formations in nature, such as stones and hills, may assume more or less geometrical form.

Such forms, corresponding to primitive action (the loop) and to primitive orientation (whirling and the horizontal plane) are the earliest development of perception. We have repeatedly emphasized that visual forms are not in the perceptive sphere alone, but also in the motor sphere of human experience. In the primitive drawings of children one might, therefore, expect that simple forms and lines would make their appearance. Since color and motion also belong to the most primitive impressions, one might expect in primitive art a pleasure in elementary color and form impressions. With

---

[1] Written with Paul Schilder as part of an unpublished book entitled *Art and the Problem Child.*

146

further development, these primitive forms may become subordinate to the perception of more complicated object forms.

The optic perception of the child is not directed solely towards geometrical forms, whether they be simple or complicated. The child has a fundamental interest in the human figure and everything connected with this human figure, as Paul Schilder has shown in *Image and Appearance of the Human Body*. To begin with, the child has no immediate knowledge of its own body. To build up the image of its own body it has to turn to the bodies of others. Even small infants before they are one month old demonstrate a lively interest in the faces, and facial expressions of those about them. The child soon tries to build up knowledge of its own body by incorporating its optic experience with all the other sensory experiences which it has gained in the observation of others. It seems that it perceives all non-geometrical forms as though they were similar to the human body. Even the forms of so-called inanimate nature are not always seen in their geometrical and physical qualities but, if one may so express it, in their human qualities.

One may venture the general statement that art often revives the primitive aspects of the world, both as regards geometry and the human form. The various art movements may be compared with specific stages of psychological development. This is a rather schematic view, and we shall return to this problem when we discuss schizophrenia. The drawings of normal children have many features of certain art movements because of their tendency to revive the more primitive attitudes toward life. It may be expected that children with defects in the intellectual sphere who also suffer from severe emotional problems, and children who suffer from an impairment of the function of the central nervous system will show tendencies to revert to primitive experiences.

Primitive color experiences are frequently found in Puerto Rican, South American Indian, and American Negro children, on a racial basis. Such trends are emphasized even more strongly when there is a mental handicap, an organic disease of the brain or a severe emotional problem. In these children it was also observed that there were primitive form principles corresponding to the primitive color principles. Mondrian-like patterns and constructive principles reminding one of the later pictures of Paul Cezanne were seen. One cannot explain all the tendencies in the drawings and paintings of children by a few simple principles. However, the simple geometrical patterns are conspicuous. Children with reading disabilities often show an extremely well-integrated sense for form, color, and composition due to the fact that they are thwarted in one approach to reality, namely reading, and choose another way to reality through highly developed color and form principles. Whenever one finds a primitive form of art expression, one should always ask what factors are driving the individual to such an expression and whether the individual does not at the same time try to compensate for this regression to primitive stages by progressive tendencies in some other direction.

It is easy to find parallels between the drawings being discussed and the work of Vincent van Gogh, Paul Gaugin, Paul Cezanne, cubism, futurism, constructivism, and many other movements in modern art. Many of these modern artists and art movements have consciously revived primitive types of sculpture and painting. Early cubism, for instance, received many impulses from primitive Negro sculpture. The tendency of the artist obviously is to go back to primitivity in order to gain a new aspect of reality otherwise overlooked. The real artist never looks back; he looks forward in the sense of richer reality. The child also has this forward-looking drive, but it cannot find the way as well as the mature artist does. The psychotic artist will be an artist only to the extent that he can use his regression so that the gleam of a richer reality shines forth.

Among the modern artists only van Gogh is known to have been definitely psychotic, but there is still serious controversy over the type of psychosis he had, with present evidence leading to the opinion that he was not an epileptic but a schizophrenic. Although every schizophrenic individual suffers from strong regressive tendencies which drive him away from reality, one can yet always find some evidence that the individual wants to return to reality. Many schizophrenic persons are, therefore, capable of real artistic production in so far as they not only go back to primitive depths of experience, but give hints of striving back from this primitive life to a more developed one. The psychopathic personality does not have access to the deep layers of human consciousness as the schizophrenic person has. However, the psychopathic individual has less difficulty in finding his way back to reality. Constitutionally inferior individuals with emotional problems may react with regressive patterns.

The following three children belong to a family of constitutionally inferior heredity and also present severe emotional problems:

The mother as well as all three children of the K. family were in the Psychiatric Division of Bellevue Hospital at the same time in 1938, after a long struggle on the part of the social agencies to keep the family together in the community. The parents were born in Greece and came to this country in early adulthood. The father was a carpenter and skilled artisan. Marriage was arranged by a professional matchmaker. The mother was an inferior person and always irritable, disagreeable, and complaining of poor health which she ascribed to her childbirths. The father not only felt superior to his wife but was convinced he could have done much better in life without her and the children. He had an excellent work record until 1933 when he began to complain more and more that he was not getting enough out of life. Finally he began to complain of poor health, and quit working, allowing agencies to support the family, until he left the country and returned to Greece, having misrepresented his family status by claiming in his passport that he was a single man. Subsequently, it was learned that he had married again, had another child in Greece, and had settled there.

The mother was unable to accept this desertion. Even with home relief support she could not care for her home because of ill health, and her emotional instability. She cried constantly and maintained that she was dying. She would keep the children awake at night in anticipation of her immediate death, or she would walk the streets with them to keep from dying. The children were Gus, age 14, Tony, 13, and Lena, 10 years. Needless to say they became problems in the schools and the streets. The boys were irregular in school attendance, were restless, inattentive to their work, and quarrelsome; they wandered the streets and got into minor difficulties, stealing anything they could. The girl was reported to have had a "nervous breakdown" in school, in which she cried hysterically, hid from the other children, felt that she was hated by everyone, and was fearful in general. It was Lena's condition that precipitated the break-up of the home.

In the hospital it was found that the mother was a mental defective with the mentality of an 8 year old child. Her emotional instability, pseudo-delusional ideas of bodily disease, and fear of death were sufficiently fixed to require a long period of hospital care. Gus and Tony were amiable, likeable boys, although somewhat infantile in their attitudes. They were on the borderline of mental deficiency, having IQ's of about 75 on the standardized verbal tests (Stanford-Binet). However, they showed average intelligence in handling non-verbal, performance or manual tests. This type of discrepancy in intellectual functions is not uncommon in constitutionally inferior children. They were distressed about their mother and sister and were liable to periods of brooding and irritability when they might become antagonistic to hospital routine and personnel, but in general they were able to make themselves happy and useful in the protected environment that seemed to meet their needs. Lena was more inferior in every way. She was of borderline (75%) intelligence on all psychometric tests. She was infantile and asocial. She could not get along with other children and needed the constant reassurance of a mother substitute. She needed prolonged institutional care, whereas subsequently Gus and Tony did well in a foster home and in special classes in the public schools.

The art work of Gus shows primitive features in two of his productions (Fig. 28a and b). In one he used dark red cubes and quadrangles piled one upon another to make a house. It is a severe composition enlivened merely by the words "Post No Bills" and "Grocery 1912," together with other short grocery store signs. The second picture is composed of a dark green arc on a dark neutral background. These are form principles of an abstract character. In this case, the low intelligence and emotional disturbances gave the boy an access to form principles which often remain hidden from a more gifted child. It is astonishing with what great capacity he worked these form principles into pictures which have a threatening connotation. In the portrayal of a waterfall (Fig. 29a), the blue of the water is almost symmetrically flanked

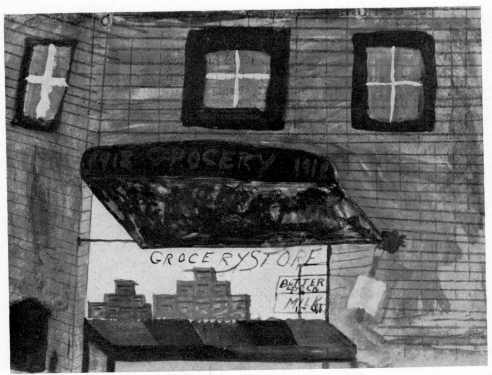

FIG. 28a. Grocery Store, by Gus (*water color*).

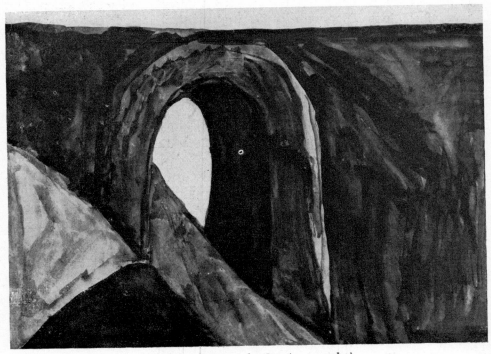

FIG. 28b. A Tunnel, by Gus (*water color*).

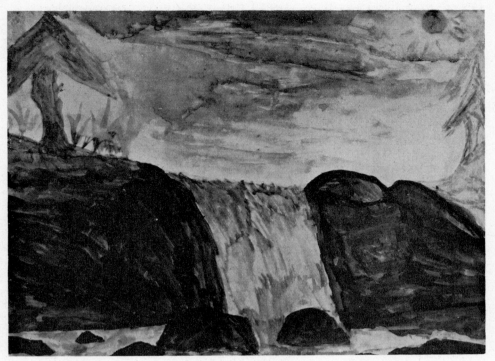

FIG. 29a. Waterfalls, by Gus K. *(water color)*.

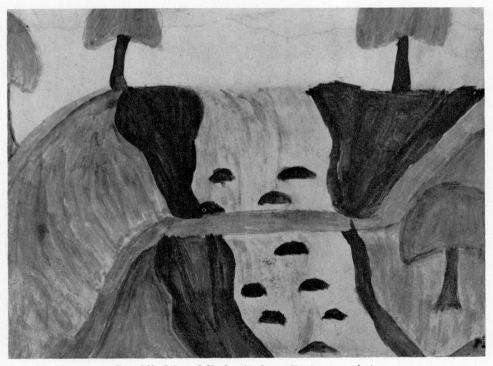

FIG. 29b. Waterfalls, by Anthony K. *(water color)*.

by black earth; two black boulders are in the center of the lower end of the waterfall. The dark green trees forming the sides of the picture are almost symmetrical. A dark red sun breaks through the bluish green of the not too friendly sky. This sombre picture is deeply impressive. It is an original creation for this child and was widely copied by other children. It made a more or less grandiose impression and they apparently found it simple to copy. However, those who copied it did not show the original grasp of the form problem.

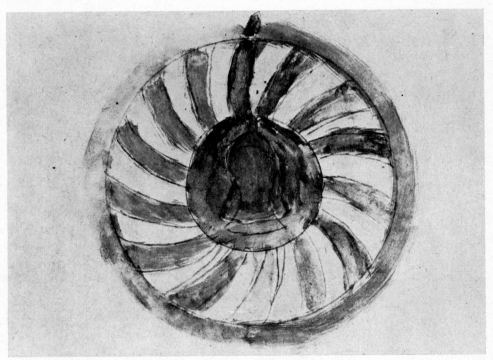

FIG. 30a. Design, by Anthony K. (*crayon*).

It has been stated that intellectual incapacity may be of value in discovering simple form principles. This is obvious in the drawings of Tony, Gus' brother. This child is younger and of an inferior intellectual level. He tried to draw the waterfall (Fig. 29b) which his brother painted so successfully; but there is no unity of form and construction. The colors are brighter, and light green plays an important part. The waterfall and boulders are unconvincing, and the harmony of the picture is badly disturbed by two red streaks crossing it, apparently signifying pathways over the waterfall. It may be worth while to keep in mind that it is probably not so difficult to discover form principles by merely regressing. However, these form principles have to be used again in an approach to reality, in which this second child undeniably fails completely. Another of his pictures is merely decorative and symmetrical (Fig. 30a). There is one picture drawn by the sister Lena, who is intellectually still more inferior (Fig. 30b). In spite of the good technical capacity, the study is completely empty and shows that the child has seen only the banal aspects of nature. It is to be noted that in none of the pictures by this family do we find human beings or animals.

We have seen that mental deficiency, which lessens the adaptive forces based upon logical thinking, liberates deep-lying energies and primitive

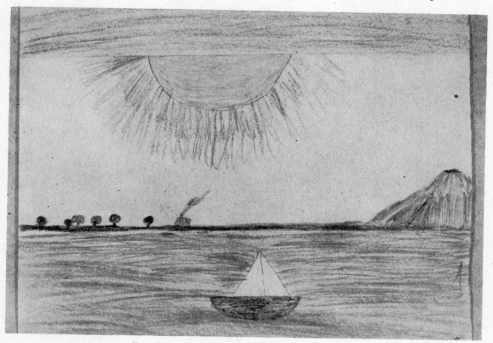

FIG. 30b. Boat Scene, by Lena K. (*crayon*).

reaction patterns. Primitive gestalten and form principles make their appearance in the art of mental defectives. From a clinical point of view it is well known that a mental defective also shows primitive or so-called infantile emotions which are liberated in accordance with the same principles. However, the psychology of the mentally defective individual cannot be fully understood by such simple formulations. The defective person not only often develops very strong asocial drives but he may also develop very strong forces in the moral consciousness at a primitive level. Out of such a conflict arise neurotic symptoms, the genesis of which is often more clearly expressed than in persons with a greater power of formulative thinking. In such cases the neurotic symptoms may be found to be of a severity and primitiveness often resembling psychotic symptoms of the schizophrenic type.

It must not be assumed that in mental deficiency only the mind is affected. Mind and emotions can be separated from each other only artificially. In the majority of defective persons disturbances are found in the emotional life which are not merely the consequence of the diminished power of logical thinking but represent a comparatively independent disturbance in the emotional sphere. Some children may show particularly strong aggressive drives

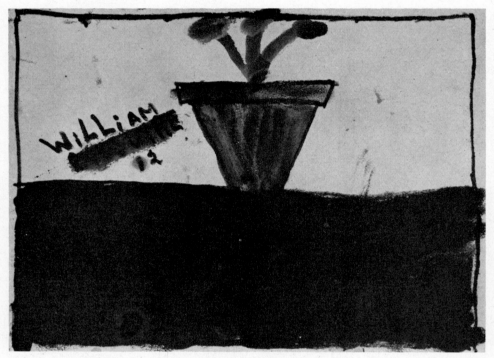

Fig. 31a. Flower Pot, by William (*water color*).

or an increase in sexual urges. In others the emotional life may be flat and the drives may be more or less diminished.

There probably exist an almost unlimited variety of primary emotional deviations in defective individuals. They may appear very bizarre at times, due to the lack of normal intellectual control. Indeed, pictures may occur which one may call psychotic and which, as R. A. Greene has pointed out, are far from being rare.

William was an 11 year old boy from an Irish family of a very low level. His father was an alcoholic who never assumed any responsibility for his family. The mother was blind and a mental defective. The oldest brother always had been a delinquent and wayward child and finally reached a reform school. Two older sisters were mentally defective and had been committed to institutions. William had been before the children's court several times, beginning at the age of 9, for minor delinquencies such as truancy, wandering the streets, and stealing. He had been adjudged "Neglected" by the judges, due to the totally unsuitable home situation. Our examination showed that William had an IQ of about 70 with the mentality of an 8 year old child. However, he was able to do only the first grade school work, showing that he had not adjusted to the schools even as well as an 8 year old boy. He was a sullen, tense, unhappy child who could not get along with other children and distrusted even the friendly approaches of

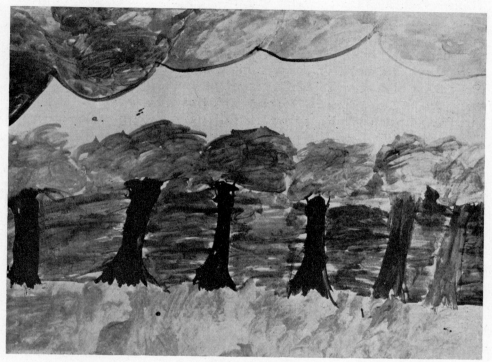

FIG. 31b. Trees, by William (*water color*).

adults. He was always on the defensive and would not respond to affection or sympathy as the normal small child will.

His unfavorable environment had made the child shy, and his withdrawal added to his adaptation difficulties. His art work may be classified in two categories: dull, unimaginative, brightly colored crayon pictures which see only a very limited part of reality, make up one group. The objects were banal, such as a boat, the face of a policeman, a house, a laundry wagon, an alarm clock, a teacup, an airplane. It is as if only a very small part of optic reality were utilized. When the same picture was drawn in water colors, darker colors were preferred and the brush strokes resisted a too schematic copying of an insignificant reality. This produced his second group of drawings. At the same time one sees more primitive form principles breaking through, as in the flower pot (Fig. 31a). The simple motif of trees in one straight row, with dark trunks and dark greenish-yellow crowns, the handling of the yellowish earth, the dark grey background, and schematic bluish-green and dark clouds—these add artistic value to the picture (Fig. 31b). This obviously is not due to specific capacity of the boy but to general human qualities liberated by his emotional unrest as well as by his constitutional defectiveness. Pathological art usually reveals otherwise hidden aspects of reality. The charm of such productions is based upon an insight which is gained not by personal experience but is almost superhuman, as if reality could present itself naïvely.

In every great artist, similar regressions to more primitive aspects of life occur. Some of the later rhythmical motifs of Vincent van Gogh such as *The Starry Night* (1889) are of a like character. However, van Gogh came to his surprising aspect of reality by a process of continuous experimentation and work on reality. Whereas the pathological artist is bound to the special aspect of reality which he displays, the true artist is conscious that there are other aspects, too, and he is capable of showing how the part of reality which he chooses to depict fits into the picture of a richer world. The primitivity of a van Gogh, a Picasso, and the surrealists therefore also points to a fully developed reality. Even the primitive art of Negroes points in some ways toward a more total aspect of the world.

Julius presented a sharply contrasting picture to William in his personality and emotional responses. Whereas the latter was always shy, alone, fearful of human beings, dull and forlorn, Julius was always in the center of a group of boys, be they bent on mischief or fun. His bubbling gaiety and surprising sense of humor deserted him only when he was once again facing judges or psychiatrists for some delinquency and he was making a futile effort to hide his identity and past record, which already was a gloomy one. He was 14 years old but said he was 11, probably in part recognizing the fact that he was nearer 11 in his mental development and partly to hide several years already spent in a reform school, which he would prefer to relate as though he had gone in one door and out the other.

He had been known to the courts since the age of 11 when he wandered the streets after his father had been sent to a hospital for the mentally ill. Later in the same year he broke into a store with a bunch of boys (he always did everything with a bunch of boys), and stole 24 cents from the cash register. He was sent to a reform school, was paroled after a year, but again broke into a grocery store with a gang of boys, and was sent back. This repeated itself year after year. The reform school had sent him to us for an examination, complaining that he did not respond to their training or to schoolroom teaching. When he was not in the reform school the complaints against him were truancy, unwillingness to work unless he was forced, and a preference for life on the streets with harmful companions.

On our ward he was our most popular boy, always entertaining the others with singing, improvised dancing, jokes, and happy reactions to every situation. Tests showed that he had an IQ of 70 and the mental age of a 10 year old boy. He also had a reading disability and could not read above the second-grade level. From this it is sufficiently evident why he truanted and found satisfaction in his own mode of life.

Like the other boy, William, this one produced pictures which showed that his world of concepts was empty and contained very little of the deeper

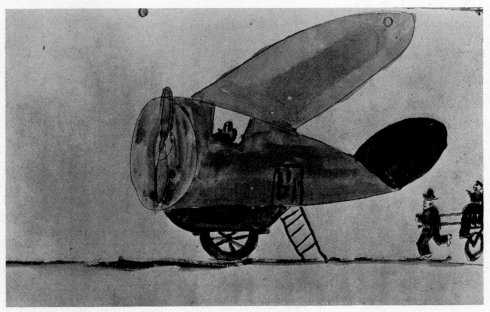

FIG. 32a. Aeroplane, by Julius (*water color*).

structures of reality. His drawings, however, are concrete and fairly realistic, as, for instance, the picture of an airplane (Fig. 32a).

There is another angle to his drawings which undoubtedly is derived from the comic strips and reveals his interest in people, what they do and what they are like. One of these is extremely aggressive, depicting the shooting of a bank robber. A great number of comic strips deal with the problems of children and adults in subordinating their general aggressive trends to a more human aspect of life. Our patient showed a strong tendency to aggression and a desire to dominate. In comic strips the tendency to dominate is often expressed in such a way that the other person is not seriously hurt but only checked in his aggression by being ridiculed, ridicule being a milder way of showing one's superiority to others. Aggressive acts which make others inferior without serious harm are the main topic of so-called funny papers and comic strips. This is a mild form of aggression in which the individual exposed to ridicule may emerge as the real hero who has been punched and laughed at but still survives. It is perhaps one important feature in humor and in comic art in general that the individual acquires the deep insight that no aggressiveness can annihilate him and deprive him completely of his human dignity. However, there is the other person who tries to show up his victim as ludicrous. The more profound artist will be capable of seeing in his victim the general ludicrousness of the human race. He will also allude to deeper characteristics of human weakness.

Our patient was humorous in a superficial way in his relation to others.

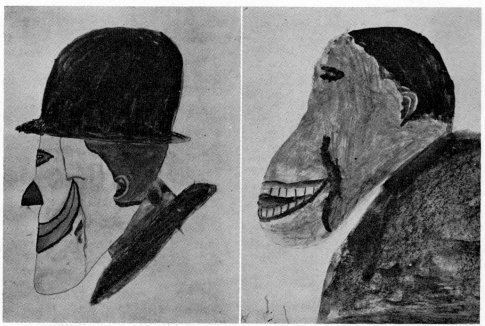

FIG. 32b. Clown, by Julius (*water color*).   FIG. 32c. Monkey, by Julius (*water color*).

He made them laugh and ridiculed them, which was one of the milder and more amiable forms of his aggressiveness. This tendency also expressed itself in some of his drawings. He drew human faces with distorted chins, ape-like, and in discordant colors of bright yellow and crimson (Fig. 32b). They are supposed to be clowns. There is also the head of a monkey very closely resembling his clown pictures (Fig. 32c). It represents a superficial aspect of the human face in its ridiculous phase. It is almost as if Julius chose merely one characteristic of humanity, and it is a more or less empty scheme of things with an exaggeration of one outstanding feature. It will also be noted that his drawings are oriented in a sinistrad direction, characteristic of left-handed individuals.

There is no question that these drawings were influenced by comic strips and cartoons. The point is, why did he choose them? They must have aroused something in him which corresponded to the more simple features of the material offered to him.[2] It has often been stated that children are very suggestible and that they are mere imitators. However, such a point of view is not justified. Children incorporate those parts of reality which they can adapt to their own needs and purposes. Without any question, every art, including that of the child and even the psychopathic child, is not isolated from cultural influences and from the persons surrounding the artist. The final product is the result of a mutual interaction, and in human interrelations pure imitation or copying does not exist.

Schizophrenia is a disease process which involves not only the psyche in the ordinary sense but also the organism. There are changes in the vegetative functioning and in the functioning of the brain. There is often interference in intellectual function with retardation or deficiency in children; sometimes there is precocious ability in language and art that may raise the IQ of the child above the expectancy level of the family. However psychic processes similar to those found in schizophrenia form the background of everybody's life experiences. Man's earliest childhood with all its strivings, yearnings and uncertainties, with all its difficulties in grasping the world and getting in closer touch with other human beings, is still alive in every human being, and it is possible that man has to go back to it whenever he wants to create. Human beings who have access to the deepest layers of human experience have a better possibility of seeing new visions of this world. They may not always find the way back to the world of their fellow men; they may seclude themselves in preoccupation with their inner conflicts. They may feel misunderstood and attacked and may answer with aggression. This is the stuff of which philosophers, poets, and artists are made. Sometimes they do not seem to be able to distinguish between the creations of their own fantasy and the real world. It often seems as if they have forgotten to check their fantasies against reality and against the experiences of other human beings. Such individuals have been called schizothym, or schizoid, or even schizoid psychopaths. The indiscriminate use of these terms, however, is not advisable.

The genius, even if he appears schizoid, is characterized by a deep respect for the community and for reality, and he merely has reverted to the creative sphere of primitive existence in order to utilize it for a better mastery of the world. This separates him from the schizoid personality and schizoid psychopaths who, in spite of their efforts, do not find the way back to the world as it is generally known. Such an individual is helpless in his undirected drives, struggles in vain with his aggressiveness, and even at the end of the journey cannot distinguish between his private world and that of social reality. He is really close to the schizophrenic, or he may be mildly schizophrenic, although he is not sick in the ordinary sense. He is a disharmonious personality and

---

[2] See Bender, Lauretta and Lourie, R. S.: *The Effect of Comic Books on the Ideology of Children;* and Bender, Lauretta: *The Psychology of Children's Reading and the Comics.*

therefore does not fall back into the complete and lasting abandonment of reality which characterizes the severe cases of schizophrenia.

Nat was a 10 year old Jewish boy, with a younger brother and a baby sister. His mother was defective and inadequate, his father, who was dead, had been psychotic. His brother was defective and was sent to a state institution for defectives. His baby sister, when she was 5 years old, was observed on our ward to be defective and schizophrenic. He was sent to us at the request of his teachers because he was restless in school and pre-occupied with other problems than his lessons. He said that his brother called him a sissy and a fairy but that he had no wings and could not fly; he wanted to know why Pharaoh killed all the babies and what was the name of the man killed by David and how did he kill him and how did the stone get into his brain and why did Samson's wife want to know where his strength lay. The referring school doctor called attention to his chorea-like motility. He was a dull child, with an IQ of 80, his best functioning being in verbal and visual motor tests.

His mother did not think there was anything to complain of in the boy, since he gave her no trouble. At home he stayed in a room by himself and read books all the time. His younger brother was mischievous and got in a lot of trouble, but Nat was a model boy. He was always respectful although he never showed affection for anyone.

On the children's ward he could not enter into the other children's play. He complained that they called him "sissy, fairy and pansy." In interviews with the physician he spent his time telling fantastic stories of mystery and violence in which he was always the central figure. He would say, "Let's talk about detectives; Sherlock Holmes could catch plenty of crooks. I like Dick Tracy, too, even though they ain't real. If there is a murder they find it out. I'm going to be a detective when I grow up. I'll catch crooks like him. If you get your man you don't shoot him, you take him by the neck and twist him; you say, 'Come on before I knock you over,' then he will tell, 'I did it.' If he don't tell, then there are guys at the window and they shoot him. Or I would get a grip around the neck and punch him in the back. I would give him a kick so he would drop his knife, and put him in jail. I would knock him off the mountain and cut his head off. I'll try to jump on him and grab his gun. I'll put my right to the heart and my left to the shoulder. If he were my stepfather (he has no stepfather) and he tried to do something to me, I would say, 'Listen here, you mug.' I would throw him over even if he were a pirate. If he were a big man I would take it easy until I got so mad that he couldn't stand against me any more."

His motility was choreic and when he talked associated movements of the hands and fingers were evident, which resembled effeminate mannerisms. He whirled on the longitudinal axis. His motor awkwardness and inhibition interfered with his manual ability, while he showed a high verbalization ability which he coordinated with his rich fantasy life. Every effort was made to help him to find some social values. His story telling and art work were highly regarded and he was discouraged from sitting in secluded places, preoccupied with sterile fantasies. After improvement, he was returned to his home and school for six months, but then was returned to us because he had regressed more deeply into his fantasy life. He was unable to keep up with his school work and had become negativistic toward his mother; he would shut himself in his room and spend the time in daydreaming and reading. He was unable to enter into a fight with other boys, but when his feelings were hurt he would be found in a remote corner shadow-boxing. He still delighted in telling fantastic stories of princesses and ogres. Thus while his preoccupations in the verbal field were more fantastic, more removed from reality, they still concerned themselves with the same problems of aggression and love.

He was encouraged to dramatize his fantasies with his physician who had to play the role of the criminal while Nat was the detective. At Nat's instruction the criminal (physician) was disguised as a woman and wore a wig. Nat (the detective) discovered and questioned him and tore the wig off, thus exposing the criminal. He pointed a gun at the criminal and accused him of robbery and murder and asked for an explanation. In a stage whisper he coached the criminal to reach for his gun and make an attempt to get away. Then in a loud voice he shouted at the criminal, foiled his escape and turned him over to the police.

From the first, art work challenged him and revealed all his inner conflicts, whether emotional-conceptual or motor. He suffered from lack of self-confidence and was continually wanting to be reassured. When a picture did not progress to his liking, usually due to his difficulties in expressing motor concepts, he walked up and down the room waving his arms or shadow-boxing. This may have been an expression of his profound difficulty in breaking through the inhibitions that were imposed upon his own motor functions. On the other hand he was never at a loss for ideas; he had an apparently inexhaustible fund of vivid story material. His technical ability, although limited, lent itself to his special problems.

The drawings which Nat made soon after admission show very primitive and stiff figures drawn in profile, but they show a trend to rhythmic repetition. At this time he displayed a strong tendency to connect persons in a group, one person putting his hand on the shoulder of another, or two persons firing guns at each other, with the path of the bullets connecting the two guns. At that time there was no tendency toward any composition. The guns already strongly suggested penises. It is remarkable that in his gestalt drawings separation played a great part. In one drawing the connected figures were spatially separated and secondarily connected by one line. This is usually seen in the work of much younger children. Interestingly, his motility at that time was described as so unusual that some of the physicians thought that he was suffering from chorea.

Several months later, when Nat's actual art work started, he drew rigid and expressionless faces consisting of only a few lines with a disproportion between head and body. He started to distort the body and a characteristic gesture appeared in which the arms seemed to be crossed. This experimentation with different postures soon led to the drawing of more or less violent movements. Characteristically, he bent the legs and let both of them swing to one side or let one swirl in the air. There was an astonishing amount of motion. The heads were always comparatively large. Emphasis was put on the hands and often something like a rod was held in the hand, which could as well be a penis as a gun. He said they were guns. Angular profiles with large eyes which were often displaced posteriorly were preferred and gave to all figures a wild, aggressive, and inhuman expression. The problem of arm posture was important to him and he was concerned with acquiring the technical ability to draw a fist in the act of hitting another person.

Nat became more and more interested in uniting several figures in one picture. In one of the pictures five smaller heads form the upper border of the picture, a sixth large head appears in the middle and upper border of the picture; only two arms are drawn. The distribution of the heads is almost perfect from an artistic point of view.

Nat's chef-d'oeuvre (Fig. 33) is a fight picture in which the whole space of a large sheet of drawing paper was dramatically filled with fighting groups. In the composition the majority of the figures are in the lower left quadrant. The upper fourth of the study contains most of the composition. There are large heads and distorted arms and legs in vigorous motion. Everything he had learned about the expression of motion in arms was utilized in this presentation. A large figure in the foreground has the usual rod-penis-gun in his hand. Other fists and arms are flying in the air. Persons are lying on the ground. The different figures are in an actual fight and really hit each other. Real contact is shown. The composition and distribution of the figures on the sheet is impressive. The drawing portrays motion, personal contacts and fighting. Nat's technical inability was no doubt responsible for the rigidity in the faces and extremities and adds to the threatening character of the picture. This becomes almost an integral part of the study. One is inclined to believe that the technical skill is not so much a disadvantage, but actually expresses the characteristic general tendencies better than would have been possible with a fully developed technique. The motif of the picture is a ruthless fight and his particular style served this motif very well.

In a picture called "A Summer Day and all the people are resting in the shade," circular lines which were practically absent in the other picture became paramount; even the faces show less of the shark-like expression.

The figures drawn by Nat have no ground. They seem to be suspended in the air. He obviously was merely interested in the figures, and a background did not exist for him. Modern paintings occasionally have the figure suspended in the air but evidently for a different reason. The floating figures in Marc Chagall's pictures have a background and this artist also deliberately changes the direction in space. The upside-down world and the upside-down position are intended to provoke the bewilderment of the spectator by expressing an uncertainty of the world. Our little artist saw in the world only the parts he was interested in and these were human figures in the act of

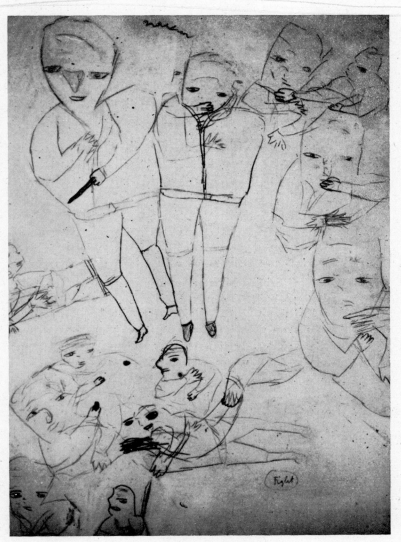

FIG. 33. Fight, by Nat (*pencil*).

fighting. The rigid and expressionless faces of his figures correspond to the fact that their personalities appear chiefly in one aspect. He often drew with rather thin lines, but this obviously had to do with the speed and haste with which he was working. This presents a strange contrast between the aggression in the content and the softness of the pencil strokes. These contrasts are the very essence of the schizophrenic personality which sees the world in partial aspects and does not bother to make a unit out of these partial aspects.

When Nat was 17 his 5 year old sister was referred to us because of unsatisfactory development. We found that she was seriously retarded and also schizophrenic. Nathan visited us and told us that he had stayed for a while in an institution for normal children. At the time he was living at home and attending a trade high school but he could not keep his mind on his work because of his daydreams, mostly sadistic, in which he "tortured torturers as they tortured their victims." He expressed a strong and fanciful transference to the psychiatrist. He was admitted to the hospital where the marked obsessional, compulsive anxiety features were emphasized. He was given electric shock therapy and discharged, but was unable to get along and returned to the hospital himself. He was committed to a state mental hospital where he had a course of metrosol shock with 20 grand mal convulsions. He remained for 5 years until 1947. The diagnosis was hebephrenic and paranoid dementia praecox. He was said to be very much improved when he was discharged, and has remained at home since then.

Among his later preoccupations was a tendency to think of people in terms of an infinite number of colors. He was afraid he would assign the wrong color to people and thus misvalue them. The more positive his evaluation of a person, the more nearly the colors would approach white; the negative values were thought of as black. The people he didn't like were big fellows and bullies. He was afraid they would fight with him and knock him out. He had some auditory hallucinations in which he was razzed and teased by such people and called "fairy." It is interesting that in his adult psychosis, the delusions and hallucinations have the same content as his preoccupations and drawings at 11 years.

In summary, the fantasy life of this boy was filled with fights and aggression. The aggressiveness expressed itself in the lines with which he drew the faces, in the violence of the movements he depicted, in the tendency to multiplication of the same motifs, and in the preponderance of sharp angles and spike-like forms. The content of his most striking drawing is a fight between men with an instrument which combines the features of gun and penis. His aggressive drives expressed themselves in the energy of the drawings and the spatial arrangement.

The artistic value of some of his pictures is considerable, due partially to the primitiveness of his technique which seemed to adapt itself almost specifically to the expression of his problems. He reminds one of caricaturists like Chaim Grosz and Peter Arno, only Nat was really interested in the fight, whereas the caricaturists substitute laughter for personal aggression.

Art is a means of expressing the inhibited aggressive drives of mildly retarded and schizophrenic children and depicts their struggle with emotional disorganization and their primitive perceptual experiences.

BOATS IN THE ART AND FANTASY OF CHILDREN[1]

THE ever-increasing significance of art work and projective methods for the armamentorium of the child psychiatrists, the problems of the standardization of these methods, and observations suggesting that the fantasy life of the child has some principle which results in symbolic structures different from those already well known in the adult; all justify a more extended study of the formal and symbolic character of the spontaneous fantasies of children. The purpose is to help map out the symbolism, to determine the maturational form problems, and to relate them to personal, emotional, and social problems. The study of the spontaneous drawings of boats by children with emotional problems, both before and during a war, has been chosen for this purpose.

A period of two months in the years 1941 and 1942 were chosen. In 1941, 128 children were on the children's observation ward of Bellevue Hospital, and in 1942 there were 122. The average daily census was 50. We try to have an unselective admission policy for any type of behavior problem child referred to us at 12 years or under who is not merely mentally defective. The art work is produced in an art classroom, without suggestion, guidance, or instruction.

All the boats produced under these conditions were collected. It is of considerable interest that, for a similar number of children over an equal period of time, a similar number of boats was produced in each year; namely, 77 in 1941 and 75 in 1942. In 1941 this represented the productions of 34 children; in 1942 it was the work of 45 children. Since the hospital is located on a large metropolitan river, we considered the possibility that the children were merely copying the boats they saw on the river. However, a statistical analysis of the types of boats drawn shows that in 1941, 42 per cent were sail boats which do not appear on the river, 7 per cent were primitive undifferentiated boat forms, and 51 per cent could be considered steam boats of which a smaller percentage represented forms identifiable on the river.

We have prepared a series of pictures showing how the development of ship drawings progresses from a simple undifferentiated primitive whorl, which has been shown in previous studies of gestalten[2] to be the basic primi-

---

[1] Reprinted in part from Bender, Lauretta and Wolfson, William Q.: The Nautical Theme in the Art and Fantasy of Children. *American Journal of Orthopsychiatry*, 13:462-467, 1943.

[2] See Chapter 4 Maturation of Gestalten.

tive visual motor configuration. At first, the figure or boat is undifferentiated from the surrounding background of ocean and sky. Then the figure or boat undergoes progressive differentiation and clarification; and only later, the background undergoes such clarification.

It is possible to check this developmental sequence by the production of experimental primitive responses or regressions. This was done by the saturation technique of Anitra Karsten and Kurt Lewin. The child was set to drawing ships until he refused to draw any more. Toward the end of the procedure small rewards might be necessary to keep him at work, but eventually a point was reached at which the child would not proceed. Characteristically, the background first showed signs of regression. It was less clearly drawn and small items which may have been present disappeared. Later on, the figure began to undergo de-differentiation. The cabins, the portholes, the men on deck, and the various identification marks were lost, and the ships began to take on a more curved aspect, in line with the primitive whorl tendency. In some cases, the differentiation between the ship and the water was eventually lost, leaving the ship as merely an additional wave on top of the water.

It is our belief that an important part of the tendency of children to draw ships lies in the fact that such drawings follow easily in their development from primitive gestalt principles, and are therefore chosen as a universal symbol which does not, in its production, arise easily from primitive configurations. In addition, as we shall show, no symbol is chosen as a universal symbol which does not fit primitive emotional trends.

There is a characteristic nautical scene found among the productions and dreams of many children and adults which may be described as follows: A ship is upon an ocean. No land or anything else is in sight or outside the borders of the picture. A bright sun beams down on the ship. Characteristically, this is a pleasant scene. The ship is safe and in general, no danger is expressed in such scenes. The scene is in motion: the waves move, the boat moves, but the motion is without direction.

One has the feeling that this picture is a solution to the oedipus problem as posed by perhaps a plurality of humans. In the pre-oedipal period it seems that for the majority of humans the mother is more important than the father; at least close physical relations are more generally to the mother. It is good also to have a benevolent father.

In these pictures the individual is generally on the deck or, more primitively, in the boat. Some of the boats have very obvious windows, although this is more probably a later feature. The wish is merely to come in closer relation to the body of the mother and to be carried by her. In the young and in regression, there is a tendency to regard the upright posture, self-sustained, as a definite burden. This is seen in some schizophrenics and in

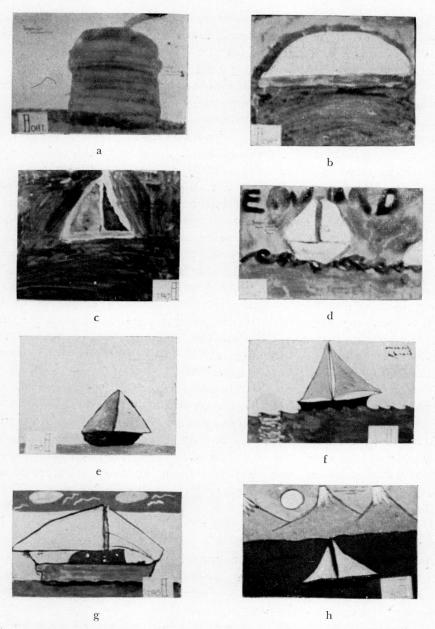

FIG. 34 (a-h). Eight boats, showing evolution of the boat form *(water color)*.

hysterical astasia-abasia. In this fantasy the individual is once again carried by his mother and not by his own motility.

The sun or the moon and any other background differentiation represents the father. We may say, therefore, that with the organization of the background and recognition of the sun in the heavens with its supportive warmth, comes the recognition of the father in the parent-child group or in the child's world. This corresponds to the structure of the child's world in which the mother occupies the central position and the father a more peripheral but nevertheless essential position. The father is partly outside the mother-child relation, but the importance of being nurtured by the father is also asserted, for the father is necessary for the complete family relation, just as the background is necessary for the figure.

In the play, *Lady in the Dark,* a central feature that is never completely discussed is the song "My Ship" which the heroine, Liza Elliott, is unable to remember completely and which runs through all her sexual dreams and fantasies. Later on, it is pointed out how aggression toward the mother and fear of competing with the mother prevent her from having proper sexual satisfaction. In the play, sexual satisfaction, analysis of the mother-child relation, and the remembering of the song, "My Ship," are simultaneous. The description of the ship given in the song leaves no doubt that it is the very one described in the art productions which we have been discussing.

Freud says, "The female genital is symbolically represented by all those objects which share its peculiarity of enclosing a space capable of being filled by something—viz., by pits, caves, hollows, etc. The ship, too, belongs to this category. Many symbols represent the womb of the mother rather than the female genitals as, for example, rooms."[3]

The use of the ship as a female symbol is very widespread in literature. Groddeck quotes an old Irish legend in which the female genitals take the shape of a ship's hull, and the male genitals take the form of the mast. An old Irish colloquial term for "clitoris" is "the little man in the boat." In *The Way of the World,* by William Congreve, and in the more modern *Infanta Marina* by the poet Wallace Stevens, are further examples which illustrate the recognition of Freud's symbolic evaluation of the ship in terms of the female genital.

Other references directed more obviously to childhood fantasies point to the ship in terms of the mother or of the maternal womb. In his book, *Lincoln: A Psycho-Biography,* L. Pierce Clark recounts the following dream. "Lincoln feels that he is in a singular and indescribable vessel. It is always the same throughout his life, and the whole substance of the dream pictures it moving with great rapidity toward a dark, indefinite shore." This dream Clark connects with the close early relation of Lincoln to his dead mother, and also with obvious regressive tendencies. In children's poems ship symbolism is seen in Eugene Field's *A Dutch Lullaby* which is the story of Wynken, Blynken and Nod; and also in Robert L. Stevenson's *My Bed Is Like a Little Boat.* The Biblical story of the flood and of Noah's Ark is re-

---

[3] Freud, Sigmund: *General Introduction to Psychoanalysis,* 1943, p. 139.

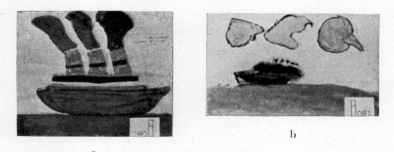

Fig. 35a, b. Two Primitive Steam Boats (*water color*).

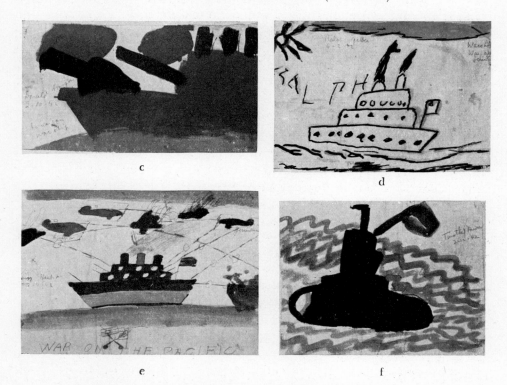

Fig. 35c, d, e, f. War-time Boats (*water color*).

peated in many folklores as the symbol of world destruction and rebirth. The Ark with its pair of animal parents has been a favorite children's toy for generations.

Eight year old Mollie was brought to our ward because of running away from home and telling fantastic stories about being abused or neglected by her parents. Her mother had died at the birth of twins when Mollie was 2 years old, and she had been cared for in various ways until her father remarried when she was 4. Mollie went to live with her father and stepmother, but the twins did not. Later a half-brother was born of whom she appeared very fond. Mollie appeared very confused in regard to her place in the family and much concerned about stories of cruel stepmothers, while she insisted that her present mother was her own, and that her stepmother had died when she was born, although she had been told the facts correctly. When asked what she thought about boats, she said: "Oh, don't ask me, I hate boats. Once I dreamt I was on a boat with my family, the boat almost went down, all the water came over the boat and everybody almost died, even my baby brother." This dream shows her fear of mothers, the threats against the mother herself, and against siblings, all implied in the idea of death at childbirth.

In the two-month period in 1942 very definite differences were discernible in the drawings and paintings. In 1941, only 6 boats showed any of the paraphernalia of war. In 1942, 50—or two-thirds of the pictures—had war paraphernalia involving the background, such as airplanes, bombs, submarines, as well as the boat itself in the form of guns, searchlights, etc. These had largely replaced the sailboats of 1941, only 11 of these remaining as compared to 34. The same form principles remained although the 1942 boats showed many more details and seemed more elaborately patterned. In particular, the 1942 boats had many more insignia. In many instances, of course, this could be considered as part of the war paraphernalia, such as the swastika or the American flag, but in many other instances it occurred as numbers or names not related to the war.

This seems to have a double significance. It emphasizes the importance of the family group and its relationship to the social order. It also appeared that the insignia replaced other father figures which were usually a part of the background, but in times of stress had rejoined the mother figure and strengthened the family unit. It is as though in times of world stress, the oedipus situation requires more consideration of the father and a stronger family unit to protect the child.

The following dreams of an unhappy child whose oedipus situation was never solved because of disharmony in the family with desertion by the mother when he was 4 years old, and subsequently by the father, will illustrate this:

Edward Johnson was a Negro boy of 10 who was difficult in every way in his boarding home and finally set the house on fire, apparently by accident. He stated that when he grew up, he wanted to be a mechanic. He hoped he could build boats and ride in them; if not, he would build trains and ride in them; if not, he would build whatever he could. Given three magic wishes, he would like a boat that goes sailing around and would take his friends with him. He has dreamed about boats. In one dream, he was in the Navy on a mosquito boat and sinking enemy boats with two torpedoes on the side of the boat, reporting it on the radio, and then going back to the harbor. It was a good dream. There were other boys there. One boy, Gerald Johnson, was a friend Edward knew in Staten Island. He was the captain. Edward would tell the captain what to do so that the captain would tell the other boys. For example, Edward would tell him there were enemy ships ahead ready to shoot. He would spy through a looking glass and look at the flag of the enemy boat.

He had other dreams of boats before the war. One was about a fishing boat. "We named the boat Columbia. We went out there in the river and let down little rowboats for fishing. Then the men risked their lives to get the fish and sometimes the fish got them instead and pulled them in the water and they died. And every year the people would go out there and throw flowers in the water for the dead people in the river." Edward always stayed on the big boat and did everything to help the men in the rowboats. He would throw down ropes when they wanted to get back in the big boat. Then they would throw back fish when they caught them and he would help cut a fish and clean it. It may be noted that his dreams before the war allow him to kill the man on the boat, presumably his father. But now, at war, the captain of the boat bears the family name and he, Edward, takes orders from him to protect the boat and themselves.

A 5 year old boy who had lost his father came to the bed of his mother with his two younger siblings and suggested: "If we had a flag and pretended this bed was a boat, maybe we could do something to make the war stop." Before the loss of his father and before the war, when he was 3, he spent many mornings pretending the bed was a boat and he and his mother were sailing the seas together. He always warned off father or younger brother with the threat that they would drown in the surrounding waters.

In general, one may discuss this problem from the point of view of universal symbolism. Time permits neither discussion of the various historically important theories of universal symbolism nor of the nature of the spontaneous activity which gives rise to universal fantasies. Two factors seem necessary for the formation of universal symbolic productions. The first is the presence of a universal repressed fantasy; and the second, not so well known, is that the symbols must conform to the psychophysiological organization of the individual.

In our discussion of children's boats, we have attempted to demonstrate both these factors. We have shown how the oedipus situation is symbolized in the boat drawings of the children. This portion of the discussion has been of relatively well-known clinical, psychoanalytic, and literary material.

In considering how our boat drawings fit the psychophysiology of the child, the first factor to be recognized is that, in providing art material for the child to work with, we are providing a relatively plastic field which may be structured by the child in accordance with his needs and psychomotor tendencies. The general relation of art work in children to results obtained by projective methods is well known. It has been found in previous studies on the genesis of gestalten that spontaneous activity in the visual motor field is primitively a circular or vortical movement. Paul Schilder[4] also emphasized that undifferentiated loops, vortices, and whorls all in motion are the primitive spontaneous activity of the visual field, that the primitive unit is to be considered a sensory motor unit, that the primitive visual activity is very closely related to the primitive motor activity, and that there is a dynamic similarity between the two. It may then be said that primitive spontaneous activity which may be seen in such art productions will tend to emphasize the production of circular figures. It has also been shown that the presence of this primitive vortical activity will distort the copying of specified figures, that is, the copies are apt to be modified in the direction of conformity with primitive organizational tendencies. Such tendencies are collectively spoken of in gestalt psychology as the internal organizing forces.

It follows that the more a production can be made in conformity with the primitive organizing forces, the more easily it will be produced. We have aimed in our series of pictures to show how the ship drawings fit into the primitive organizing forces and are, therefore, easily developed from spontaneous activity; it must be remembered however that any universal symbol must conform to these principles.

From the point of view of a thorough-going gestalt psychology, the need-structure is to be considered an integral part of the internal organizing forces and therefore the demonstration that the universal symbol corresponds to both psychoanalytic and gestalt principles may be reduced to the statement that nothing will be produced which does not conform to the internal organizing forces of the visual motor functions, the emotional experience, and the social environment.

Given a number of pre-adolescent children with emotional and behavior problems, in general unselected, who have an opportunity freely to produce pictorial art, a certain number will be compelled to draw boats. This probably represents children with particular problems in the oedipus situation due to serious disturbances in the parent-child relationship during the oedipus period. These children will also dream about boats or furnish other fantasy material about boats. Such boats will follow certain laws of progressive development depending upon the maturation level of the visual motor field configurations; also upon the personality structure and the specific emotional problems which will, in turn, be related to world-wide social problems. The boat is the mother, the child is inside of it. The primitive level is a simple whorl-like undifferentiated boat form on an almost undifferentiated background consisting only of ocean and sky. There is a constant

---

[4] Schilder, Paul: In Search for Primitive Experience, Chap. I in: *Mind, Perception and Thought in Their Constructive Aspects.*

interplaying motility. Differentiation in the background permits the appearance of the father on the scene, most characteristically as a sun. The individual child's problem is easily woven into the general pattern by a simple integration into the picture of action or movement, which is the basic principle of all sensory patterns. In war time there is much more organization of the background and a strong tendency to add insignia, often to the ship in the form of the flag. These, nevertheless, are background phenomena and represent the father. Thus is revealed the child's need for the father and the stronger family unit remaining intact in time of war. In adult fantasy the ship represents the female genitals and sexuality.

This work emphasizes the value of combining the use of projective techniques, gestalt psychology, psychoanalytic technique and social orientation in a genetic study of the fantasy life of the child to give a deeper understanding of the emotional problems of childhood, the genesis of symbolism and the special problems of the child in war time.

❧ 11 ❧

ANIMALS IN THE ART AND FANTASY OF CHILDREN

THE recurrence of animal figures in children's phobias, totemism, myths and fables, indicates that animals have certain attributes which furnish the human mind with an excellent medium for the displacement of repressed drives.

R. E. Money-Kyrle, in discussing the relationship between animal phobias in children, and totemism, says "Many children develop not only a great respect and dread of certain animals but also a marked tendency to identify themselves with the very animals they are afraid of. In other words, they invent for themselves something very like a private system of totemism; they are spontaneous totemites."[2]

The universality of animal fantasy is well illustrated in the myths, fables and fairy tales in the literature of every country. This is emphasized by Anna Freud who in discussing the individual animal fantasies of two of her patients, states that these themes "are by no means peculiar to these particular children: they are universal in fairy tales and other children's stories."

For the psychiatrist, children's animal drawings are of particular interest. A collection of about 75 animal drawings, gathered over a number of years on the children's observation ward of Bellevue Psychiatric Hospital, has been studied.

The children whose drawings are included in this report ranged from 7 to 13 years of age. The sex difference of the children who drew the pictures was the usual one on the ward: there were more boys than girls.

After reviewing the material it soon became apparent that we were dealing with two groups of pictures, as well as two clinical types of cases. Broadly speaking, the pictures could be divided into aggressive and non-aggressive looking animals. Included in the pictures of non-aggressive animals were the domestic animals, such as ducks, horses, birds, rabbits, cats and dogs, while the pictures of the aggressive animals contained beasts of the jungle and forest, and several that belonged to the bird and insect family, namely eagles, woodpeckers and a bee. The snake, because of its symbolical import, was classified with the aggressive animals. Upon further analysis of the case records, we observed that the pictures of the aggressive-looking animals were

---

[1] Reprinted from Bender, Lauretta and Rapoport, Jack: Animal Drawings of Children. *American Journal of Orthopsychiatry, 14:*521-527, 1944.

[2] Money-Kyrle, Roger: *Superstition and Society,* 1939, p. 58.

174

those associated with psychoneuroses, while the mild behavior problems were those connected with the non-aggressive animals.

Sigmund Freud in *Totem and Taboo* pointed out that one reason why "bearers of the soul" were portrayed as animals in primitive times was because of their association with movement which they showed by "their extreme motility and flight through the air and other characteristics". In our series of drawings birds were commonly drawn by children from broken homes who were impulsively getting away from some unpleasant environment by truancy or vagrancy. Although we had a good series of horse pictures, in no case did this animal take on the phobic role that it did in Sigmund Freud's case of Little Hans. The same clinical picture was found in children who drew horses or birds. It seems that in both these instances the animal was one which represented movement to the child. The cat and dog pictures usually had a direct reference to the home and frequently stood for the children in the home. We had a small group of duck pictures and some excellently drawn ducks, together with ducklings. One assumed that the ducks stood for a mother figure. It was therefore interesting to find that most of the ducks were drawn by children whose mothers were aggressive and in conflict with their children. The pictures of the non-aggressive animals were far more numerous that those of aggressive animals.

However, it was in the group of aggressive animals which made up only 10 per cent of all drawings that we found our best correlation with clinical material, as all these children suffered from a severe neurosis. We divided the group into four types—the first of these contained pictures of very aggressive animals and the clinical pictures were equally severe. In all three cases of this type there was an obvious inverted oedipus complex with severe anxiety. The third type contained a picture in which the child was identified with the attacking animal. The fourth consisted of a picture in which the animal drawn appeared to be connected with a phobia formation. The following case histories and pictures are those of the children who drew aggressive animals:

Type I contained wild animals which nevertheless looked benign:

The first case is that of Daniel, a 13 year old white boy, of dull normal intelligence. He was sent to Bellevue by the court on the father's petition because he stole and stayed away from home. The father was an alcoholic who had a prison record and was very abusive to the boy. He made him shine shoes and then used the money for liquor. The boy said he was given a beating a day. He was bad every day until punished, after which he was able to get along. Punishment was followed by a period of absolute dejection in which the boy felt that he was no good. He drew a picture (Fig. 36a) of a circus which contains an elephant, a rhinoceros, and a giraffe which give the appearance of being friendly. From interviews with the boy, it was obvious that he was very fearful of his father. The mother volunteered that she fre-

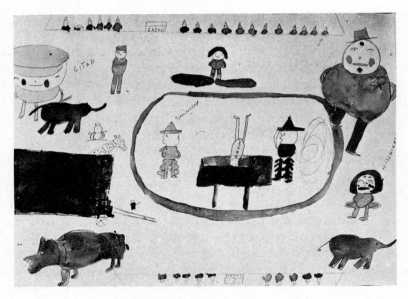

Fig. 36a. A Circus, by Daniel (*water color*).

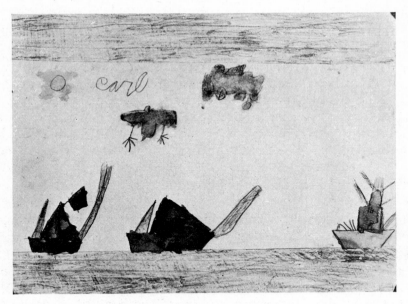

Fig. 36b. Eagles in a Boat Scene, by Carlos (*water color*).

quently had to protect the child from his father. The boy was intimidated, depressed, and his aggression was not manifest. In spite of our every effort, this boy was subsequently committed to a correctional institution following what appeared to be compulsive delinquent acts.

The next case is that of Carlos, a 7 year old boy of average intelligence. He was sent to Bellevue because of temper tantrums, destructiveness, and poor adjustment in school. His behavior was further aggravated by a reading disability. The mother rejected the child. The father went to prison when the boy was 2 years old and the child has not seen him since then. Of his father, the boy stated: "He's a bad man. He was born in Germany. He used to hit me all the time. First he'd hit me and then he'd give me money. When I was 5, he went back to Germany. Sometimes I'd like him." The boy was depressed and anxious. He drew an eagle flying over a boat (Fig. 36b). Of the eagle he said: "It's good; eagles are American. They bring letters like pigeons. I drew it because it stands for the United States Army." He stated that he was frightened of all jungle animals but the elephant. During one of his interviews, this boy played with soldiers. He had the Americans outnumber the Germans ten to one. Then he proceeded rapidly to destroy all the Germans. During this play, he stated that when he grew up, he wanted to be a soldier. When asked why, he replied that he liked to fight and because he wanted to fight the Germans. His pictures contains an eagle which probably stands for a good father image as contrasted with the bad German father. As we have learned in the previous chapter, the boats in the picture probably stand for the mother.

The third case is that of Samuel, an 8 year old colored boy of average intelligence, with a reading disability. He was referred to Bellevue because of poor adjustment in school. His mother was a mental patient in a state hospital; the nature of her illness was unknown. The boy was cared for by several aunts who lived in the neighborhood. The father was an alcoholic who punished the child for his poor school work. The boy stated: "I'm afraid of my father; he hits me." His behavior on the ward was characterized by aggressiveness, antagonism to authority, marked feelings of inferiority, with a tendency to compensate for this by bullying. His antagonism to authority seemed to be a reflection of the home situation in which the father was antagonistic and abusive. This boy drew a picture of a forest with a reindeer, lion, and elephant (Fig. 37a).

We know that children, like primitives, identify themselves and their parents with animals. This knowledge has been emphasized in our puppet show themes.[3] In the group of pictures just shown, there is the suggestion that depressed rejected children who suffer from feelings of inferiority find it necessary, when the conflicts become intense, to identify themselves with large animals whose aggressiveness is modified. There is a close association here with primitives. "The totem of a savage clan," says R. E. Money-Kyrle, "is a parental, most often a father symbol." Geza Roheim has stated that children play at being dogs or horses because "they pretend they, themselves, are dogs or horses. They have reached the stage at which they have overcome animal phobias and introjected their oedipus complex in a symbolic fashion

---

[3] Chapter 15.

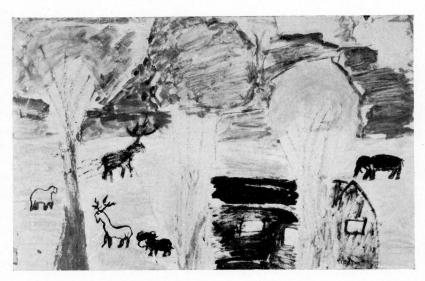

FIG. 37a. Forest Scene, by Samuel (*water colors and crayon*).

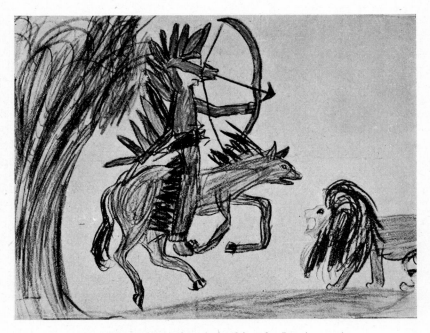

FIG. 37b. Indians Shooting a Lion, by Ira (*crayon*).

in play."[4] It is possible that what Geza Roheim suggests about animal play is also true of this type of animal drawing.

Anna Freud brings out a similar point in discussing the animal fantasy of

―――――――――

[4] Roheim, Geza: *The Riddle of the Sphinx*, 1934, p. 157.

a 10 year old boy. She says after discussing the fantasy: "Once more, the stress laid on the former savageness of the animals indicates that in the past they were objects of anxiety. Their strength and adroitness, their trunks and uplifted finger (referring to elephants in the fantasy), obviously were really associated with the father. The child attached great importance to these attributes: in his fantasy he took them from the father whom he envied and, having assumed them himself, got the better of him."[5] This is probably seen best in the boy who drew the eagle. And finally, the size of these wild animals must be another reason why some children identify themselves with them. Gigantean and Lilliputian dreams follow a similar pattern. Sandor Lorand, quoting S. Ferenczi, states the following: "Ferenczi believed the cause of such dreams to be that they are a residue of childhood recollection dating from a time when because we ourselves were so small, all other objects seemed gigantic. . . ."[6]

Type II was characterized by the frightening aggressive animals.

The first case in this series is Ira, a 9 year old, colored boy of average intelligence, with a special gift for drawing. He was brought to the hospital because he was restless, disobeyed his mother, found it difficult to fall asleep and because he talked to himself at bed time. He was frightened of the dark and was enuretic. He had been a problem child since the age of 2. The father, who was dead, separated from the mother when the child was 2 years old. The mother remarried when he was 5 years old. Early development was normal. He walked at 9 months but he did not talk till 3 years. As his mother worked, he was always cared for by someone else. During psychiatric interviews the following facts were revealed: He was interested in the problem of Life and Death, and God. He was frightened of going to sleep and did not fall asleep until 11 P.M. While trying to fall asleep, he thought about a good fairy, Mister and Mrs. Twiskey, an androgynous figure, who performed good deeds. He wanted to be a girl but would rather be a white boy. He tied a string around his penis to avoid wetting the bed. He called the penis a "nasty thing" and wondered why girls did not have one. He expressed the wish to cut it off. Later, he changed his mind about this because "it was the only one," and if he lost that he would die.

He was hypochondriacal; for example, he stated that he could not get along in school because of his goiter which made him weak. It wiggled around in his throat and made him wiggle. He was frightened and complained of the aggression of other boys. He had anxiety dreams of falling off high buildings or of tumbling into the ocean or of being blown by a strong wind. His ambition was to be an artist, and a cowboy so he could shoot. He did not like his teeth and wanted to bite off the middle part of his lip because other children did not have it and because it did not look nice. His picture (Fig. 37b) of an Indian on a horse shooting a lion with an arrow

---

[5] Freud, Anna: *The Ego and the Mechanisms of Defense.* 1937, pp. 81-82.

[6] Quoted in Lorand, Sandor: *Fairy Tales, Lilliputian Dreams and Neurosis.* 1937, p. 459.

probably could be interpreted as the boy shooting his father. One should recall that his ambition was to be a cowboy so that he could shoot. He returned to the hospital at the age of 15 when it was evident that he was schizophrenic, and he was transferred to a state hospital.

Hyman was a 10 year old boy, of dull normal intelligence. His school complained that he was erratic in his work and that he visited the toilet too frequently. The boy complained of nightmares of a sexual nature and was preoccupied with sexual matters. He was enuretic and had sexual activity with other boys and with his brother in which he played the passive role in rectal intercourse. He dreamed of fellatio being forced on him by other boys, and of being bitten by mice. The father worked at night so that the children did not see him very often. The father was a quiet unassuming individual who took little responsibility for the direction of the family affairs. The mother who was quite neurotic, frequently punished the boy. He was obsessionally concerned with the fear of the death of either parent. The boy expressed a preference for the father. He was frightened of animals, particularly of snakes. His picture (Fig. 39a, Plate III) shows a number of snakes which point to either the mouth or anus of horses or Indians. The boy's fear of snakes would suggest that he was frightened of the penis, while he is probably identified with the horse and the Indian. This boy and his brother were subsequently sent to a cottage-type institution, where he received considerable psychotherapy and developed as a highly neurotic personality.

Stanley, a 10 year old boy of average intelligence, was brought to the hospital because he was disobedient, refused to go to school, and was a feeding problem. The mother stated the boy liked to wear her dresses. The boy looked and acted effeminate and was preoccupied with the problem of masculinity and femininity. He said he wanted to be an artist designer of women's clothes. He played a game of kings and queens in which he was usually the princess. His human drawings were frequently concerned with women. He believed both men and women have a penis and testicles but that women's genitals differ only in shape. At one time he said, "I'd die if my penis were cut off but I'd look like a girl then." He had a dream in which he shot his father because the father hit the mother. "I shot him through the heart and he was dead, and I was glad. Then I awoke feeling scared because I thought I shot my father." Although the boy produced many drawings of females with whom he was obviously identified, the two drawings (Fig. 38a) of the bee, and the woodpecker are of the type of aggressive animals we associate with a frightening father. It is interesting also that he used water colors for the animals and crayons for his other drawings. This boy is also described in: *"Impulsions, a Specific Behavior Disorders in Children."*[7] In adolescence, he became a severe schizophrenic.

These three cases have the following in common: They have very severe psychoneurotic problems (this is also characteristic of the schizophrenic

---

[7] Bender, Lauretta and Schilder, Paul: *Impulsions, a Specific Behavior Disorder in Children.*

child);[8] they have an inverted oedipus complex; in each case the pictures demonstrate an oral aggressive trend. Melanie Klein in comparing the cases of the Wolf Man and Little Hans, points out that the probable reason for the better prognosis in the case of Little Hans was that he had overcome his anal

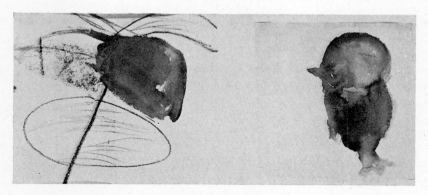

FIG. 38a. The Bee and The Woodpecker, by Stanley (*water color*).

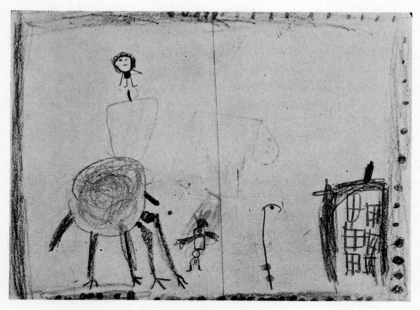

FIG. 38b. A Ride on an Elephant, by Ann (*crayon*).

sadistic stage and had reached the genital stage. The Wolf Man, on the other hand, never overcame his early anxiety which was associated with his oral aggression, consequently he was frightened of a devouring wolf which really stood for his father.

[8] See Bender, Lauretta: *The Problem of Anxiety in Disturbed Children.*

Type III which contains one case is characterized by the ferocious animal which is identified with the boy and is helping him to destroy the father.

Emilio is a 12 year old, colored boy. He was referred to Bellevue because he was thought to be retarded intellectually. The examination showed that he had a reading disability with an IQ of 110. His fantasy life was apparently about wild animals which might kill men, undoubtedly his father, and this was probably the basis of his compulsion to draw. His father was abusive and the boy called him "bad, mean, crazy." The boy imagined in play that he was the wild animal and accompanied his play "with strange sounds resembling the grunt of a wild boar or some other beast." He freely wished his father were dead and even said he would kill him. At other times, he elaborated the fantasy in which he threatened to kill his father but at the last moment said, "I wouldn't kill him because I don't kill anybody." In this boy's picture (Fig. 39b) two men are being attacked by wild animals. The boy is apparently identified with the animals who seem to be attacking father figures.

This patient's drawing is similar to the ones in the previous type where the animal was both frightening and aggressive, except that in this instance the child is identified with the frightening animal which attacks the father figure instead of being terrified by it.

Type IV contains an animal drawing which shows phobic features:

It is that of a 7 year old girl, who was brought to the hospital because her compulsive questions and behavior were driving the parents frantic. She bit and beat her younger sister, screamed, and tore her mother's clothing. Ann drew a picture (Fig. 38b) of a little girl on top of an elephant and of a peculiar looking man whom she called the fat man. Ann stated that when her father took her to the zoo, he told her that the fat man was the fattest man in the world. From her associations, it was obvious that the little girl in the picture was Ann herself while the elephant stood for the father. Although Ann enjoyed riding on the elephant she expressed the fear that she might fall down and be kicked by it. She was also frightened of the monkey because it bit. These fears were apparently the result of the projection of her own aggression.

This case illustrates another type of animal picture which is, in a sense, a pictorial representation of an animal phobia. It shows the following characteristics of a phobia formation: Displacement of fear from father to animal; reversal of aggression. Melanie Klein postulates an intermediate step in which a mild phobic animal is employed instead of a wild ferocious animal, for example, as seen in our Type II.

We have described the analysis of a group of animal drawings, collected over a number of years. We found that the pictures could be divided into two large groups: Pictures of non-aggressive animals, including such pictures as

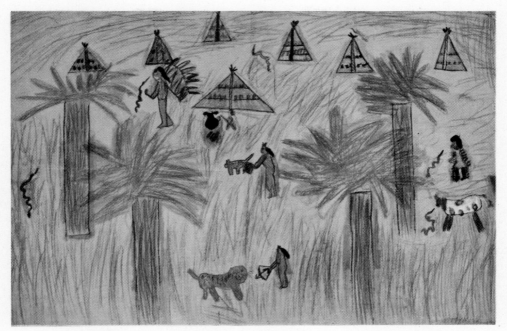

FIG. 39a. A Field of Horses, Snakes and Indians, by Hyman (*crayon*).

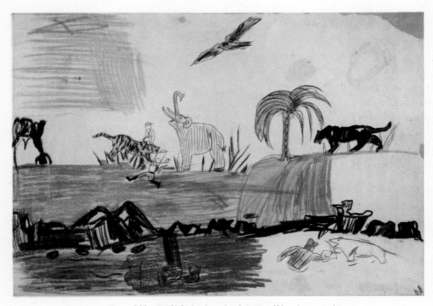

FIG. 39b. Wild Animals, by Emilio (*crayon*).

horses, birds, etc.; pictures of aggressive animals. It was our impression that attributes of motility were an important factor for the choice of the animals in this group. Children who drew horses and birds frequently gave a history of truancy and vagrancy. Cat and dog pictures appeared to symbolize children in the home and were drawn by children who came from broken homes. There was a small number of such pictures which seemed to portray a contented mother with her children. Such pictures were interesting in that the mothers of the children who drew these pictures were aggressive and rejecting. The non-aggressive animal drawings made up the great majority of the pictures.

The pictures of the aggressive animals, considerably fewer in number, were even more interesting. They were divided into four types according to the aggressive animal portrayed. Type I consisted of jungle or forest animals which were nevertheless benign in appearance. The psychodynamics of the children who drew these pictures showed depression and feelings of inferiority which were associated with a punitive or an absent father. The identification of the child with the strong, peaceful animal seemed to be on the basis of an attempt to reconstruct in fantasy the kind of father the child did not experience in reality. Type II contained ferocious attacking animals. They seemed to stand for the punitive father. The clinical picture in each of these cases was based on an inverted oedipus complex. Type III also contained attacking animals. However, in this type the child was identified with the aggressive animal. Type IV contained an animal picture showing phobic features.

Sigmund Freud has pointed out that the child's ability to replace the father by a phobic animal is facilitated "because the inborn traces of totemistic thought can still be easily reviewed. . . . Children do not as yet recognize or, at any rate, lay such exaggerated stress upon the gulf that separates human beings from the animal world. In their eyes the grown man, the object of their fear and admiration, still belongs to the same category as the big animal who has so many enviable attributes, but against whom they have been warned because he may become dangerous."[9] Our drawings likewise revealed this totemistic type of thinking which enabled the child to replace the father by the symbol of an animal. Further, the type of animal employed was intimately connected with the psychodynamics of the individual case.

From this study it may be concluded that some of the children from our psychiatric ward who draw aggressive animals suffer from a severe superego which leads to a displacement of the fear of the father onto an aggressive animal. The aggressive animal may stand for a big, protective father in contrast to the real father's aggressive behavior; the severity of the superego may

---

[9] Freud, Sigmund: *Analysis of a Phobia in a Five Year Old Boy.*

lead to the acceptance of the inverted oedipus situation with a fear of a devouring animal; or the child in a similar position may attempt to overcome the painful situation by identifying himself with the aggressive animal and turning against the father; finally, the child may choose an aggressive animal to whom it may display its ambivalent feelings, as has been seen in the case of Little Hans.

GROUP ACTIVITIES ON A CHILDREN'S WARD AS METHODS OF PSYCHOTHERAPY[1]

THE children's ward of the Psychiatric Division of Bellevue Hospital is a residential service for the children of New York City who need examination, observation or treatment for any type of behavior disorder, psychiatric or neurological. The ward has a capacity to care for fifty children of both sexes from 1 to 12 years.[2] In general the service was organized like the service for children in the New York State Psychiatric Institute and Hospital, as it has been described by Howard W. Potter. But while Dr. Potter looked upon ward life as a means of observation, treatment, and re-education of the individual child we have emphasized the use of ward activities for observation of the child as a part of the group and for group psychotherapy.[3]

Our emphasis on group psychotherapy has been due in part to the necessity of treating a large number of children on a city service with a limited staff of psychiatrists. But we have also found that group activities are the more successful way of communicating with children, of getting them to express their emotional problems, of giving them full play for their impulses for aggression and affectionate relationships, and of relieving them of anxiety and apprehension. Finally we have tended to emphasize the specific value of group therapy as a means of aiding the needs and drives of the normal child and of the child with a behavior problem in becoming a more successful social personality.

The essential needs of any normal child are food, clothing, warmth, support from falling (until he has learned to walk), protection from an aggressive world, and demonstrations of love from the persons who give him these things. Children also need an opportunity to identify with these people and an opportunity for self-expression and independent action. Upon the satisfaction of these needs the personality is built. The essential drives of the child are for free expression of his own impulses to be aggressive or active,

---

[1] Reprinted in part from Bender, Lauretta: Group Activities on a Children's Ward as Methods of Psychotherapy. *American Journal of Psychiatry*, 93:1151-1173, 1937.

[2] The author's experience on this ward started in the fall of 1934. The children's ward has been functioning in its present location since May 1933, and since 1921 in the older buildings. Until April 1937, when separate wards were organized for them, adolescents were cared for with the children. See Curran, Frank J.: *Organization of a Ward for Adolescents*.

[3] See Chapter 1, p. 25 for survey of more recently organized in-patient services.

to love, and the chance to exercise the growing functions of his physical, intellectual, emotional, and social personality.

A deprivation in the satisfaction of the needs of the child or of the demonstrations of love which should accompany it, results in developmental retardation, apprehensions and fear, prolonged infantile behavior, and attention getting mechanisms. A repression of the drives results in feelings of inferiority, anxiety, and guilt.

Behavior problems, psychopathic or neurotic reactions, and conduct disorders arise from deprivations in the satisfaction of the child's basic needs and drives due to a failure on the part of parents or parent substitutes, or to constitutional weakness or organic disease in the child. Behavior problems are associated with mental deficiency, epilepsy, organic brain disorders or somatic diseases, in part because such children find it difficult to obtain or accept the satisfaction of their needs, especially as the needs may be greater than normal, and because such children find it difficult to express their own impulses or exercise their growing functions.

I. THE THERAPEUTIC FUNCTIONS OF A WARD FOR CHILDREN'S BEHAVIOR PROBLEMS

The therapeutic activity of a children's ward caring for behavior problems should satisfy all the child's needs for physical growth and health, and the needs for exercising its expanding physical, intellectual, emotional, and social functions. But in addition it should strive consciously to supply the special needs of a child with a behavior problem. These are demonstrations of love and tenderness and approval from the adults who are serving him; free expression of the child's feelings of affection; free expression of the child's impulses for aggression; free expression to the psychiatrist and other therapists of the child's neurotic complexes; relief from feelings of anxiety, guilt, inferiority and insecurity; opportunities for the child to become socially at ease and socially acceptable at his own value; crystallization of the child's ideologies which are suitable for himself and the social milieu in which he lives.

At the same time it is essential to arrive at a diagnosis or a complete formulation of the problem from both an etiological and a mechanistic point of view, considering all the biological, personality and environmental factors. Sound therapy in a medical setting must be determined by such a full understanding of the problem. However it will be noted that all techniques which are available for therapy also contribute to the better understanding of the child's problem and thereby aid in a dynamic, etiological, diagnostic, and prognostic formulation. This emphasis on a dynamic and etiological formulation or diagnosis preceding or at least running in conjunction with therapy is in contrast to the practice of many child guidance clinics.

II. STAFF PERSONNEL

It must be recognized that the children will look to every adult member of the staff or personnel as a possible donor or recipient of affection or aggression. There need always to be both men and women on the staff. This allows for a choice of father or mother substitutes. The younger children may be more prone to accept the woman physician as the good and loving mother or the severe and threatening mother, depending as much on their relationship to their own mother as on the actual experiences with the physician. Children in the latency stage are more or less indifferent in their relation to the mother figure, except to the extent that they have remained infantile and dissatisfied. Children in early adolescence are inclined to react strongly for and against the physician of one or the other sex, due partly to budding erotic interests. There is often a more or less strong negative transference for the first physician whom they contact or the one who is the senior physician. This physician often aids the child to become oriented but does not receive his confidence; the child looks to the second physician as the arbitrator.

Nurses, teachers, and other members of the staff often serve as the arbitrators between the child and the physician and should be freely utilized as such. The tendency for the child to throw all of his anxiety and apprehension upon the person of one physician and all of his admiration and confidences upon another person should be openly recognized. Active treatment can often be performed through some other member of the personnel, once that person has received the child's attachment. Teachers with whom the child spends several hours of the day are often the recipient of such attachments, and the physician may be able to guide the therapy through the teacher far better than he could perform it directly, at least for a part of the treatment program. Special identification processes often play a role. Attractive nurses usually win the heart of the young adolescent boy and can do more under the guidance of the psychiatrist to relieve the child's emotional stress than the psychiatrist in his daily psychotherapeutic hours.

One medical student, on hearing of the difficulties in treating the psychopathic child[4] who is not able to form deep attachments or feel any guilt or anxiety, suggested that one of two physicians should be severe and punitive and that the other should love the child, console him and protect him from the severe psychiatrist. Something like this does occur when the child feels that the physician in charge who represents the hospital, writes to the judge, and talks to the parents, may be a severe punitive parent and the other physician a loving understanding parent. Free expression of affection, small gift giving, granting of special favors by the person who is the recipient of the child's affection and confidence is freely encouraged on the ward, especially for the neurotic child who is full of feelings of his own inferiority,

---

[4] See Bender, Lauretta: *Psychopathic Behavior Disorders in Children,* 1947.

anxiety and guilt. It should be discouraged only in those children where it is known that such contacts stimulate erotic impulses previously aroused by seduction by an adult.[5] In these children other means of satisfaction should be cultivated through all kinds of social activities and interests in productive activities without physical contacts.[6] The hyperkinetic child who is continually grasping and clinging to adults, just as he is continually aggressive towards children, needs to have his impulses directed towards more clearly patterned activities such as he may obtain in different types of shop work, music, schoolwork, etc.

III. STAFF CONFERENCES

Numerous conferences with the various workers on the ward (including junior psychiatrists, social workers, psychologists, teachers, nurses, consulting physicians, occupational therapists, reading tutors, artists, puppeteers, musicians, medical students, volunteer workers, and attendants) as well as personal supervision by the physician are necessary to encourage all of the personnel to be alert continually to the individual child's needs, to the means for meeting these needs, and to the underlying principles which advance our knowledge in diagnosis and therapy. From the beginning it is most important that everyone should have an objective attitude towards the child's problem and should help him get the same attitude.

The questions are: Why is the child in the ward? What has gone wrong to cause him to be socially rejected and put in the hospital? Who put him there and why? Who is to blame? The child will nearly always say at once that he is to blame, that he has been bad and deserves it. He believes that it is punishment. The first step in treatment is to clear up this misconception in the minds of both the child and the staff. Psychiatric observations and psychotherapy are not punishment.

The second step is to get both the child and the staff to realize that the effort is first and foremost to determine the cause of the behavior difficulty and to give an understanding of the cause to the child in as clear and objective a way as possible. Any specific treatment which meets the special needs of the child should be sought for. The next step is then to relieve the child of his feelings of guilt, of inferiority, of shame, of rejection, and of apprehension for the future. The final step is to give him new and satisfying experiences and social relationships.

---

[5] Bender, Lauretta and Blau, Abram: *The Reaction of Children in Sexual Relation with Adults,* 1937.

[6] See Bender, Lauretta and Cottington, Frances: *The Use of Amphetamic Sulphate (Benzadrine) in Child Psychiatry,* 1942.

IV. BODY INTERESTS

It is justified to place a strong interest on the wellbeing of the child's body while he is in the hospital. This may be accomplished in the most natural way by utilizing the usual hospital routine and physical examinations. Every effort should be made to improve and promote the child's physical health. Tonsils, teeth, eyes, posture, weight, skin should be considered, and abnormal conditions corrected when possible. Furthermore every effort should be made to improve the appearance of the child's body and to give him or her a feeling of satisfaction in this improvement.

The culture of body beauty is an appropriate interest for young girls, and attractive young nurses are the best teachers. The girls' dressing room is a suitable center where the girls can gather several times a day to learn to bathe themselves, care for their hair, teeth, and fingernails; to learn the use of cosmetics, the care of their clothes and the choice of such ornaments and ten-cent-store jewelry as may be available. It is the proper place to concern themselves with problems relating to menstrual periods, and such problems pertaining to sex as they wish to discuss with the nurses. It also happens often that this is the place and time for them to discuss and consider with the nurses many problems of conduct and behavior that have arisen during the day, partly because they realize that the nurses are the ones who write daily reports of their behavior.

We do not try to cultivate the children's tastes above their social and economic level. Simplicity, cleanliness and ten-cent-store equipment are the proper standards. David M. Levy[7] has emphasized what he calls the psychiatric-physical approach, which is a frank approach to the child through the doctor-patient relationship of examining, discussing, and evaluating the child's body. Paul Schilder has made an analysis of ideologies as a psychotherapeutic method especially in group treatment. He emphasized the attitudes towards the body in terms of beauty as one of the basic problems and its consideration among adults as one of the justified means of clarifying ideologies in group psychotherapy. The same holds true for children.

Paul Schilder and David Wechsler have shown that the small child's concept of the inside of his body is that it is full of food.

When we ask a child what a mother is good for, he will invariably say "to give food." The food-giving mother is therefore the first symbol of the loved object. It is accordingly not surprising that among the most active centers on our ward are the diet kitchen and the dining room. One of the greatest privileges which can be given to any child is to allow him free access to the diet kitchen. The diet kitchen maid's interest in the children's food,

---

[7] Levy, David M.: *A Method of Integrating Physical and Psychiatric Examinations and Body Interests in Children,* 1929.

her efforts to please each child as much as possible, her patience in letting them come into the kitchen to help wash the dishes (especially with the electric washing machine), to polish the steam table, and prepare the dishes and food for meals, can play an important role in any children's service. The kitchen maid can also save little tid-bits of food to be dealt out as a favor to the children who help in the kitchen and she is also the guardian of the fruit brought by the parents for the children's between-meal snacks. These things are mentioned as examples of how the normal needs and interests of the child may, on a residential service, be met and how in the most natural way they can contribute to a sound therapeutic program. The personnel should be chosen with the qualifications in mind which will allow each one to play his or her part in the therapeutic program.

V. WARD ROUTINE BASED ON NATURAL RHYTHMS

The ward routine, if properly planned, is something more than merely an economical and convenient means of caring for a number of children. It is important to emphasize the value of the rhythm of routine in contrast to the tendency to allow the child to follow his own undirected impulses. Though much may be said in line with modern progressive educational methods in the individualization of the child, routine group activities may be a justifiable means of socialization when the routine is based upon the natural rhythms of the child's growing organism and the environment. It should be based upon the normal rhythms of sleeping, eating, resting, and physical, intellectual, and emotional activity. The pediatricians' newer methods of self-regulation of infants' feeding, sleeping, and elimination express the effort to find the rhythm most suitable for each infant in his environment. This not only promotes their physical but also their mental and emotional wellbeing.

For older children the rhythm must adapt itself to the physical age level, to the intellectual maturation, and to the motility or impulse pattern. It is determined also by the natural environment, day and night and the season, and by the social environment. On a ward in a city hospital it seems necessary to adjust the routine to the nursing and diet kitchen regimes which require that the children get up and go to bed and eat their meals at relatively early hours. There is nothing arbitrary about such a routine, as it obeys its own laws which can be understood even by the child.

In a group of children who are predominantly hyperkinetic or neurotically restless it is important that the rhythm of the routine should be in short waves. This is by all odds the one most valuable disciplinary and socializing factor of the ward organization. Every effort should be made not to allow the rhythm of the routine to be easily disturbed. All members of the staff should be impressed with the value of routine for its own sake. In the life of insecurity and uncertainty in which many problem children live, the ward routine is in itself an experience which gives many a child a new feeling of certainty, and a chance to relax.

We have long known of the value of a rhythmical routine in the treatment of mental disorder in adults, where the disturbance in the normal rhythms of life is one of the outstanding features of a mental illness. We have recognized that a severe disturbance in biological rhythmicity is specific for the psychoses and organic brain disorders of children, and is especially evident in earliest infancy.[8] The value of a rhythmical routine in the training of deviate children and in the treatment of behavior problems is even more striking. Such children are characterized by poor habit patterns, feelings of insecurity in an uncertain and often unfriendly world, strong feelings of guilt in relation to their own behavior and reactions; they have rarely had any experience which has given them any personal satisfaction or feeling of accomplishment. They are bewildered and distrustful of the immediate situation and are filled with fear and apprehension for the future.

For the child to find himself quickly and easily experiencing a rhythm which has meaning in itself, which can be depended upon, which gives a continual satisfaction without much chance for failure and which makes him an acceptable member of a group, is a new and satisfying experience. To the majority of our children, the only disciplinary method that is needed is to be dropped from the routine briefly. If a child makes himself unwelcome in any group, he is removed to the nearest quiet room or corner by himself until that activity is over, or if he wishes to return sooner he may do so without explanation. Rejection from the routine does not carry over into the next activity unless the behavior does, and this does not occur often.

Where more serious behavior difficulties arise, it is possible to show that such difficulties are due to the accumulative effects of anxiety on the part of a seriously neurotic child or to the uncontrollable behavior of some organically disordered or psychotic child—so-called organismic panic. The behavior of one such child in a group may arouse the anxiety of the whole group until it is recognized and corrected, after which the routine will resume its usual rhythm.

VI. GROUP ASSURANCE TO ALLAY APPREHENSION FOR FUTURE INSECURITY

A child should be told as soon as it is known what the future holds for him, and to what extent his behavior can modify his future. It should be the unshaken faith of the children that the staff will play square with them in regard to both the present and to what is promised for the future. This is

[8] See Bender, Lauretta: *Anxiety in Disturbed Children,* 1950.

not always easy to accomplish on a ward where the admission and discharge rates are rapid and where the children come and go through all sorts of agencies including the children's courts, and where each child's stay is of relatively short duration. One of the most important means of accomplishing this, of course, is to have the confidence of the outside agencies and children's courts so that it will be possible to foretell for the child what the outcome will be, following recommendations.

When a child must go to a situation he cannot accept, the reasons for it must be clearly understood not only by the particular child but by all his companions. On one occasion a group of children stormed the psychiatrist's office, one of them literally waving his fist in the psychiatrist's face, shouting, "What do you make Whitey go home for? He don't want to go home. He don't have to go home if he don't want to. You ought to send him to school or something. You know his dad is crazy or something. He says he will run away from home again if you do. Whitey don't want to go home." It was explained to the whole group that Whitey had to go home but only for a little while, and that then his mother could arrange to take him to children's court so that the hospital could recommend that the father be examined to see if he was "crazy."

Whitey himself was a little too full of anxiety and fear to accept this himself, but several of the other children understood and took him off to console him and encourage him. In major emotional crises, it is nearly always better to work with a group than with a single child who is too overwhelmed with his emotions to be articulate about them. In a group of children there are enough who can simultaneously threaten and revile the physician or authority without the individual child himself having to feel too much guilt and anxiety for the revolt. Besides, if the revolt is not justified someone in the group will surely sense it and express it for the group.

VII. SPONTANEOUS ORGANIZATION TO RELIEVE GUILT AND ANXIETY

There have been episodes when the group has become self organized on the basis of mutual and overwhelming feelings of anxiety and fear, often on the basis of sex tension on the ward or of apprehension as to their destiny when they leave the ward. These are group phenomena, and should be recognized and treated as such. They are apparently more likely to occur among a group of behavior problems than in a normal school or camp group. In a large group of children individual treatment would never cope with the problem and would show an essential failure to understand the group phenomena among children of this age.

Group guilt and anxiety have been observed, on occasions, when the group has been organized on the basis of guilt and punishment. A highly moralistic epileptic child, John, and a compulsively neurotic child, Eddie,[9] who stole, ran away from home and attempted to compensate with a highly righteous attitude and an ambition to become a priest, organized a "Purity Club." It was a secret organization and rapidly developed great influence on the ward. Those children who were not accepted into membership were ostracized on the ward. Very soon new children were waiting around in deep distress to find out if they would be accepted. The members were recognized by a white bracelet on the wrist which was made by braiding strips of white muslin. The aim of the organization was proclaimed to be purity and goodness in thought and action and to help all the other children to attain the same. Physicians and nurses were advised that the need for any supervision or discipline would be eliminated.

The organization reached a climax when a committee of four children called at the physician's office with a report which read,

"Bernice S.   A Record.

She stuck a shoe in her No. 1. She says the more we do it the faster we go home. She says she told Patty. She lies. She stuck a pillow in it—No. 1. Signed Operator 48, 42, 29, 31."

The children refused to attend classes with her, and abused her so that she had to be removed from the ward for a few days, until Eddie's individual therapy was advanced and, John, the epileptic child had the treatment he needed. Once the situation was recognized (which was done by an interview between the physician and the worst offender), it was explained to the group of children as a whole that they were punishing this child because they felt guilty themselves. They were told that the other child was sick, not because she masturbated, but just because she was sick and for that reason she found it harder than the rest of them to get interested in other things.

It is customary to tell the children when one child is obviously mentally sick. This is the best way to solicit interest and consideration of the other children and to allay their anxiety. The most seriously psychotic children can be kept in a group of children if this technique is used, to the great benefit of the sick child and with no detriment to the other children.

VIII. SUPERVISED ACTIVITIES REVEALING GUILT AND ANXIETY

Practically all of the spontaneous organizations among the children have shown, in the same way, that they grew out of the dominating emotional attitudes in the group which are anxiety and guilt especially in regard to sex

---

[9] See Chapter 13 and Fig. 40a, b and c for Eddie's case history, drawings and therapy.

phenomena, and apprehension for the future destiny of the child. For this reason spontaneous organizations on the ward have been discouraged whenever they have been recognized. Similar phenomena have been observed among the girls alone. Even efforts to organize the children into something similar to the monitor system in the schools or the scout organization has come to disaster among our children. There was an organization of G-men who were given badges marked "G-men" which was supposed to stand for "Gaylord's" men after the admired male nurse on the ward. The G-men were voted in by means of a ceremony each night and were to change office rapidly in the hope that thus abuses might be prevented. But as we have always found in such organizations, the G-men took upon themselves justification for aggressive and abusive acts against other children which they seemed to see as their own bad behavior justly punished. One boy of 6 was found heartily slapping a smaller child and jumping back with joy after each slap. He did not seem at all concerned when the physician approached. He said proudly, "I'm the G-man today." When told that he could not be the G-man any more because he hit the other child, he cried bitterly, "But I want to be the G-man. It is all right to hit if they are bad when you are the G-man." One thus sees that the organization gives the child the false sense of being able to express his own aggression freely and at the same time to relieve himself of guilt for his own wickedness by punishing the other child. Paul Schilder and Lauretta Bender in their studies on aggression in children have shown the same concept in the child who says he wants to be a G-man (in the usual sense) so that he can catch and kill the gangsters which is right, because the gangsters are bad and kill good people.

IX. ACTIVITIES DEVISED TO RELIEVE ANXIETY AND GUILT AND GIVE FREE EXPRESSION TO AGGRESSION AND AFFECTION

With these problems in mind it is evident that we need group experiences by which the child can express his aggression without feeling guilty and can otherwise find relief for his many negative emotional attitudes of guilt, anxiety, apprehension, uneasiness, inferiority, and insecurity. He must also have means of being articulate about his positive emotional attitudes of identifying with others and of trying to orient himself positively and constructively in the physical and social world. It is obvious that this is possible partly through play, sports, shop work, useful housekeeping or ward tasks and errands, school work, reading of suitably chosen books, nature study, etc. Such activities may be sufficient for normal children. But for emotionally disturbed children there is a need for activities and projects that more nearly meet their special needs because of their anxiety, insecurity, and difficulties in articulation and orientation. We developed group activities based on the graphic and plastic arts, puppetry, dance, and music.[10] Clearly there is almost no limit to the number of projective techniques[11] that can be developed depending on the talents and interests of the staff personnel. The same techniques have been developed widely also by the progressive schools under the influence of John Dewey's philosophy. Herbert Read of England has also developed the thesis that the most natural and ennobling form of education will be through the development of artistic expression. This he maintains is especially important in a democratic society.

X. GRAPHIC ART

At all times on the children's ward, spontaneous art work is encouraged. Pencils, crayons, and water paints on all kinds of paper were originally utilized as a specific art class activity with specialized art teachers. The same activities are carried on in the regular school rooms;[12] at other times nurses and volunteer workers have conducted group art classes or encouraged individual children to draw and paint. And of course psychiatrists and psychologists in examination, research, and therapeutic situations have used the art activities of the children freely.[13] These projects were employed not only as they are in progressive schools for their educational and socializing values, but specifically as a psychiatric approach to the understanding and therapy of the child's emotional and mental conflicts and problems.

In our art classes the aim has not been to teach children the technique of art, to develop any latent artists, or to evaluate the finished product for its esthetic content; notwithstanding that, an occasional child with latent ability has been trained intensively, and social readjustments have been accomplished in this manner. Incidentally, the creations of some of the more interesting children, particularly in the schizophrenic group, have proved of unusual significance artistically and psychologically, as may be seen from the work of Francine.[14] The aim is to encourage the children to project their own inner fantasy life and their naïve reactions to their life experiences. Children find this easy to do and indeed get great satisfaction from such activities.

---

[10] We received the greatest help in developing these projects from the Works Projects Administration from 1935 to 1940 when we were furnished with many talented and professionally trained workers in the various fields of art and education.

[11] Lawrence Frank formulated the concept of the "projective techniques" in 1939.

[12] See Chapter 17 on *School Room Techniques*.

[13] Finger painting has frequently been employed but in our hands has proved less useful than the more spontaneous forms of art activities.

[14] See Frontispiece and Figures 20 and 21. There have been several demonstrations of the children's art work at the Museum of Modern Art, The American Orthopsychiatric Association, 1939, and The Fifth International Congress of Pediatrics in New York, 1948.

Art productions often offer a contact with a child who otherwise may be unable to express himself to the physician for reasons either of language inadequacy or of emotional blocking. The art productions afford an excellent means of expressing and revealing the unconscious life of the child, his emotional conflicts, and his fantasy life. The technique once established may be used either alone or in conjunction with any other method as a specific technique for psychotherapy. Children may be sitting and drawing while they discuss their problems with the physician, or they may illustrate their fantasies revealing much more to the psychiatrist, and at the same time crystallizing their own problems and ideologies. It is not permissible for a child to play at being a gangster and beat up the other children on the ward, nor to withdraw into day dreaming aggressive fantasies. But art productions having the same content seem to satisfy their drives and produce interesting pictures which can be studied and admired by the art teacher and the psychiatrist.

Other children who see them experience the same fantasies and at least in part get some satisfaction for their normal aggressive drives without suffering from guilt. We have had pictures painted of the hospital being smashed by giants, burned down by fires, and destroyed by bombs from airplanes killing the doctors and nurses. The production of such a picture by the child, having it admired and laughed over by the very physicians, teachers, and nurses who are destroyed in effigy tends to free the child of those feelings of anxiety and apprehension which are connected with the hospitalization.

XI. PUPPET PROJECT[15]

The puppet work will be fully described below. Here it will merely be stated briefly that by means of puppet shows we are able to present all of the problems of childhood in relation to aggression and social relationships at every level from the primitive oral aggression to the ambivalent aggression of a child toward his sibling, or the open aggression against an unkind stepfather. We have found that the value of our puppet work lies in the fact that every character is identified by the child with himself or one of his parents or some part of them or a sibling. Thus Casper, the hero, is the child himself, the part that we may call the ego, while Charlie, the monkey, is the more primitive animal part of the child. The bad boy in the play is the bad part of himself. The baby sister is both the sibling and the baby part of the child in the relationship with the mother. The policeman is the good father and the giant, the wizard, etc., are the bad fathers; the witch is the bad mother. The much hated and feared alligator is oral aggression both by the child and against him.

---

[15] See Chapter 15.

With such an array of characters we are able to present before the children plays which include every type of problem which concerns children, dealing in the main with various satisfactory and unsatisfactory relationships within the family life. We are also able to discuss solutions. The children enter freely into the spirit of the plays, advising or reviling or encouraging the different characters. This gives them an excellent chance to express their aggression openly without fear of punishment, without any need for feeling guilty, and with the encouragment and approval of some fifty other children about them as well as of those who are in authority.

The technique may be varied by giving only half of the play at one time and allowing the child to finish it in the course of the week either in group discussions, in the puppet classes where they are learning how to make and play with puppets, or in individual interviews with the puppeteers or one of the physicians. Group discussion on the various problems which are brought out in the puppet play have been most successful in getting expressions on problems both of aggression and of love. Such problems are discussed as "Does the mother still love Casper after the new baby comes?" "What is Casper's mother good for?" "How would the witch (the bad mother) treat her children?" "Is it right to kill the alligator?" "Should Casper marry the princess and why?" "Should the father or the mother beat Casper?" All sorts of problems can be discussed in terms of Casper, with whom the child freely identifies himself. The puppet shows are also an excellent source of material for the physician to use in individual treatment, which may be used as dream material is used. The child never retells the puppet show as it is produced, but modifies it in the telling to suit his own emotional problems. Furthermore, the puppet classroom affords an excellent workshop where the child can utilize any material to express his problems from clay to the actual putting on of a show by the child.

XII. MUSIC PROJECT

Music activities of various types are of great value. The music projects which have been used on our ward have varied from year to year depending on the gifts and interests of our staff personnel. At times we have had the children formed into regular classes taught by two musicians, one a pianist for the accompaniment and one a singer and teacher. At other times the music activities consisted largely of group singing, a rhythm band, and singing games for the smaller children. The teachers should be real musicians, able to give something to the children and to hold their interest without being disciplinarians.

From the point of view of group treatment and as a socializing factor the music activity is found to be most valuable for the younger children. There is a group of children passing from childhood into the latency stage who are making the transfer badly due either to constitutional inferiority, hyperkinesis, deprivation of any adequate maternal care and affection, or other neurotic factors which tend to keep them infantile. They are thus unwilling to accept the schoolroom situation, to make any new attachments, or to start to develop those emotional and social functions which characterize the latency stage.

These children are usually first appealed to in the music class. The rhythm band is of special value. The fascination of its instruments, the noise making, the aggressive activity of beating or pounding the instruments, and the contagious rhythm, win the children over. They are thus beguiled into a type of training under a sympathetic "mother" which gives them a pattern for activities and a sense of accomplishment and satisfaction. Furthermore they are forced to accept the group or social situation. Only after success in the rhythm band do many of the more difficult children enter into the singing of the songs, and gradually carry over what they have experienced in the music class into the schoolroom and other activities.

Music therapy is one of the most valuable means of training the hyperkinetic child whose main problem is one of direction, attention, concentration, motivation, attaining a goal, and patterning of impulses, all of which are disorganized in the hyperkinetic child. The fundamental, almost primitive organic nature of the disturbance in the hyperkinetic child which resolves itself into an overflow of unpatterned motor sensory behavior best adapts itself to the primitive rhythms of the band involving as it does a complicated but primitive motor sensory pattern and almost always including a human relationship and social adjustment. We have already shown that form or patterning is one of the fundamental principles in play in children.

The rhythm band is not assigned to certain children but every child who comes to the hospital learns to play not one instrument, but all of them. They play rhythm accompaniments to such pieces as the *Barcarolle* from *Tales of Hoffman;* the *Blue Danube Waltz;* Mozart's *Minuet* from *Don Giovanni;* Beethoven's *Rondo;* a simplification of Haydn's *Clock Symphony,* and the *Andante* from Haydn's *Surprise Symphony.* All are much reduced of course and perhaps Mozart or Haydn would not recognize them, but the kernal of feeling for good music is planted, the ear is developed, and the response is always gratifying.

It has long been known of course that the defective child responds to music both actively and passively when he cannot respond to any other activity. Many of the more defective of our children who cannot be assigned to any other activity, spend many quiet and happy and well directed hours in the music group. Singing games for these as well as for the smaller children of good intelligence have proved of value.

The shy, withdrawn, depressed, homesick, and inferior-feeling child finds a chance to take part in group activities in the music room which fascinate and beguile him and give him a new sense of satisfaction. Folk songs are taught together with the folk lore that proves of interest. Our music room overlooks New York's East River and its fascinating river life which interests the children for hours every day. Tales of the Erie Canal and of the Cape Cod country enrich the lives of the children from the Lower East Side of New York who have had few experiences which tended to emphasize the romantic or the beautiful. Sometimes the children have learned and sung quite well many of the songs from *Pinafore*. At Christmas time the ward life not only during the music classes but all day long is full of Christmas carols. At Easter time, Easter music is learned and sung.

For the self-conscious, growing child with awkward motility and strong feelings of inferiority the music classes combined with rhythmic games or dancing, have their obvious value. The creative dance with percussion music is discussed below.[16] Now that we recognize how closely motility is related to the emotional state and the ideation of the child, it is clear that there must be a conscious effort at integrating the motility with the emotions and the concepts of some common means of expression.

Any and all spontaneous ideas for a living tableau or play or so-called pageant are welcomed. For example, one 10 year old boy worked out a pageant between two warring Indian tribes that presented the war dances and appropriate music with the instruments, until finally they all sat and smoked the pipe of peace. Entering the game at this point, one marvelled at how long that group of restless children could sit and smoke the pipe of peace, with appropriate body postures and facial expressions of calm. The boy who originated the pageant had episodes of aggression so ferocious that he had actually killed a little girl before his admission to Bellevue.[17]

Besides the professionally supervised music projects where the children learn to perform and enjoy the best music within their reach, they also have an amateur hour at party times or in the evening under the guidance of the nurses where they are allowed and encouraged to demonstrate any impulse to sing, dance, tell stories or otherwise "show off" under the guise of an "audition." Many of our Negro children especially show no small amount of native ability. Every child is encouraged to take part and many a child in this way learns to sing and dance spontaneously without adult direction. Popular songs and dances are also encouraged.

---

[16] See Chapter 19.

[17] See Bender, Lauretta and Curran, Frank, J.: *Children and Adolescents Who Kill*. Case II—Adolf, 1940.

XIII. SCHOOL ROOM ACTIVITIES

Any residential program for children should be organized around the school program since school makes up the largest part of the organized and supervised activities of most normal children. The philosophy and techniques of teachers who deal with problem children in a program such as ours are fully discussed below.[18] Some of our early experiences in the class rooms on the children's ward are worth considering briefly.

We divided the children into two groups, an older group of the fourth grade and up, and a younger group usually of the first to third grade level. The young group represents children who have not made the necessary social adaptation to the school room either because they are intellectually handicapped by mental deficiency, specific reading disability[19] or speech, hearing or visual defects, or because of neurotic problems which make it hard for them to give up their babyhood and enter into the group demands of the latency period. The group consists also of a number of hyperkinetic children who are under observation to determine if the hyperkinesis is controllable.

One of the functions of the teacher of this group is to entice each child into experiencing the satisfaction of learning. The thrill and joy of the child who is first learning to read has not been sufficiently emphasized. To have seen a child safely through this experience is to see him through one of the critical periods of his life. The child however who is placed in the classroom with other children having this experience and who cannot get it himself is doubly distressed by his own lack of joy, his failure to become one of the group, and his overwhelming feeling of inferiority. A child with such an inability is entitled to careful analysis and study. If the child does not have the mental level of 6 to 7 years which is one of the requirements for reading readiness, he should have other activities which will give him satisfaction. If he has a special reading disability, this must be analyzed and properly tutored by whatever specific or remedial techniques are indicated.

To accept the teacher as authority and as a mother substitute, to take part in group activities, to be active when his group is active, to direct his impulses and drives in accordance with the group pattern, and to be able to accept the rivalry of other children of his own age is a necessary part of growth. Many a child is brought to us because an inadequate relationship in his home before he went to school made it difficult for him to accept the new relationships in school. But if he could be helped at least to be happy in the schoolroom and could see in his teacher an adult who is happy in his

---

[18] See Chapter 17.

[19] A special program for the diagnosis and training of reading disabilities is a necessary part of any educational and therapeutic program for problem children.

presence and likes doing things with him and for him, he then has something to compensate him for the home inadequacies.

The teacher of the older children from the fourth through the sixth grade has a different type of problem. She must constantly readjust her classroom activities to fit an ever changing group of children with different needs, and yet must make the group feel that they are working as a unit. Every child must get some sense of accomplishment, however small. This usually necessitates that the work be so arranged that the child can get a good mark or its equivalent in deserved praise for the first part of his stay in the room; he then learns to accept harder work with less success.

Nearly all of the children brought to us are over-graded in their own schools and are struggling against impossible odds. The schoolroom work is organized around a nucleus of common interest in some project, so that several children of even different grade placements can be organized in a common problem, and can do work of value for their own level of accomplishment. It has been our experience that the sense of class unity attained in the schoolroom often results in free and open discussions of the children's behavior and emotional problems, including those which lead to hospitalization. Composition topics are assigned which encourage the child to express his fantasy life and to project his emotional problems. This after all is the major concern of the children as long as they are in the hospital. Such topics include "Once I had a dream that—" or "If I could invent a new world according to my own fantasy—" These compositions can be read in class and lead to group discussions. At the same time it is not forgotten that the children should as much as possible keep up with their regular school work, especially those children who will return to the community school or to special schools.

XIV. GROUP DISCUSSIONS

Our success with group therapy in various activities has led us to realize that there is an actual emotional advantage in having several children with similar problems, and most of the children do have similar problems, deal with these problems together. We have found that even the most intimate problems of the child are best discussed in groups. This is comparable to the group therapy used by Paul Schilder[20] for adults. A group of adolescent girls will discuss their sex problems, describe their own experiences, talk about masturbation, and ask more questions in groups than they will individually.

A male or a female psychiatrist can handle such a group satisfactorily and do more to relieve tension among a group of girls than can be done in many

---

[20] See Schilder, Paul: *Results and Problems of Group Psychotherapy.*

hours of individual work. Similarly a group of boys will discuss all problems freely. A shy, repressed child can be added to such a group, can benefit by the experience and gradually start to take part when no other method so quickly puts him at ease. Children will talk freely in each other's presence and to the physician if they realize that the other children have had experiences similar to their own and that the physician knows about children's experiences, and does not disapprove.

Group studies of pre-adolescent delinquent boys were made by Pauline Rosenthal on our children's ward in 1940-41. After observing the tendency for spontaneous group formations on the ward she attempted to isolate certain of these groups and to organize them into group discussions. She concluded that "the group technique corroborates the usefulness of Franz Alexander's application of the psychoanalytic theory of neurotic symptom formation to the study of the pre-adolescent delinquent as well as to the adult criminal. It relates the fantasy content to the early rejection and to the present symptoms, such as stealing. It makes possible a relatively rapid orientation to the entire group. It is offered as an aid to accurate diagnosis, without which prognosis, therapy, and disposition can be nothing more than rationalization or speculation."[21]

XV. GROUP PLAY TECHNIQUE

Play technique with small children in groups also has some distinct advantages. A group of three little boys of 6 to 8 years was brought together in a play session. One was a stammerer who had been made very neurotic and unhappy by a neurotic mother obsessed with the idea that his masturbation caused his stammering. A second child had a habit tic and was full of phobias and fearful fantasies. The third was a mute, blocked child whose father had been in a hospital for the mentally sick but had escaped from the hospital, terrifying the mother and the child with the possibility of his return to the home. The three children and the psychiatrist at first sat around a table for meals talking freely, and later played with all of the miniature toys. The advantages of such a technique cannot be appreciated until it is tried.

The children naïvely told what they noted in each other. Each child in turn was jibed by another for his own peculiarity, which made it possible to discuss these things freely, to laugh over them and to let the tormented child know that the physician understood and sympathized. The two talkative children in the group actually said that maybe the mute fearful child was "crazy." Since the child's real problem was a "crazy" father with whom he had to identify himself, he flushed with anguish. It opened up the way however

---

[21] Rosenthal, Pauline: A Group of Pre-Adolescent Delinquent Boys. *American Journal of Orthopsychiatry, 115:*126, 1942.

to talk about "craziness" and "crazy" people: What one would do if one had a "crazy" father and how one would protect one's mother from a "crazy" father.

A psychiatrist talking with the child alone would never have had the courage to have attempted such a discussion. The stammering child was jibed for the way he talked. He said it was because "I play with myself, my mother said so." The second boy with the phobias looked interested and said he did that too, but it was dirty and "the mummie with the big eyes" came through the window after him when he did it. There was talk about masturbation, and why mothers worried about it, and whether "mummies" were real. The child with the phobias told one of his fantastic stories. It amused the other children very much.

All enjoyed the story and the boy with the phobias and tics did not jump around so much. This was noted by the stammering boy, who suggested that the active one had a spring in the seat of his pants that made him jump. The boys and the psychiatrist looked for the spring but did not find it. Then it was suggested that they examine the boy who did not talk to see if he had a tongue. Everyone stuck out their tongues to see how far they would go. Then one boy said there was a little tongue in the back, maybe that was missing, so they looked further. Then everybody tried yelling to see who could make the most noise. The boy who could not talk could do almost as well as the others (including the psychiatrist), although he was a little shy. Then the boys put the miniature toys on the table and everybody played soldiers with shouting and loud talking, including the boy who would not talk. Next time he talked even more.

There is practically no limit to the usefulness of such group activity. The group or social situation rather than detracting from the value of the treatment adds a new factor of freer and more fertile associations and better catharsis as well as the opportunity of experiencing the emotions of the other members of the group and of finding that one's own experiences have social value for the other children and for the psychiatrist.

XVI. GROUP TREATMENT IN STAFF OR STUDENT CONFERENCES

An excellent method of group therapy for children may be used in presentation before staff conferences and groups of medical students or nurses.[22] In this method the group of children are chosen for the similarity of their problem, although of course there are individual factors and reactions. The children should be allowed to be present during the discussion. The value of

---

[22] Karl Bowman in *The Psychiatrist Looks at the Child Psychiatrist* also discusses the value of this technique.

such conferences becomes evident when it is realized that in dealing with disturbed children one problem is to relieve the child of an overwhelming sense of his own guilt. One conference on the "Delinquent Boy" centered around eight young boys who were sent to us for running away from home and associated stealing. These boys were charged with delinquency in the children's court and by implication threatened with reform school. A discussion directed at the staff on the reasons why boys run away from home and steal, with a presentation of each boy, was enlightening to the boys themselves. Even though they could not be objective about their own problems, they could appreciate the problems of the other boys, and they could get from the lecture what was of value to them. A similar conference on a group of children with sibling rivalry was of equal value to the children. The same can be said of almost every problem which confronts children. Such techniques are of value chiefly in orienting the problem child to his problems, and help to prepare the children for whatever long time program of training or psychotherapy may be planned for them.

XVII. CONCLUSIONS

In a children's ward which is used for the observation and treatment of behavior disturbances, the group psychology is determined by the psychology of the children constituting the group and by group phenomena. Behavior problems such as we find in the Psychiatric Division of Bellevue Hospital often occur in children who are psychotic, have an organic damage of the brain, or who are congenitally deviate. The majority of the children have neurotic behavior problems even when they also have one or more of the other problems. They are filled with fear and apprehension because of insecurity in their family relationships with inadequate or unsuitable expressions of love from parents or parent substitutes. They are filled with anxiety and guilt for their own behavior difficulties arising from aggressive impulses, sexual impulses, and the need to attain personal satisfactions.

The hyperkinetic child usually tends to increase the anxiety of the group by his open display of aggression which demands retaliation and defensive aggression on the part of the group, by his unrestrained sex play, or by his frank play for attention. The occasional psychotic child tends further to increase the anxiety of the group by his specific overwhelming anxiety and his bizarre behavior and his difficulties in identification and orientation. All of the children are insecure and fearful in regard to their future on leaving the hospital.

From these situations spontaneous group emotional crises arise. As a result there may be revolts against authority with anxiety and guilt which can be allayed by individual and group assurance that the staff is essentially concerned with the problem of re-establishing the child in the family group most suitable for him. Group revolts are best handled in groups. There may be group demonstrations organized through mutual feelings of guilt and anxiety which are usually directed against some unrestrained or hyperkinetic child who like the sacrificial lamb receives the whole burden of the children's guilt, hostility, and hatred. Supervised organizations on the ward similar to the monitor system or the scout movement very quickly tend to assume the same role. The tendency for group phenomena must be recognized and gratified; this is best done with group projective activities.

The staff personnel must understand the psychology of the group and be encouraged to allow and give a free expression of affection and reassurance to replace aggression, anxiety, and fear. The routine of the ward activities should be based upon the needs of the growing child and the normal biological rhythms of the child and of the environment. Such a routine is of fundamental importance in establishing a normal rhythmic pattern in the disorganized deviate child. As such it gives the children a sense of security and of personal satisfaction, and it reduces the need for aggressive discipline from the staff.

Some group activities are especially adapted to allow free expression of aggression or affection and the resolution of emotional complexes. These include the puppet projects, the art projects, music, dance, and drama. Many others could be devised. The value of supervised play and shop work has long been recognized in education as a means of expression of aggression and controlled competition. Experiences in the various classrooms of personal accomplishment which are recognized by group standards compensate for or eliminate feelings of inadequacy and guilt. Opportunities for group experiences of rhythmic patterns in perceptual-motor, and emotional-social fields are accomplished in part by the music and dance classes. Group expression is freer and encourages the individual child to find relief from his anxieties and fears by the sharing of mutual experiences and by the conviction of social approval or understanding. The group psychology adds a definite quality which may tend to increase anxiety or fear or to diminish it, depending upon the control of the situation by the psychiatrist. Intensive individual treatment, where it is indicated, progresses more rapidly against the background of organized group interests and group activities.

❧ 13 ❧

THE USE OF GRAPHIC ART IN PSYCHOTHERAPY[1]

THE specific value of artistic expression in its relation to the therapy of emotional and behavior disturbances of children is the subject of this chapter. Art work has been used by other psychiatrists interested in the treatment of the abnormal child. John Levy (1934) employed art as an adjunct in the psychoanalysis of children who for a period, at least, found it easier to express themselves in pictures than in words. He used this technique for handling material below the level of consciousness, and as a help in overcoming resistance. He emphasized that interpretations of the pictures were essential and that the child had to develop the technique of verbalizing while he was drawing. R. E. Appel also used a drawing technique as an aid in the study of personality difficulties in children. He asked the child to draw a house, its inhabitants, and their activities. He interpreted the drawings for the child freely and dramatized as much as possible to suggest to the child the idea of playing a game. He found that this gave an insight into the child's personality problems and the background of his personal life and interests. Edward Liss called attention to the synthetic value of graphic art as well as to other forms of art, as aids in the technique of psychotherapy. These workers each emphasized a specific technical procedure and the importance of the interpretation.[2]

In our art projects, we have observed a variety of ways in which the art work may be of value in relation to psychotherapy, and we are inclined to believe in the value of every art production without attempting to standardize the conditions under which it is produced or always to give interpretations.

Graphic art is a means of establishing rapport with children who are not spontaneously expressive; who have speech or language difficulties, who are reluctant to discuss their intimate problems, or who are taciturn or withdrawn.

It is a means of obtaining insight into the child's unconscious life. In his drawings a child may unwittingly reveal his fantasies, emotional drives, com-

---

[1] Reprinted in part from Bender, Lauretta: Art and Therapy in Mental Disturbances of Children. *Journal of Nervous and Mental Disease*, 86:249-263, 1937.

[2] Since this paper was written (1936) there have been a number of other contributions on the use of graphic art in psychotherapy of children. Many psychotherapists take it for granted as an adjunct to their treatment of children. See Despert, J. Louise: *Technical Approaches Used in the Study and Treatment of Emotional Problems in Children;* and Naumburg, Margaret: *Studies of the Free Art Expression of Behavior Problem Children.* See also Chapter 1 for other references.

plexes and conflicts of which he is himself unaware, or for which he has no other medium of expression. This knowledge may be used in formulating psychotherapy or plans for the child's social readjustment. Often, however, it seems that the mere expression of unconscious fantasies is of psychotherapeutic value, although we realize that there are other workers who insist that the acceptance by the child of the verbal interpretation of the drawing is the essential component of the treatment.

There appears to be definite evidence that the graphic expression by means of acceptable art work of the aggressive impulses in the young child, and often, also, of sexual drives in young adolescents, has definite psychotherapeutic value. Children who are able to produce vividly aggressive pictures which are admired and cherished by the art teacher, the psychiatrist, and the other children, and for which the child suffers no feelings of guilt, frequently as a result exhibit less aggression in their behavior. There are some children who seem to be relieved of much sexual tension by being able to produce drawings which are at least symbolically sexual. The possibility of stimulating erotic tensions in groups of children by frankly sexual productions has also been noted.

Art classes are in many ways a socializing force. The significance of group therapy has already been emphasized and will be especially evident in our experience with puppet shows. Group activities appear to be especially valuable in children in the latency period since they are inclined to express themselves more freely in groups than individually. The experience of one becomes the experience of all. When one child produces an aggressive picture which expresses the fantasies of other children, they all benefit by the experience. The relief of most inhibited, inferior-feeling children that they cannot draw or paint is readily overcome in the group. The child who has produced something of value which he can share with the group or give to his psychotherapist or teacher has won for himself social approval, admiration, and love.

There is therapeutic value also in the opportunity to express the impulses for motor activity and in the creation and experimentation with forms regardless of their ideational content. We have already seen the experimental tendencies in the maturing child in the form principles of play, in sidewalk drawings and games, and in reproducing all kinds of configurations.[3] For the very young child, the mentally defective, the severely neurotic or schizophrenic child who is struggling to understand the world of reality, a pencil-paper play with the repetition of the simplest of forms probably gives considerable satisfaction to impulses for patterned activity. Experimentation with simple form productions may represent the beginning of integrated

---

[3] Billy (see Chapter 6) seemed to get some relief from his compulsion to draw significant figures and form his aggressive impulses when he was motivated to draw the figures daily to the point of saturation.

activity. A similar function is often served by music and dance in children who present the more primitive behavior patterns.

Finally, we have found that our art productions have given us a particularly valuable clinical record of certain types of behavior difficulties in children, of their progress and, often, of their improvement under psychotherapy.

Brief case histories of five children will be presented to illustrate these various points.

Eddie was a 12 year old boy when he was brought to us for stealing and running away from home. A careful analysis of the boy's own story showed that he did not want and never planned to steal, but whenever he saw money about the house, or was given money by his mother to make some purchase, he had an overwhelming impulse to take the money and run away. The impulse was immediately associated with a tight sensation in the left side of his body, which grew in intensity if he attempted to resist the temptation, until it became a severe and unbearable pain which could only be relieved by his taking the money, leaving home and wandering about the streets until the money was spent for necessary food and he became exhausted. Then he would return home full of remorse.

His parents were inclined to consider this story a rationalization to excuse his theft. We however had no reason to doubt the reality of his suffering. They attempted to correct him by imbuing him with the ambition to become a priest and to live a good and holy life free from his temptation. They also attempted to fortify him against temptation by leaving him alone to do his homework with money on the table before him. Needless to say, he suffered much from these corrective procedures; he also developed a sanctimonious attitude.

The parents insisted that in other respects the home life was ideal. They explained, however, that the mother was really a stepmother, but they did not think that Eddie knew this, although his mother had died when he was 5 years old, and there was evidence that he had some memories of his own mother. He had been placed in a boarding home when his mother died, and was told that she was sick. When his father married the stepmother, Eddie was brought home and told that his mother had recovered. He remembered that his own mother had been fatter, but he was told that he remembered his mother when she had been pregnant with his little brother. Actually the mother had lived six months after the birth of the younger sibling, and had died suddenly of pneumonia.

Eddie had a great facility for making pencil sketches. He would sit and draw pictures by the hour illustrating his remarks while he discussed his problems with the physician (Fig. 40). First, he was asked to draw anything that he liked and he drew a picture (Fig. 40a). This appears to be a very realistic picture of one of the rooms on the children's ward. All of the details in the room are correct. It includes the picture of a little patient, Joe, who was being treated for a burn on his back, therefore he is lying prone, with the covers over him in a tent formation; a nurse is standing at the head of the bed. One would not think that this was in any way related to the child's unconscious life. However, when he was asked to draw a picture of his recollections of his

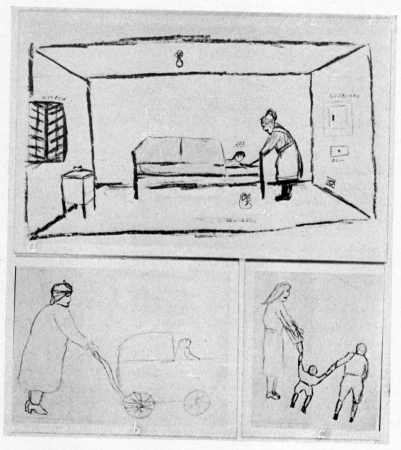

FIG. 40a (*top*). A Scene in the Hospital, by Eddie (*pencil*).
FIG. 40b (*left*). Early memory of his mother with his baby brother, by Eddie (*pencil*).
FIG. 40c (*right*). Later memory of his stepmother with himself and brother, by Eddie (*pencil*).

mother before she was ill, he drew the picture (Fig. 40b), which is almost identical in its general patterning, to the other drawing. The mother manifests a marked similarity to the nurse, standing in the same position grasping a baby carriage, and the form of the baby is also similar to that of Joe.

From these two pictures, we observe that when the boy was asked to draw whatever he liked, he used the everyday material of the ward but patterned it after his earliest and most significant memory. We may say that he sees in the routine events of the hospital wards, patterns similar to his earliest significant memories. We also learn that he does not remember his mother as pregnant, but as caring for his brother. Later he was asked to draw a picture of his "mother" as he first remembered her after she had supposedly reunited the family following her sickness, and he produced the picture seen in Fig. 40c. It is clear that this is not the same woman who played a part in his earlier memory; this picture really depicts his stepmother. The father was persuaded of this when he saw these pictures, and admitted that his first wife was a more obese woman than his second. He also was persuaded to tell the boy the truth about his mother and his stepmother.

In a similar way, the boy continued to reveal to the physician and to himself a great deal about his problems, conflicts, and special interests. It became evident that his compulsion to steal money or suffer a pain in his left side was due to the feeling of loss of his own mother, to doubt concerning his own identity, to doubt concerning the sincerity of his father and stepmother, and to doubt concerning their identity; all resulting in a compulsive drive to go out and seek his mother and settle these problems. After the real identities of all members of the family were correctly explaind to him, and after two months' participation in psychotherapeutic sessions, which included drawing with the physician, he returned to his home. He had no real ambition to become a priest. His best drawings consisted of horse races and his keenest interest was in sports which were denied him at home because he was not trusted to leave the house. It was not possible to furnish him with intensive psychotherapy through a clinic which we thought he needed although he had some supervision through a social agency. He apparently controlled his stealing fairly well until three years later at the age of 15, when he appeared in children's court on a charge of petty thievery and was sent to a correctional institution.

Luther was a bright little Negro boy of 6 years who persistently ran away from home. He was the illegitimate child of his mother who probably cared more for him than for anyone else in the world. During his early years she devoted herself to his care, doing house work during the day to support him. Then she married a stepfather for Luther, so that she might stay home. He seemed to accept the stepfather fairly well because he now received more attention from his mother, but when the first baby came he began running away from home. He told a policeman who found him alone on a dock one night that his mother did not love him any more because she had a new baby that kept her busy. When she became pregnant a second time he ran away even more frequently, although at that time the stepfather deserted the family. Luther was very homesick in the hospital because his mother could not visit him often, due to her baby and the advanced stage of her pregnancy. One day he painted a picture of his dream in vivid colors (Fig. 41a). Later, he also produced the same scene in colored clay. He described the picture as a jungle with a snake running after the mother and the child. He said that if the snake catches them it will eat them up. Then it will burst and they will be free again. He told us that it was really the child that was running away, the mother was running after him, and in the end they would be safe together.

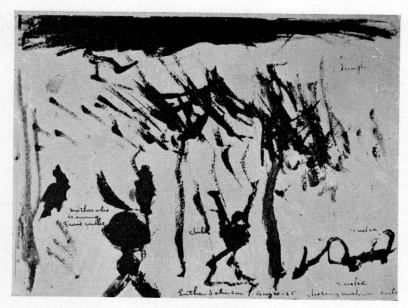

FIG. 41a. A Dream, by Luther (*water color*).

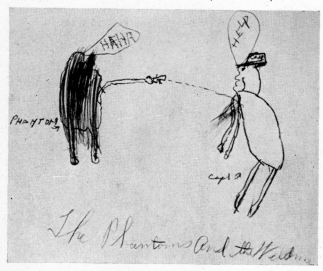

FIG. 41b. The Phantoms and the Wild Man, an illustration
for a story by Jacob (*crayon*).

It is usually considered that the snake is a penetrating phallic symbol.[4]
Among our children, however, we have found that the snake may be a symbol of oral aggression. It is really a primitive animal with a threatening

[4] See Chapter 14 for discussion of the meaning of snakes in children's graphic and plastic
art production.

mouth and a large gut or belly. It usually represents the child's primitive concept of his fear of the threatening parent, either father or mother. In this case the snake represented Luther's concept of the stepfather who had threatened his happy love life with his mother.

We kept Luther with us until after the new baby was born, in order to help him accept his siblings and to help him to understand how much his mother would now need him to help with the babies, especially since his stepfather had deserted the home. Because the mother was able to get financial aid for her children under supervision from a welfare organization, this was a reasonable program to offer the boy.

However the next winter when he was 7 and in the second grade at school he was returned because of the persistent running away from home and truancy as well. The mother had not been able to cope with two babies and this boy. It had also developed that he had not learned to read as rapidly as he should have. Psychometric examinations showed that he had an IQ of 119 but was a reading disability. We started a program of remedial tutoring and recommended foster home care which was arranged through a child placement agency. We have frequently observed that children with reading disabilities often show compensatory adeptness in artistic ability to make articulate their emotional and social problems.

Jacob was an 11 year old boy who had a neurotic tic in which he made a loud barking noise, which disturbed the other children in school and even the other members of his family, so that neither his school nor his home could tolerate him any longer. In addition, he had an infantile, unhappy, hostile personality, making for conflict with other children as well as with his own brothers. Wherever he went, he made himself unpopular and he soon realized that he was unwanted. On the children's ward he was in constant trouble. He was a strong and healthy boy, and on the slightest provocation and often without apparent cause, he would strike at and abuse other children, none of whom he liked; but when hit in retaliation, he would start yelling and running to the nearest adult, a woman if possible, complaining that he was hurt. He was also hypochondriacal and always had some imaginary ill, for which he needed attention.

He was the second of three boys. The mother had never wanted her children and never loved any of them, but she depreciated this one especially, often in his presence stating that she had never had anything but trouble from him since the day he was born. It became evident that his unhappy personality was the result of an effort to obtain some maternal attention and love, and that his aggression against all other children was an expression of his antagonism toward his two brothers who got what little maternal affection was available in the home.

Effort to make any psychotherapeutic approach to this boy failed at first. Then it was learned that he was attempting to terrorize the children by gruesome bedtime stories. He was encouraged to tell these stories to his psychiatrist, with whom he had a good relationship as a substitute for his mother. He illustrated these stories with drawings. He was able to provide a different story with illustrative drawings each day. With this procedure, in conjunction with the usual group activities and the socializing effect of the ward routine, his tic gradually diminished, and his aggressive behavior was less marked. On days when his psychiatrist was not able to arrange to see him, his behavior would tend to return to its former pattern. The technique appeared to be a fairly satisfactory release for his emotions.

Figure 41b illustrates Jacob's story of *The Phantoms and The Wild Man*. His pictures were always hastily and crudely drawn. They always expressed an aggressive idea. He never used any color except red to indicate dripping blood.

THE PHANTOMS AND THE WILD MAN[5]

"I was walking on the street and met a man. He was running away from town. He said he wanted to go away from town. He said, 'I'm the captain.' I brought him on the ship. I told him if he wants to go to the country and capture some wild men. He said the only one he should catch is the Thing— the Phantom. Next they get shipwrecked and they find an island and there is all kinds of fruit and everything. They see a shadow. They see this shadow every place on the island. One man took out his gun and shot at the shadow and he didn't die. He shot the shadow of the shadow. The shadow shot the captain. The captain was wounded and he died. Next the other guy, he began to walk away. Next he meets a lion and he shoots the lion and sees the lion turn into a black thing. All lions turn into Phantoms if you shoot them. Next he saw the Phantom. He didn't have no tools to shoot. He ran away. Next he saw other phantoms. The good guy he says, 'I want to make myself a hypnotizer or a magician.' He learned a couple of days hypnotizing and being a magician and a lion came and he hypnotized the lion, but the lion didn't go to sleep. He sprang on him and he had a broken arm. He made the magician thing and turned him into a phantom, next a skeleton—he changed into a lot of things.

Next day he came to a phantom and he shot the phantom. The phantom died. Next he goes in a cave and sees a lot of phantoms. They say, 'Here's a man that's killing all of us.' The next morning he is still in the cave. They all search for him and they can't find him. They said, 'Let's go back in the cave; maybe he's still there.' They couldn't find him. He stands right next to them and socks them over the head. He sees a snake coming out and kills a Phantom. Next he sees the good guy and wants to kill him, but the good guy changes into a great big man and says, 'Kill the man over there.' So he killed all the men. Next he says, 'Now to find wild men.' He goes out and sees a couple of wild men. He sees a big one. The big one he gets the things. Next they want to make a lot of money and that's the end."

---

[5] Shorthand transcription as Jacob told the story impromptu.

This may appear to be a very confused story in which everyone is killed. But it is really a very significant recitation, and completely explains Jacob's problems. The story may be interpreted as a fantasy in which Jacob returns to his mother's womb, of the happiness which such a life affords, where he is able to kill all his mother's unborn children, including his two brothers. The story begins with Jacob as the hero, and he uses the personal pronoun "I," but soon he changes and refers to the hero as the "good guy" in the third person. He goes to the island to seek happiness and kills all the shadows, and the shadows of shadows, and phantoms, and animals, and wild men. There is a snake in his story, too, which is probably the symbol of both his inadequate father and his aggressively abusive and rejecting mother. He is then born again, big and strong, and is able to kill all the men who oppose him. Finally, he is a successful business man.

The value of therapeutic measures of this kind lies in the actual expression of his aggressive tendencies, fantasies and conflicts, in the transference relationship with the psychiatrist, in the interpretation which is given to the boy, and in the socializing factors implicit in the group activities of the children's ward.

The picture shows a phantom killing the captain. The captain must be Jacob, as he lives in this world without adequate protection from his mother and who is constantly threatened by his brothers.

Actually while Jacob was in the hospital, his mother deserted the home. Arrangements were made to place all three boys in an institution for normal boys where Jacob was able to get psychotherapy. He got along well enough and volunteered in the marines in World War II. However while on active duty there was evident anxiety and a return of his tic which led to a neuropsychiatric discharge. Jacob came back to us, at that time, asking if he could get any treatment that would make it possible for him to return to military service. He was referred to a clinic for treatment but was not able to re-enlist.

Morris was a 10 year old boy. When he came to us he was a pathetic child. He had a neurological condition especially in his legs which made them feeble and produced chorea-like movements. Before admission it was said that at times the movements were so severe that he had to be carried about, and on occasion they became so intense that they were thought to be epileptic fits. This diagnosis semed reasonable especially since his mother had epilepsy and was being cared for in an institution for epileptic patients. Morris had been living in an orphan home which was thought to be inadequate to care for a boy with such difficult problems. Morris had had some very unhappy experiences. Even before his mother had been separated from him, she would often become psychotic and at such time she would chase Morris with a knife and threaten to cut off his feet, saying his feet were not any good and were making him have fits like hers. He told us that on one occasion he hid under the bed just in time to avoid losing his feet.

When he came to the hospital his legs were weak, clumsy, and awkward. There was definite evidence of a slight choreiform disability and poor muscular development, especially in the left leg. There was however never any indication of epilepsy. Morris was very self-conscious of his disability and tried to conceal it by clowning. He tried to play the role of Charlie Chaplin. But

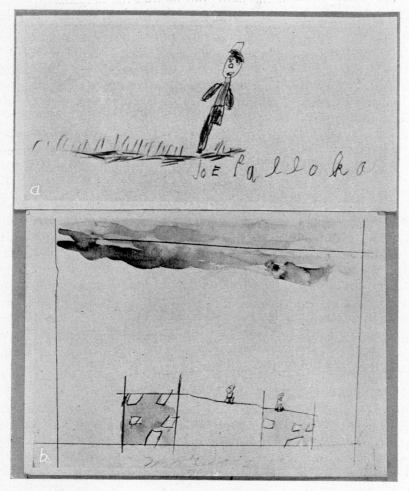

FIG. 42a *(top)*. Joe Palooka, by Morris *(crayon)*.
FIG. 42b *(bottom)*. Tight Rope Walker, by Morris *(pencil and water color)*.

among the children he felt very inferior and could not compete in their active play and fights.

When asked to draw pictures of a man, he drew a one-legged man and called it Joe Palooka (Fig. 42a). When he was given the miniature toys which we used for psychotherapeutic work, he always had his soldiers riding to battle in trucks, because he said they did not want to walk. During the weeks that he spent with us he was given active orthopedic treatment and physiotherapy for his legs, psychotherapy by play technique, as well as group work in the art class. We could follow the progress of his improvement in his art work. Soon his men had two legs instead of one, although at first they were still always riding in carts. Later, they were walking on the ground, and soon they were climbing ladders. Finally when Morris was ready for discharge we got the picture (Fig. 43b) where a man is walking a tight rope between two buildings. When Morris left he was not secure on his feet and in his ability to compete with other boys in active play. He was placed in a boarding home and arrangements were made for further orthopedic care and psychotherapy which utilized his ability to express himself in art. He joined a boys' club where he participated in an art class and a class in jujitsu. His physical condition, posture and gait improved steadily. At 15 he returned to the home of his father's family, together with his father, while his mother was still in the institution. With his growing motor coordination and interest in sports he developed good social success despite his limited intellectual endowment.

Marty was a 6 year old boy who was referred to us because of his very disturbed and autistic and regressed behavior. As he showed all of the typical features of a schizophrenic child as described by Howard W. Potter,[6] we considered him to be a case of childhood schizophrenia. When he was first brought to the children's ward, he was almost completely out of contact with the world of reality. He was mute, resistive, inattentive to what was going on about him, unconcerned about other children or even about his own physical needs. He would not keep his clothes on and had to be spoon fed against great resistance.

He had not always been an abnormal child but had developed normally until 4 years of age. He had shown a change in his behavior associated somewhat unclearly with minor episodes which seemed to have frightened him. For example, he had dropped a roll of toilet paper in the toilet causing it to choke and run over, and his mother screamed at him. On another occasion he was slapped by a neighbor for slamming a door.

When Marty first spoke on the ward, his speech was incoherent and bizarre. Thus he might say, "The blood is coming from the red eyes of a fish." Our treatment of this boy included the usual socializing activities of the group projects of the ward, attempts to utilize fleeting contacts with several members of the staff, and efforts to bring out the normal aggressive tendency of the 6 year old by encouraging him to play the role of a cowboy. We furnished him with a cowboy suit and gun.

Marty's drawings, only a few of which are shown, record his improvement under therapy. His gestalt drawings are seen in Fig. 15 and the discussion of them is in the accompanying text. His first drawings, which are not

---

[6] In 1939 the diagnosis of childhood schizophrenia was not frequently made. Marty was one of the first of our subsequently extensive series of cases of childhood schizophrenia. Howard Potter's criteria for the diagnosis of childhood schizophrenia were published in 1934 and were used in the diagnostic evaluation of this boy.

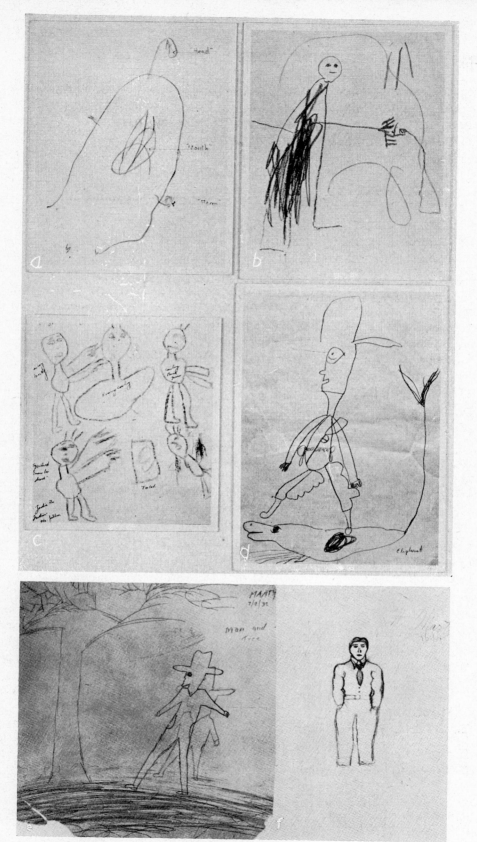

FIG. 43 (a-f). Drawings of a man, by Marty, at ages 6-4 (*top, left*), 6-7 (*top, right*), 6-10 (*center, left*), 7-6 (*center, right*), 9-11 (*bottom, left*), 15-4 (*bottom, right*).

reproduced, represented the simplest, most primitive scribble which characterizes drawing activities of 1 and 2 year old children. But even they may have been of value to him as a motor activity which produced a creation which had some hint of a world of reality which he tended to lose hold of so readily.

Fig. 43a shows his first recognizable picture of a man, but it also reveals the bizarre dissociations which characterize schizophrenia. The mouth is not in the head, but where the stomach should be. This is very primitive production and was drawn about a month after he entered the hospital. Three months later, after the cowboy treatment had been started, he began to draw the pictures which characterized a considerable period of his treatment. Fig. 43b shows a cowboy with a smoking gun in his hand. The hand that held the gun was always emphasized and the smoke coiled around the background. Three months later, he was able to draw pictures of significant emotional problems in his life which were used by his psychiatrist for interpretative purposes during a period of active psychotherapy.

Figure 43c shows a number of cowboys and Indians. The Indians are the enemies of the cowboys, their eyes are usually shut because they are dead. They represent his father, for whom he began to express an open antagonism. It is to be remarked that Marty's illness began at the period when the oedipus complex is most significant in the emotional development of the boy. We also see the toilet which figured in one of his early infantile frights. A dead Indian is being thrown down the toilet to be flushed away. Subsequently it was possible to discharge the boy to his home and readmit him to public school, although it was still evident that he was not a normal boy.

A year after his admission to the hospital he drew the picture in Fig. 43d. By the Goodenough score this is better than average for a boy of 7 years. We were surprised that he called the animal an elephant. To us, it resembled one of the alligators in the puppet shows which Marty often saw while he was in the hospital, and which terrorized him for a long time before he could be persuaded that the alligator was not real and would not devour him. To us, the picture signified Marty himself who has conquered his fear of the unreal alligator. But even in this picture Marty indicated that things did not appear to him quite as they did to us. It will be noted that his "elephant" tends to resemble his earliest drawings of a man except that it is in a prone position.

When Marty was 10 years old we arranged to have him return to the hospital for metrazol shock treatment. His drawing of a man, Fig. 43e, lower left, clearly resembles the one he drew at 7 years. This man is standing on the earth near a tree, but he has a shadow of himself behind him which may suggest something of the way Marty felt. The only details of the clothing are the pockets, although at 7 years there had been elaborate details to indicate a cowboy suit. At this time his Stanford-Binet test gave him an IQ of 92.

After the metrazol shock treatment, Marty was somewhat more responsive and active and related better to reality. He continued with his school work until he graduated from high school at 19. He was a slow, shy, withdrawn boy whose school work was mediocre. The school authorities considered him dull and a day dreamer. He was protected throughout his boyhood by his sister two years his senior. The two of them visited the hospital or clinic at frequent intervals in Marty's interest. His thought content seemed largely dominated by his sister. When he was 15, his psychometric scoring was 79 on the Bellevue-Wechsler test with a great deal of variability in test responses. He was in the 2nd term of high school.

At this time his drawing of a man shows anxiety and a rigid posture. The hands are deeply buried in the pockets. The great effort at control is shown here as it was in the gestalt drawings (Fig. 15d).

On one of his visits his sister, who was then 17, accompanied him. She showed grimacing, was anxious, and expressed ideas of mystic powers whereby she could understand and care for Marty and his sex life. She had become schizophrenic herself, although as a child she had never shown any of the schizophrenic features which Marty had. She was subsequently hospitalized and received shock treatment but at 23 years of age was still seriously disturbed. Marty was living at home and earning a fair living as a salesman although he still showed many childhood schizophrenic features such as whirling on the longitudinal axis, manneristic motility, emotional inadequacy, marked dependency on his mother, and an immature handling of his sexual problems.

This review of several case histories has been presented to indicate different ways in which graphic art productions of children may be adapted to psychotherapy.

Art is of course only one of many adjuncts which may be utilized in psychotherapy of children, but in some instances it is a very valuable means. There are many ways in which it may be useful to the child who is struggling with emotional problems. These include the motor impulse to activity, producing a realistic creation with a pattern which is appropriate for the level of maturation of the child; the opportunity to express instinctual impulses, such as aggressive and sexual drives, in the form of artistic productions which are acceptable to the group, and admired by those from whom he wants approval; the group experience of observing other children drawing similar pictures or some picture which the individual child might not have the ability or courage to draw; the production of drawings which reveal the fantasies and unconscious life of the child, not only to himself, but to his psychiatrist who may thereby be guided in the psychotherapeutic program and in suitable situations may offer interpretations to the child.[7]

----

[7] It is of interest in this connection that Harry B. Lee has stated that the creative work of artists is a self-discovered psychotherapeutic procedure which makes it possible that the particular kind of personality of the artist may "convalesce from a neurotic depression brought on by the effects of having hated too much," or that "various esthetic states of mind occur in particular kinds of personalities in order to relieve acute psychological emergencies due to the activation of destructive rage which is not being efficiently repressed."

CLAY MODELING AS A PROJECTIVE TECHNIQUE
IN CHILD PSYCHIATRY[1]

MOST investigations into the creative ability of children have emphasized their graphic accomplishments, and indeed so far in this book we have interested ourselves largely in the use of the graphic arts as projective techniques in child psychiatry. Significant investigations of the child's manipulation with plastic materials may be found in the German literature. Otto Krautter made a careful analysis of his own important work and reviewed the work of his predecessors.[2]

Interesting analogies in the maturation processes are found in comparing the art expression of children in plastic and other media. Important differentiations become evident which are due to significant differences in the medium upon which the child's maturation processes play. Some insight is also gained into the psychogenesis of the creative processes which are of importance in the study and treatment of behavior problems in children.

Otto Krautter and those who preceded him tended to emphasize the objective side of the creative functions in the normal maturing child. David M. Levy and J. Louise Despert in their techniques have used plastic material as approaches to emotional problems in children. The present study will investigate the correlation between these findings and our own observations regarding the personality development of the child. Special considerations have been given to emotional and social problems presenting themselves in those children who came to the children's ward for observation and therapy.

Each maturation process takes place within its own specific cycle, although there are close correlations between them. Krautter and others have shown that the plastic maturation cycles as compared with the graphic maturation cycle is a much shorter and therefore a much quicker one. However, like drawing, it is initiated by the sheer love of motor activity directed at the material. The child's treatment of the material is an expression of his drive for motility, and a reaction to sensory and tactile stimuli which arise more from the motor than from the optic field. Krautter calls this first stage

---

[1] Reprinted in part from Bender, Lauretta and Woltmann, Adolf G.: The Use of Plastic Material as a Psychiatric Approach to Emotional Problems in Children. *American Journal of Orthopsychiatry,* 7:283-300, 1937. Throughout this chapter "clay and "plasticine" are used interchangeably.

[2] Krautter refers to the work of Buehler, Lay, Rouma, Kopky, Wulf, Bergmann-Koenitzer, and others.

the kneading period which corresponds to the scribbling stage in drawing. There is no intention as yet to copy or to create a form. It is an exploration of the external world by rhythmic activity out of which patterns are built. We have shown[3] that these same form principles occur in the play activities of children. Any form that a child has made himself may be called a "man," a "tree," a "mother," a "baby," and so on. It is not necessary that there exists a resemblance between the form and the interpretation given to it, as long as the form can carry out the role it has been given by the child. These creations, unintentionally made, therefore become carriers of a meaning.

Aside from the quicker maturation cycles, plastic material offers other advantages. Plasticine, a nonhardening clay that has been used by most of the other investigators as well as by ourselves and by schools and nurseries all over the world, lends itself especially well to the repetitive aggressive destructive type of behavior which, as studies on aggressiveness in children have shown,[4] seems to characterize the normal development in children both in their play activities and in their verbalizations. Similar principles which take place in the sensory motor patterns have been demonstrated in the study of sidewalk drawings and games of children. Our experiences with children's reactions to puppet shows reveal related principles in the emotional patterns.

Technically, plasticine is easier for the child to handle. Instead of holding one medium such as a pencil or crayon in one hand and using it on the second medium such as paper, the child in plastic work manipulates the medium directly with both hands. Such handling is based on correlated motility patterns of both hands adapted to the material. The motility problems seem to be similar to the grasping reflex of the newborn. Furthermore the child can experiment with three dimensional patterns and depth without technical difficulties.[5]

Otto Krautter's observations, which are substantiated by our own independent investigations, show that the next higher stage is a more integrated rhythmic rolling which replaces the non-specific treatment of the first stage. The rolled cylinder appears to be the "gestaltungselement" in creative plastic work. It is comparable to the loop, whorl or circle which form the primitive units of the visual motor gestalten made with pencil and paper. Both arise from motor drives and motor functions in relation to the medium offered. Together with the creation of primitive geometrical forms the child

---

[3] See Chapter 2.

[4] Bender, Lauretta and Schilder, Paul: *Studies in Aggressiveness: Aggressiveness in Children,* 1936.

[5] We have further encouraged the third dimensional activity by giving the child, together with the plasticine, a wooden implement or "armature" such as sculptors use in modeling figures or heads. This follows from the fact that our plastic activities were an outgrowth of our puppet activities. In an effort to teach our children the technique of puppet making, armatures and plasticine were given them as one stage of making puppet heads.

begins his first attempts in object representation. At this point there appears a resemblance between the created form and the child's concepts. The plastic creative work of the child is no longer a mere symbol but the representation of a real object.

With the appearance of representative interpretation, emotional values are attached to the creation by the child. By the attaching of emotional values, the fantasy life of the child enters into his plastic creative activities. The child's plastic work becomes a means of expression and crystallization of his fantasy life. This is one of the reasons why plastic work is so valuable in the observation and treatment of behavior problems in children. It gives us a means of investigating the fantasy life of the child and at the same time enables the child to clarify more freely and bring to conscious levels his own fantasies. Krautter emphasizes that the plastic creative work of the child begins with rhythmic movements which finally lead to the representation of objects. We are inclined to carry the analysis of the process further by showing that at the same time the child's plastic creative work is also an expression of his own motility pattern, his aggressive investigation into the world of reality, his drive to produce patterns on the receptive material with which to express his emotional and social problems, and his tendency to solve many of his problems through these experiences.

Bergmann-Koenitzer[6] demonstrated that during one stage in object representation the human form is emphasized. Following the teachings of Paul Schilder[7] we regard this as an active investigation into the body image or postural model. Krautter also relates the creating of forms in plastic work to the studies of the gestalt school, quoting especially Kurt Koffka to show that in the creation of gestalten, growth occurs by a process of structured differentiation of form. The object representative stage, as it occurs in children and as we have been able to observe it, may be summarized in the following stages: 1. Form as produced by motor impulses. 2. Form reproduced as seen or in imitation of other children. 3. Form which is projected from the body image or postural model of the body and its manifold sensory and conceptual experiences. 4. Form as an expression of fantasy, and of emotional and social problems.

The method employed in letting the children on the children's ward work with plastic material is a very simple one. A group of approximately five to eight children are each given an armature and a lump of plasticine. They are told to make anything they wish, to create freely. The examiner sits near the children and observes the entire process of creating. This is necessary for the following reason: In graphic creative work once a line has been drawn on paper, it remains visible and fixed. With plastic material every touch or pres-

---

[6] See Krautter, Otto, for discussion of Bergmann-Koenitzer's work.
[7] Schilder, Paul: *Image and Appearance of the Human Body.*

sure upon the material produces changes in form which might lead to a different interpretation by the child. In other words, a child may start out with one intention and change it a number of times before the creation is completed. To illustrate, the following observations were made of a 7 year old boy whose first creation in clay was a revolver. After considerable "shooting" he discovered that the rectangular shape of his creation also resembled the handle that flushes the toilet. He immediately remodeled the gun into a toilet. No interpretations should be made of any forms created by a child until the child has told the story which completes his work. Often we find that the plastic creation is only a picture segment ("Bildausschnitt") brought to a real, visible, and tangible level.

The first stage of nonspecific treatment of clay was observed in our nursery group, which is composed of children from 2 to 5 years of age, and also of older children who are mentally retarded, emotionally blocked or otherwise handicapped so that they cannot make the necessary motor, intellectual, emotional or social adjustments of the school child. Their approach to plastic material is that of an experimental investigation. They examine the plasticine by looking at it, smelling it, poking and hitting it, by putting it into their mouths, trying to chew and swallow it. They may drop it on the floor, throw it away or merely watch the other children. One or two children will take the armature stems and begin to hit the plastic material. Soon the others will follow. First each child will hit the clay in some kind of rhythm characteristic of his motor pattern. Before long, several children will coordinate their individual rhythms into one steady group beat. While this is going on, new discoveries are being made. Because of the repeated hitting, the plasticine lumps will take on a flat shape. One child will suddenly stop and exclaim, "Look what I made! I made a cake!" These activities are repeated over and over again. Once the children have released their undifferentiated motor drives, they soon become interested in the plastic material itself. They take it apart and put it together again. Other children may push holes into the plasticine or even use their fingernails or teeth to make indentations. Various forms and shapes are thus made. A flat piece of plasticine will be called a "cake." A polymorphous lump of clay with a little piece protruding from it is identified as a mouse.

The children are happy about their discoveries. They show them around and enjoy having their creations admired by the group. On one occasion, a 6 year old girl attached a piece of clay to one end of the armature stem. On top of this, she put another piece of plasticine in the form of a rolled cylinder. She called her creation a "baby." She showed it to a 3 year old boy and said, "You can't hit my baby." No sooner had she said this when the boy took his armature stem and began to hit her baby. Instead of being angry or upset, the girl laughed and screamed with joy whenever the boy touched or hit the clay baby. After it was completely destroyed, she made another one and this play activity was repeated over and over again.

The social implications are especially interesting in this instance because this little girl was on the observation ward together with her 18 month old brother. The two children were rejected by their mother and showed clear signs of sibling rivalry for the scant bit of maternal affection that the mother had to share between them.

At this stage we notice also the possessive nature of the child which has been emphasized previously. It seems that the children are never satisfied with the specific amount of plasticine given to them, and try to get as much as possible from the other children. Although they are working alongside of each other and observing each other's activities, they do not as yet work in social groups. This non-social stage of community activity has been observed and discussed by Charlotte Buehler, Jean Piaget, and Susan Isaacs.

The stage of cylinder formation by rhythmic movements and object representation are shown in 5 year old Stanley's "Snakes and Fish" (Fig. 44a), and 8 year old Barbara's "Chinese Town" (Fig. 44b). Stanley's picture shows a number of rolled cylinders of which two are in an upright position. The rest of them are bent into loops. Two upright pieces are called mice; the loops are called snakes and one irregularly shaped piece of clay is called a fish. Barbara's creation shows a number of loops and rings, both forms being derivatives of the rolled cylinder. What Stanley calls a snake becomes a bridge in Barbara's creation. What both pictures have in common is that they represent some kind of fears. Stanley is afraid of snakes and fish because they might kill and eat his parents. Barbara's loops and rings represent a Chinese town which was connected with fears in her fantasy life.

Marion, an 8 year old girl, gave the following story to her plastic creation (Fig. 44d):

"This shows three worms and stones. The stones are to hit the kids that touch the worms. It's bad to touch the worms because they bite you. If they bite, you'll get killed." Marion was mentally retarded, emotionally blocked and awkward in her motility. In her modeling she also showed the developmental stage of a younger child. Her discs and cylinders were the results of her limited motility functions. Nevertheless they were integrated into a well expressed story of aggression which because of her limited social adjustment were her only means of contact in this difficult world, as all of her behavior suggested.

The stage of preoccupation and investigation into the body image and postural model of the body is well known in graphic art and as has been stated has been used as a maturation test by Florence Goodenough and as a projection of personality and body image problems by Karen Machover. All of its implications in the psychic development of the child and as an actual

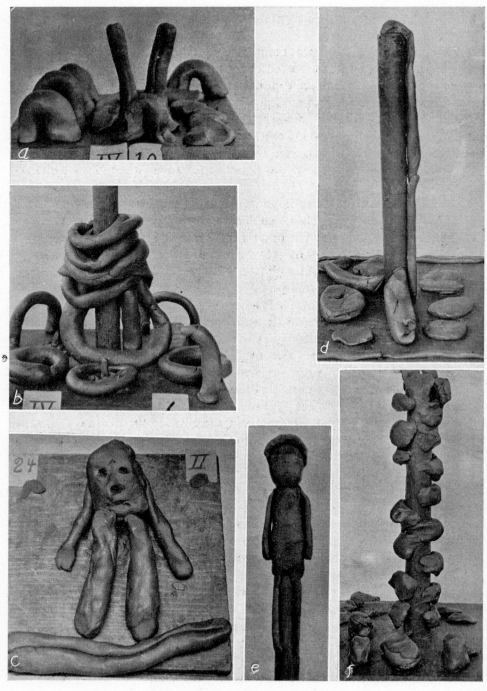

FIG. 44. Photographs of clay modeling.

FIG. 44a (*top, left*). Snakes and Fish, by Stanley.

FIG. 44b (*center, left*). Chinese Town, by Barbara.

FIG. 44c (*bottom, left*). Casper and the Snake, by Abram.

FIG. 44d (*top, right*). Worms and Stones, by Marion.

FIG. 44e (*bottom, center*). Man, by Ellery.

FIG. 44f (*bottom, right*). Ladder, by Michael.

means of investigating the child's own body model have not however been fully realized. A child with a deformity of the body will for example usually express it in his drawings of a man. The actual processes of producing a human form in plastic material has been outlined by Krautter.

Abram, a retarded 6 year old boy, produced a very primitive model of a man (Fig. 44c). His creation resembled what Krautter calls "Kopffuessler"; there is no body and the arms and legs protrude from the head. The significance of the snake in his production and his story about it will be discussed below.

Ellery, a defective 12 year old girl, made a very primitive plastic figure of a man (Fig. 44e) although details of a decorative nature were added. We often find that our defective children decorate their finished products with unimportant details. Similar findings in the graphic drawings of a man in the Goodenough test for defective children have been described by J. Israelite, Dorothy T. Spoerl, and E. W. McElwee.

It need not necessarily be the human body as a whole with which the child experiments. Functions of the body are experimented with as well, as shown in the creation of Michael, a retarded 7 year old boy, who suffered from progressive muscular dystrophy (Fig. 44f). He was very weak and physically handicapped. We had to break up the plasticine into small pieces for him. His creations were always the same. He would place these small pieces against the armature stem until the entire stem was covered. He called his creation a "ladder." He used to run his fingers up and down the "rungs" imitating the movement of climbing. In other words, a physical activity which he was unable to carry out any longer was experienced over and over again in his clay work.

Most young children are interested especially in the genital and anal regions of the body. Plastic material seems to lend itself very well to this type of investigation, first because these regions can be reproduced in actual resemblance to nature; second, unconsciously, plastic material may satisfy the child's early repressed desires to play with faeces which plasticine resembles. As a matter of fact, these investigations from time to time become a serious problem in clay class. One child will start it. His creation will soon be imitated and excelled by the other children until actual orgies of all types of perversion may find expression if the children are not controlled in some way.

Figs. 45a, b, and c show the independent creations of three boys of 6, 10 and 11 years of age. The picture of the first man shows a small head, small feet and no arms. The child's preoccupation with the anal and genital regions is expressed by the attachment of a very large penis and an anus which reaches from the nape of the neck to the hips. After finishing his creation he put small pieces of clay into the anus and removed them. In this repetition

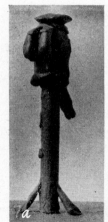

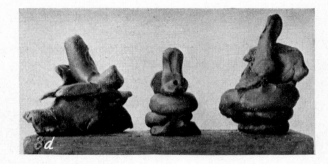

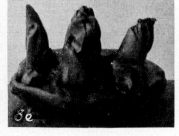

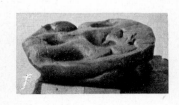

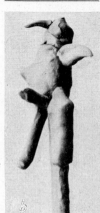

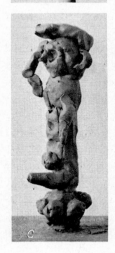

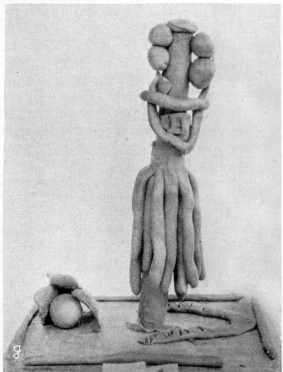

FIG. 45. Photographs of clay modeling.

FIG. 45a (*top, left*). Man, by Walter.
FIG. 45b (*center, left*). Man, by Billy.
FIG. 45c (*bottom, left*). Man, by Oscar.
FIG. 45d (*top, right*). Three Toilets, by Gordon.

FIG. 45e (*center*). Community Toilet, by Peter.
FIG. 45f (*center, right*). Community Toilet, by Peter.
FIG. 45g (*bottom, right*). Banana Tree, by Barbara.

he was probably playfully re-experiencing the process of elimination. The outstanding characteristics in the second creation are an exaggerated nose and a large penis.

We often find that experimentations with body parts are not limited to the genital and anal regions alone. In this case it is also the nose which undergoes some changes. The third creation shows a man with a penis. Around the penis this boy placed six testicles which to him was another way of experimenting.

Figs. 45d, e, and f show the experimentation two 7 year old boys with toilets and the proper body posture one should maintain in the process of elimination. One 6½ year old boy was very careful in attaching a raised cover to the toilet because, as he explained, without this raised cover one cannot sit down properly. Whereas this boy made an individual toilet for every member of the family, the 5½ year old boy experimented further by creating a "community" toilet. He made five holes in a piece of plasticine and attached five rolled cylinders to these holes, calling them "father, mother, two sisters and a baby." The top ends of these human figures were slightly twisted because, using his own words, "they turned their heads away while they sit down there." We find here an excellent combination of curiosity towards the anal region which embraces the necessity of elimination to which is added an experimentation of proper body posture, communal activities and ideologies.

An 8 year old girl showed her preoccupation with sex matters in a more symbolic way. She made a house with a clay ball on the inside (Fig. 45g). She claimed that the house belonged to a lady and the ball to a boy. Next to the house, she made a banana tree and a horse-shoe. She said:

"The horse was running so fast that it lost its shoe. The horse was scared because it is seeing something. I think it is a ghost. The horse belongs to a man. The lady in the house takes the bananas. It's her tree."

The next series of cases under discussion deals with more specific emotional and social problems.

A 6 year old boy was sent to us because he presented a conduct behavior problem. His mother had deserted him shortly after his birth and the boy had spent most of his life in an orphanage. When the father remarried, Eddie was taken back into the family. However, he failed to adjust.

His plastic creation (Fig. 46a) shows a number of small and large clay lumps in upright positions. When questioned about his creation, he told us that they are supposed to be mothers and children. The large piece of plasticine on top of the stem is the good mother. We are certain that this boy was trying to express his problem of his poorly regulated family life. Interestingly enough, no fathers were included.

A most instructive case, because it shows several stages of emotional evolution, was that of John, 9 years old. John had been exposed to all sorts of

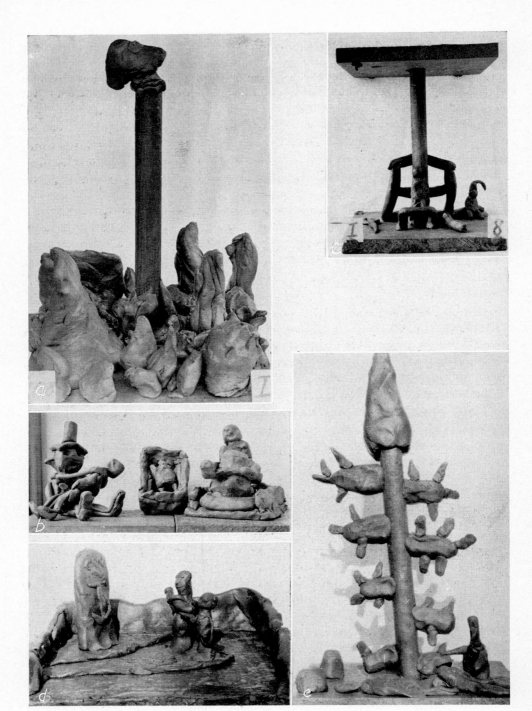

FIG. 46. Photographs of clay modeling.

FIG. 46a (*top, left*). Mother and Children, by Edward W.
FIG. 46b (*center, left*). Father and Son, by John W.
FIG. 46c (*top, right*). House, by John W.
FIG. 46d (*bottom, left*). Cemetery, by Jack W.
FIG. 46e (*bottom, right*). Lovers Near a Tree, by Isabelle W.

sexual scenes, not only between his parents but also intimate scenes between his mother and other men. When placed with a home-placing agency he did not seem to understand how to adjust to parent substitutes or to other children. On the ward he was hard to care for in the group. His behavior towards the other children consisted either in repeated attempts to see their genitals or in aimless aggression. He swore and in general used foul language with many sexual implications. He was given extensive individual therapy, partly to keep him from disturbing the other children.

John's first creation in plastic work was a human figure with an attached penis. With a small piece of cloth he covered the penis and said, "This is my mother with bloomers on." Next to the "mother" he placed a "father" also with a penis. He drew pictures of his parents, each with a penis. When we gave him puppets to play with instead of handling them like the rest of the children, he put what he called the "father doll" on top of the "mother doll," both puppets facing each other. John would then pretend that he was asleep. Suddenly he would wake up, spank both dolls, saying, "You dirty dogs! What are you doing again?" He would then deposit both puppets into a wastepaper basket and gleefully tell the examiner that both were in the toilet, urinating at each other. These activities were repeated over and over again in many similar patterns.

After a few weeks these activities stopped. John would become very irritated and abusive if anyone mentioned the word "mother." His next cycle of experimentation dealt primarily with aggression. He would make one man after another. These men were always carrying large guns. After a duration of two weeks John entered into the third stage of changing behavior. He began to make fathers. Next to these fathers John would place little boys (Fig. 46b). One picture shows a father holding a son in his arms; the other shows a father playing "piggy-back" with his son. Whereas John's behavior towards his various clay, paper and puppet mothers had been very abusive and aggressive, he now would speak about the father in most affectionate terms. Every visiting day he would find another excuse for his father's failure to visit him. Either his father was sick, or had to go away on business, or had been in an automobile smash-up, and so on.

A month or so later, John began to build houses and showed no signs of sexual preoccupation. He produced more than fifteen of such creations. His houses always looked more or less alike. A second armature base would provide a roof. Pieces of cloth constituted the walls. The occupants of these houses were always Casper, the hero of our puppet shows, and Casper's mother and his father. Interestingly enough, Casper's mother would always occupy the center of the room. Casper either would be sleeping or eating. The father would play a minor role in the family set-up. While John experimented with clay houses, his verbalization underwent a great change. He would revert to infantile behaviorism and talk "baby-talk." Whereas formerly his behavior

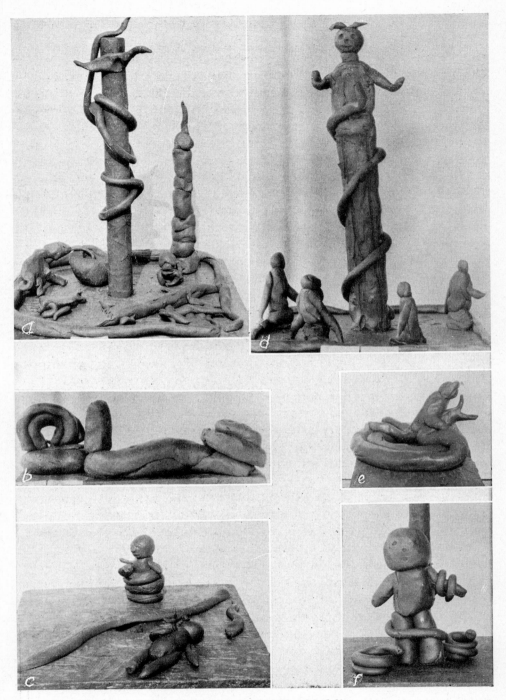

FIG. 47. Photographs of Clay Modeling.

FIG. 47a *(top, left)*. Jungles and Animals, by May.

FIG. 47b *(center, left)*. Snakes and Wagon Wheel, by Amelia.

FIG. 47c *(bottom, left)*. Snakes Punishing a Crime, by Lambert.

FIG. 47d *(top, right)*. Snakes Biting a Man, by Louis.

FIG. 47e *(center, right)*. Man Killing a Snake, by Raymond.

FIG. 47f *(bottom, right)*. Lady Snake Charmer, by Thomas.

had been quite boisterous, he now showed signs of insecurity and fears of annihilation which clearly manifested themselves in his reactions to the puppet shows. Instead of speaking in terms of the puppets, he himself became the central figure of the show. He would tell us that a bad man was going to kill him, that the giant would carry him away, that the witch would destroy him or that a dog would eat him up. This stage very clearly shows how insecure and bewildered John felt in connection with his own home situation and the task of making the readjustment which lay ahead of him. His clay work, together with his verbalizations, made it comparatively easy to apply proper psychotherapy.

The next case is that of Jack, an 11 year old boy who had difficulties in adjusting in the family. Jack was a middle one of nine siblings of domineering and unaffectionate parents. He held his father responsible for the large family and openly resented and hated his brothers and sisters. He would steal and get into street brawls for which his father would become very abusive towards him, beating him severely. He, as well as others of his siblings, were long known to school authorities and other social agencies for their asocial, aggressive behavior. On the ward, Jack would invariably come to blows with the other children and also break down in tears at very slight provocations.

His plastic creation (Fig. 46d) shows a cemetery with a tombstone in front of which stand Casper, his mother, and a sibling. This sibling belongs to Casper's step-father. From the story Jack told us, we learned that Casper's good father is buried there. Casper has a step-father but he is not as good to him as his real father was. When Casper was small, his real father played with him, gave him money and took him out for good times. The step-father, however, is very cruel to Casper. Later on in the story, the step-father is killed by a Japanese for apparently no good reason. His creation might indicate that this boy is attempting to solve the problem of a large family of unhappy children, and fantasies his father as a good father with only one child. The step-father represents Jack's relationship to his real father.

Problems arising during adolescence are also well represented in creative plastic work. A 13 year old girl, Isabelle, made a creation (Fig. 46e) showing a girl sleeping beneath a tree. Her lover stands nearby with outstretched arms. The girl dreams that the boy is asking her to marry him. When she awakens, the boy immediately proposes and "they lived happily ever after." Apparently, this girl had accepted her feminine role in life.

We cared for a 14 year old girl, May, who came to us with a history of severe premenstrual cramps. Because of inadequate enlightenment, menstruation came to her as a physical and mental shock. As a consequence, she ran away from home. When she came to us she was in a bewildered, hysterical state with many fantasies expressing her anxiety. In clay class she created a jungle scene (Fig. 47a) full of wild, aggressive animals. An Indian totem pole with phallic characteristics stands in one corner. The child said she would not live in such a place because there is nothing to eat, no place to sleep and there are continuous threats of annihilation.

In comparing the creations of the two adolescent girls, the first one seems to be satisfied to take her place in the world as a woman. Her clay work points toward anticipation of marriage and the establishment of a family. The second girl, however, is apparently confused and bewildered. Her creation shows a world full of aggression, hostility and danger, a world from which she tries to escape by running away.

Let us now reconsider the case of 6 year old Abram, whose creation (Fig. 44c) has already been shown in connection with body image models.

Abram was brought to us by his father with the complaint that the boy was neglected since the sick mother was unable to care for him. Abram was a very sickly child. He suffered from asthmatic attacks. Most of his body was covered with eczema. The asthmatic attacks and the itching of the skin kept him awake many nights, thereby disturbing the sleep of his parents; also on account of this they had been very abusive to the child and punished him physically. Two years previously he began to stammer, which seemed to be a reaction to the unaffectionate and impatient care at home. Abram was very shy and withdrawn on the ward and, at first, made very poor contact.

Towards the end of his stay with us, he made a clay model which he called Casper. As mentioned before, Casper is the hero of our puppet shows with whom the children readily identify themselves. Next to Casper, Abram placed a snake and told us the following story:

"Casper sleeps. The snake comes and bites him in the leg. Casper wakes up. He kills the snake and eats her up. The snake comes alive in Casper's stomach and crawls out from Casper's behind. The snake eats Casper. Then a truck comes and runs over the snake. Casper wakes up. He takes a knife and cuts the snake open. Then he crawls out and calls an ambulance. The snake is taken to the hospital and Casper goes home."

From the stories Abram told us about the puppet shows he had seen, we gained some insight into the meaning of the snake in his story. Once Abram told us that Casper's mother is run over by a truck, taken to a hospital and put away in a dark room. We surmise that in his clay creation, the snake represents the bad, aggressive parents. Abram's reaction to the situation is counter aggression carried however only to a certain point. The aggressor is not killed but after punishment is given a chance to recuperate. Abram reverses his home situation. He knows that his parents are glad to have him away from the home. In the story the snake is hospitalized and Casper is able to live at home in peace.

The introduction of the snake into the last case brings us to a special topic. The snake seems to play a very important role in the fantasy life of the children. At least 25 per cent of all the finished models include a snake in some manner. This constant reappearance of the snake in the clay work can be explained partly as follows: The rolled cylinder constitutes the first basic, elementary form the child masters once he has reached the stage of object representation. By rolling a piece of clay with his hands, an oblong, snake-like object is the inevitable result. This explanation covers only the formal aspect but not the emotional contents which point toward a diversified use of one symbol. Some of the snakes made by our children seem also to be phallic symbols. The creation by a 7 year old girl, Amelia, shows a snake and a wagon wheel (Fig. 47b). Amelia pushed the tail of the snake into the center of the wagon wheel saying "Now the wheel is closed."

In the case of Abram, the snake seems to represent the aggressive parents. Very often the snake appears not only as an aggressive animal but also as an animal that punishes. In most of these cases, the snake punishes a man who has either taken money, from another man or killed another man. The creation of a 13 year old boy, Lambert, shows a man with a dagger through his chest (Fig. 47c). A snake is coiled around the murderer. Lambert calls this snake the mother snake. The father snake is placed in a diagonal position between the murderer and the murdered man. Near the dead man is a baby snake. Lambert gave the following story:

"This man here (rear) killed that man (front) so the mother snake kills him. The snake is killing him so he tried to get away from the snake. The big father snake (diagonal) is waiting. In case the man gets away he can grab him. This little snake is going over to see the dead man to see if he is still alive. The men had a fight about money. One man had more money than the other. While this man wasn't thinking, the other one pulled a knife and killed him. The snake there was watching. The snake saw him when he killed the man. The snake don't know that he killed the man. The man walked where the snake was so the snake jumped on him and killed him."

In the creation of Louis, an 11 year old boy (Fig. 47d), an old man is killed by a snake because—

"the man gives the snake no food to eat. That's the reason the snake wants to kill him. The four men try to stop the snake by trying to pull it off. The man on top feels sad because the snake is going to kill him."

Fights between men and snakes were depicted by Raymond, a 13 year old boy (Fig. 47e). There were also creations where the snake is tame and not at all aggressive to humans (Fig. 47f) which shows a "lady snake charmer" made by Thomas, a 12 year old boy.

In anthropology and mythology, according to James G. Hassal, "the serpent has been given many qualities and has been worshipped because of them." These qualities include "wisdom, the power of healing, guardianship and protection, paternity, fertility and hostility." Barbara Renz points out that changing interpretations about life, nature and the world, which influenced religions and cults, have pushed the snake back from the high position it had occupied. By reversing values and interpretations, good snake gods were turned into bad demons. For instance, "schachan" in the Babylonian language, means the life-giving snake god. The Jews reversed this word to "nachasch" which means the bad devil-snake in the story of Adam and Eve. In other words, different times and different races have used the snake as a symbol for different contents. The snake as a healing agent is known from the figure of Aesculapius. The punishing snake is best represented in the well known "Laocoon" group, now in the Vatican. The snake

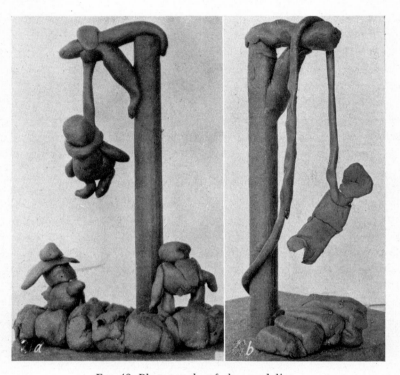

FIG. 48. Photographs of clay modeling.
FIG. 48a (*left*). Hangman's Scene, by Anthony. FIG. 48b (*right*). Executed Kidnapper, by Sol.

as the giver of life appears in the story of the brazen serpent in the desert as told in the twenty-first chapter of Numbers. The story of Adam and Eve does not need further comment. G. B. Lessing in the second chapter of his study on "Laocoon" points toward the snake as a symbol of adultery. Sigmund Freud, in his *Interpretation of Dreams,* states that the snake is a particularly important symbol for the phallus. This brief summary might be sufficient to guard us against any hasty interpretation of snakes created by children. In each case an individual study should be made as to what the snake represents.[8]

_____

[8] For further examples of the snake in graphic art, see Fig. 39a and accompanying discussion of Hyman; also Fig. 41a and accompanying discussion of Luther.

The aggression of the small child is individual and direct. With progressing maturity the child learns to subdue his own aggressiveness and to acknowledge socially accepted forms of aggressiveness, such as incarceration and execution. Therefore, a number of our children's creations in a clay work deal with executions, especially with hangings (Fig. 48). The children seem to choose hanging scenes because the armature as such seems to invite the creation of gallows. Secondly, killing by choking is much more obvious to the child than destruction by electricity, for instance. Hanging scenes also provide very interesting experimentations with gravity. Once the body is strung up it can be swung back and forth like a pendulum.

Since all the children work in groups, all the inherent benefits of group therapy apply also to our group work in clay class. While working in a group, it occasionally happens that one child may be influenced by the creation or motility pattern of another child. In all such cases the creation of the first is merely a stimulus for the others. The children modify the original creation according to their mental and motility development and their emotional needs. Objects or characters are added or deleted, so that the finished product even though suggested by another child is essentially an individual creation.

In summarizing our observations, we find that when a child works with plastic material, a definite intention to create specific objects is not always present. The activities based upon motor patterns may lead to forms suggesting definite objects which may be elaborated with secondary intent. When a plastic object is created it is not merely considered as an image with more or less similarity to the object, but it is also endowed with function. This function might be a passive one and the object might be merely played with. It might also take over the role of aggressiveness; its creator may indicate that it talks and acts. In this way, the plastic figure becomes an object of importance in the child's life. The child is given a chance to "create" his conception of the world in a visible and tangible form. Consequently, these activities constitute a real emotional release for the child.

Plastic material is an excellent medium for motility expression of children. It has the advantage over graphic creative work in that the movements of both hands are coordinated and active. Plastic material constitutes a suitable outlet for aggression, counteraggression, destruction, and construction. It has specific possibilities in helping children solve problems such as body posture and body function, especially in relation to genital and anal regions. It serves as a medium through which the child expresses problems of his own in relation to his body, to the family and to society. The child can be easily brought to an insight into his self created symbols, thereby gaining access to the social reality.

~ 15 ~

PUPPET SHOWS AS A PSYCHOTHERAPEUTIC METHOD[1]

PUPPET plays and puppet classes have proved to be a particularly effective psychotherapeutic method for use with a large number of problem children who need an opportunity freely to express their aggressive tendencies, their anxiety and their feelings of guilt, and to clarify their relationship to their mother, father and siblings, and the world about them. Puppet activities have special advantages due partly to the fact that they are natural group activities which can be added to all the other ward activities and any indicated individual therapy. The puppet plays are especially adapted to allow for free expression of infantile aggression, and to encourage a facile identification with the puppet characters. Puppet plays are especially suitable for dealing with the problems of children. Fundamental problems in the psychology of the child center about frustration, aggression and anxiety of the child; the child's fear of the aggression of its parents, siblings, or the outside world; and the child's love relationship with its parent and siblings.[2] These problems are, of course, intimately interwoven.

The puppet plays have proved to be an excellent way to express these problems, since the symbolic characters can give a free expression of aggression without causing fear and anxiety in children; they can also give a free expression of love. The latter should by no means be overlooked. There seems to have been a trend in child psychology to emphasize the aggressive, destructive and negative tendencies in children in their relationship to their parents and to neglect the equally strong loving, constructive and positive tendencies. Puppet plays for children can and always should be presented so as to emphasize the positive tendencies and they should always end with a happy or constructive solution.

The puppets which we have used were hand puppets; they are more direct in their action, more convincing in their movements, and capable of more direct aggression than string puppets. The hero of our puppet plays has been Casper. Originally a product of German folklore, he is identical with the

---

[1] Reprinted in part from Bender, Lauretta and Woltmann, Adolf G.: The Use of Puppet Shows as a Psychotherapeutic Method for Behavior Problems in Children, *American Journal of Orthopsychiatry, 6:341-353, 1936;* and Woltmann, Adolf G.: *Children's Reactions to Social Situations as Expressed in Responses to Hand Puppet Show* (unpublished lecture).

[2] See Bender, Lauretta: *The Treatment of Aggression; Genesis of Hostility in Children;* and *Anxiety in Disturbed Children.*

English Punch, the Italian Punchinello, the French Guignol, the Russian Petrushka, and the Turkish Karagoez. They all trace their ancestry back to the oldest known comedian entertainer. From the beginning of theatrical activity in India, through the Greek and Roman stage, up to the present, the type of the comedian entertainer has persisted, although somewhat modified in dress and concept. The symbol of the comedian was a phallus which modified by Christian influence has been reduced to a mere stick. The stick belongs to a character like Casper. It is the symbol of aggressiveness, of fertility and an excellent medium for settling an argument in a way that appeals to primitive people and children.

From the Middle Ages till now in Germany, Casper has been the ideal and the hero of the masses. He spoke their language, he portrayed their natural desires, he fought their battles. His "lust for life," his abundant vitality, his aggressiveness and his humor appealed to them. Heavily taxed by their sovereigns, pressed by lack of money and ungratified wants, constantly fearful of the police and judicial authorities, they turned to him. Casper would show them how to outwit a policeman, how to make a fool out of the judge, how to give the slip even to death and devils. He takes their troubles and in his way shows how to solve them. They had the satisfaction of seeing symbolically that there was such a thing as justice, that there was a figure representing them who could have his way and get away with it. He was a product of folklore, endowed with all the hopes, wants and philosophy of the creative masses.

In other words, Casper was the symbol of the ordinary man, aggressive when attacked, who likes his food and drinks, who curses and swears when necessary, who has a keen sense of humor. Most of the time this humor is rough but harmless and not insulting.

The character of Casper, his tradition and his history, have qualified him to play the role of hero in our children's ward. Of course he was changed and considerably Americanized, but he has remained true to the concepts and characteristics that have kept him immortal for centuries. In all of our work, Casper has played the same role. He is active, curious, sociable and uninhibited; he is immune to any real harm and in the end he finds the solution to his problems. At the same time his appearance and his name are sufficiently different from those of the average American child so that he is an impersonal character. His nonmasculine clothes seem to make it easy for even the girls to identify themselves with him, at least partially, although it must be admitted that the girls' problems have probably not been adequately handled.

Hand puppet play is at its best when the audience takes an active part in the performance by making suggestions, giving advice and warning of threatening danger. Casper's disregard of the advice and of the warnings of impending danger up to the very last moment provides great excitement and suspense until the happy ending restores the balance and lets the audience relax. Of all the devices invented by mankind for dramatic entertainment such as the opera, the theater and the movies, the hand puppet show is the only one which not only permits but forces the onlooker to participate. The children have been greatly benefited by this. Instead of merely taking in everything quietly, they can immediately release their emotional feelings physically by jumping up and down, shaking their fists, and expressing their desires and dislikes verbally and thus helping Casper to find the proper solutions.

Although the puppet plays are often very dramatic and provide great dangers for Casper, real anxiety seldom appears in the children who watch the show. The comic element which is the basis for the puppet play may be partly responsible for this. Besides, the life of puppets cannot be endangered because they have no life of their own. This carefree feeling toward the puppet and his doings makes it possible for children especially to enjoy such a show completely.

Casper and most of the other characters, as well as many of our most successful plays were not created or even modified by any studied psychiatric influence. They are the outgrowth of folklore. We have learned by careful observation and detailed study of the children's reactions and attitudes that puppets are especially well adapted to child psychology with its need for free expression of aggression, for free identification of the child with the puppet characters, and for the projection of the child's problems into the play. Casper has therefore gone about his business in a manner best known to himself and determined only by the centuries of human experience that have led to the creation of his specific personality; the children have participated and benefited, and we have sat by and observed.

We have learned, for instance, that every successful character whether it be an animal character like the alligator, a fantastic one like the witch, or a realistic one like the policeman, becomes identified by the child either with himself, with his mother or father or some feature of some one of them, or possibly with a sibling. Even sibling identifications are in part identification with the child himself. Such things are learned by observing the children at the time of a show, or by hearing what they have to say afterwards either in groups, in response to questionnaires, or in individual interviews with the psychiatrist or the puppeteers. We found that the puppeteers tend to play a special role in the ward life of the children, since the children identify the puppeteers not only with the characters they play, but as the makers of the puppets and, therefore, as the solvers of problems. Yet at the same time the puppeteers do not represent authority and discipline in the same way that the ward physicians sometimes must.

Folklore reveals how closely puppets are identified with the unconscious life. They have been used throughout the ages not only for entertainment but for religious, social and political propaganda and satire. An old Indian legend relates that the god Shiva fell in love with one of the puppets his wife played with and desired her so much that he brought her to life. There is another tale to the effect that during one of his travels, the Chinese King, Mu-Wang (1001-951 B.C.), met an actor who put on a puppet show before his court. His puppets were able to move their eyes and acted in such a natural manner that the king took them for actual human beings. He thought they were flirting with his wife and the ladies of the court, and ordered that the puppet player should be executed. The puppet player saved his life by taking his puppets apart, thus proving to the king that they were merely creatures of wood, leather and glue, painted in various colors.

In our experience one of the most successful plays, both for the purpose of allowing the children free expression of their emotions and of enabling the psychiatrist to get an insight into their problems, has been a play which the puppet unit had formerly used successfully for entertainment. It is called *Casper in Africa.*

Casper is traveling, and finds himself in a new country. He is very hungry and looks for food. He finds bananas growing on a tree, and takes one but puts it down for a minute and turns his back. A monkey comes out and snatches the banana. Casper turns about, is surprised to find the banana gone, but gets another and this too is similarly taken by the monkey, unseen by Casper. This is repeated many times. The children tell Casper that the monkey is taking the bananas, and advise him to get his stick. Then there is a frequently repeated play with the stick and the banana between the monkey and Casper. First, Casper knocks the monkey down with the stick and while he goes for the banana, the monkey gets the stick and knocks Casper down. Finally, they have a wholehearted fight and in the end Casper asks the children if he shouldn't let the monkey be his friend so he can help him get food. The children readily acquiesce and Casper names the monkey Charlie.

Charlie wanders off and Casper finds a treasure for his mother, a feather broom, and lays it down; an alligator comes in and swallows it. When Casper returns and finds the broom missing, he blames Charlie, although the children defend Charlie. Charlie comes in and Casper beats him. Then the alligator comes and tries to eat them both. The children advise Casper to get his stick, and Casper and Charlie try to hit the alligator. There is again considerable repetition of the hitting and biting until the alligator is killed by Charlie. Then while Casper is resting from his labors, two native cannibals come on the scene and carry on some native dances and speeches. When they see Casper they try to kill him and he is advised by the children to get his stick and call Charlie, and again there are frequent repetitions in which one or the other is about to win until Charlie again saves Casper from the natives.

This story seems to represent most of the infantile problems. The child immediately identifies himself with Casper. Casper here represents the infant starting out in a new world. He is first and forever hungry. As in all the plays, he is eager, searching, curious, freely expressing his wants; active, responding to his inner needs, without feelings of guilt or anxiety; only wanting what he wants and determined to get it. He is aggressive if necessary, he is bound to succeed and he cannot be hurt, and after each adventure he is always ready for the next. He is reasonably brave, but does not hesitate to run away when it is advisable. He also has a strong sense of his own superiority and no feelings of inferiority because there is always help at hand when

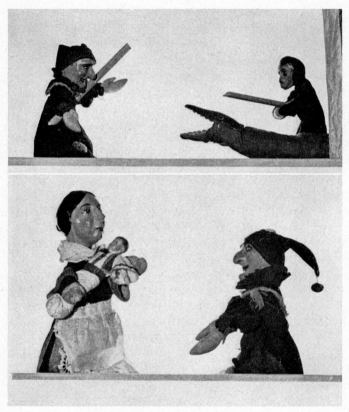

Fig. 49. Photographs of puppets.
Fig. 49a. (*top*) Casper and the Alligator and the Monkey.
Fig. 49b. (*bottom*) The Mother and the Baby and Casper.

he himself is too weak for any situation. In other words, Casper represents all that the child himself would like to be.

Casper represents something of the "ego ideal" in the Freudian psychoanalytic sense. He may also be compared with the "persona" or "mask" of Jung, signifying a person's ideal of himself, in the social situation or in relation to other persons. Of course, at best, any of these characters or the concepts which they denote are incomplete and represent only a part of a living personality. For example, Casper himself has much agility in adapting himself in different plays to different demands upon him. Certainly, different children project into him different personality qualities.

Occasionally it appears that some children give to Casper the significance of a sexual symbol. One little girl, age 10 years, whose chief problem was a sexual one stimulated by a sexually perverted father and only partially inhibited by the conventional morality of a boarding home, said that Casper was a good boy because his face was not red from rubbing, and that Casper married the monkey, and the monkey was bad because he stole a banana. Careful analysis showed that she identified herself pretty completely with the monkey and felt that he was a very guilty character, while Casper was good because his face showed no signs of masturbation. However, this type of interpretation is not the usual one. Most of the children agree that of all the characters they would only want to be Casper because he is the best one or because he always comes out all right or because he killed the alligator or because he made friends with Charlie, etc.

In his wanderings Casper first comes upon the monkey. In all of Casper's experiences with the monkey, it is clear that the monkey is dearly beloved by most of the children. Next to Casper, he is the favorite. A certain amount of fighting may occur between Casper and the monkey, but in the fights the two should be pretty well matched. If Casper gets too rough or aggressive with the monkey, the children complain and tell him not to hurt the monkey. The children know that his name is Charlie from the beginning and they insist on that name at all times, even in one play where the monkey temporarily is a girl in disguise. They say that they like Charlie because he can do what he likes, he can climb trees and steal bananas and run all around the forest, because he is Casper's friend and gets Casper food to eat and saves Casper's life and because he is funny. They think it is an advantage for a girl to be turned into a monkey for a while because she can climb trees without tearing her skirts, she can beg for food, she can talk to strange men, she can stay in the forest all night, she can fight, she can hit people on the head with sticks and run away, while as a girl she could not do any of these things. The children seem to favor the monkey because he can do what he likes and he is good to Casper, which means that the monkey can react to all his animal impulses without feelings of guilt. In other words, the monkey represents that part of the child's own personality which is defined by Freud as the *id*. However, the children agree that they would not want to be a monkey for very long, because a monkey might get caught and locked up in a cage, or put in the zoo or get shot. These of course represent external dangers which produce the emotion of fear but not feelings of guilt or anxiety. The children like Charlie because he can do what he wants without being bad.

After Casper and the monkey become friends and Casper is well fed, his next adventure is to meet the crocodile. The meeting is at first indirect. Casper finds a treasure that he is going to take home to his mother, but the crocodile gets it and eats it up. Casper blames Charlie and hits him in spite of the children's protestations. The crocodile comes to eat Casper. The monkey comes to the rescue and the crocodile is satisfactorily killed.

Each step of this must be repeated many times. Repetition is a very important feature in child psychology. It probably represents the natural primitive rhythm of life with which the child is experimenting until finally the proper solution for each new situation is reached.

In the first scene of this play Casper and the monkey have many little fights until with the help of the children they come to the solution that they are friends. In the second scene, Casper and the monkey fight with the alligator; sometimes in the confusion they fight each other until it is settled that the alligator is the mutual enemy and he is killed. He must even appear dead several times and come to life and be killed again. The repetitions are, of course, never real repetitions; there are always slight variations. This same feature is seen in all children's activities: play, drawings, early speech, games, sports, learning, etc. The alligator is the child's most primitive enemy because he represents oral aggression, oral aggression both by the child and against him. The alligator, therefore, produces both anxiety and fear in the child. Casper is safe only when the alligator is killed.

The greatest amount of excitement is shown in reaction to the alligator. Of all the hundreds of children who have seen our shows, the only ones who showed excessive fear or anxiety were three small children with very severe neurotic reactions. They had to be removed from the show because of anxiety and fear caused by the alligator. They said that the alligator was bad because he bites Casper and eats him up. The older children agree, too, that Casper always is right in killing the alligator because he bites too much, because he is always hungry and because he wants to eat everybody. That he also represents the child's own oral aggression is shown by such phrases as "I don't like him, he eats me up myself," and by the excited response of a child while the alligator is swallowing the broom, "Eat it up for me."

In several of the other plays, the alligator significantly belongs to the witch. We find that the witch represents the bad mother and we must suppose the bad mother is that part of the mother who wants to destroy the child because of his oral aggression, or the mother who denies the child the full satisfaction of his oral desires, or that part of one's own self which denies the full satisfaction of one's oral desires and punishes one's self for oral aggression.

However, now that Casper has made friends with the monkey and has satisfied his hunger and killed the alligator, he lies down to sleep and during his sleep two natives or cannibals come out and carry on mysterious talk and dancing rituals.

These cannibals can well represent the infant's primitive concept of his parents. The attitude of both Casper and the child towards these cannibals is definitely ambivalent. There are the usual repetitions of fights between the cannibals and Casper and the monkey. The implied fear is that the cannibals will eat up Casper and Charlie if they do not protect themselves with sticks, which they do to the best of their ability. It is thus seen that in this play all of the child's most primitive problems are dealt with. The child may identify himself in part with every character and may project some part of his problems into each one.

We also find that the child who has a special emotional problem will later retell the story in a modified form to conform with his own problem. A 9 year old boy who was under observation for an emotional reaction after killing a 4 year old girl with a stone and burying her body in the forest, retold the story as follows: "Casper killed the alligator with a stone and buried it in the forest." Several weeks later, when his own psychic mechanisms were trying to help him forget his own experience, he related this story differently. He left out the scene in which the alligator was killed and even when reminded he denied that there was any alligator in the story.

Several other puppet plays have other additional characters. There is Casper's good mother and also the witch, which as we have already stated, is identified by the child with the bad features in his relationship to his mother, or to the "bad mother." There is a policeman which in one play is Casper's father. There is also the wicked giant and the magician who appear to be identified with the bad features of the father or the "bad father." There is a little girl who plays different roles as Casper's sibling, as the feminine features of himself or as the image of his mother in the girl he wants to marry. With these various characters in mind any number of new plays can be written to present different emotional problems. These can be presented very realistically or with various amounts of fantasy and symbolism.

A puppet play called *Rock-a-bye Baby*[3] was written by us to present the problem of sibling rivalry. It is a realistic play but is helped out at a critical point by the use of a symbolic character, the witch.

Casper is 5 years old and enjoys getting all the attention possible from his mother. He likes to have her play "choo-choo train" with him and to have her wash him and unbutton his pants and to baby him. Now the time has come when she tells him he must not be too rough with her and that he should learn to help himself because she has another baby inside herself which will come soon. His father who is a policeman tells Casper he must grow up now and not be a baby any longer. Casper does not want a new baby in the house. But the baby comes and Casper finds that it needs most of his mother's attention and that he, Casper, must be quiet most of the time. The baby is left for him to look after and he declares that he does not like it, that it is de-

[3] For the complete script of *Rock-a-bye Baby* see: Woltmann, Adolf G.: *The Use of Puppetry as a Projective Method,* Anderson, Harry H. and Anderson, Gladys L., Eds., 1951.

priving him of his mother's love and care, that it wets itself and is a dirty brat, etc. Casper asks the children what he should do.

Many of them agree with him that the baby is no good and Casper gets a good deal of hearty advice to throw the baby out the window, to drown it or throw it in the furnace, etc. Some of the children cry out that it is a sweet baby and Casper should like it. The children get very excited and sometimes there are open fist fights among them, especially if there happen to be two siblings in the group.

However, in response to Casper's expressed wish to be rid of the baby, the old witch comes. Casper tells the witch with the help or objections of the children, that he does not like his baby sister and wishes the witch would carry it away. The witch offers to help him by making the milk turn sour which Casper then gives to the baby and makes it sick. When the mother comes back she carries the baby off to the hospital in obvious distress. Then Casper is sorry. He tells the children that he did not want to make his mother feel bad, that she must love the baby as she loves him, and maybe she will not love him any more if anything happens to the baby, and that he would not like anyone to give him sour milk, etc. Then Casper sends for the witch to come back. But she refuses to help him by making the baby better since she can only do bad things to children. So Casper gets his stick and beats the witch until she is dead and her power is also dead.

The mother comes home with a well baby but remembers to bring some ice cream for Casper, too. Thus she expresses her love for him. The father comes in and tells Casper that he hopes that Casper will now be the little policeman that will protect his sister from harm. All the family dance together to show how much they love each other and how happy they all are together.

Even those children who do not obviously have a problem specifically related to sibling rivalry, or those who do not have younger siblings, are intensely interested in this play. Those who do have specific problems due to recently born siblings may show evidences of some acute anxiety. Such children are inclined to retell the story in a distorted way.

There was one 8 year old boy who had shown an unusual amount of infantile behavior following the birth of a brother three years earlier when the mother had clearly transferred most of her love to the younger child and had openly threatened to institutionalize the older child because she felt that she could care for only one child at a time. This boy said the mean old witch nearly killed the baby; that Casper loved the baby but the witch wanted it to die and that Casper saved the baby's life by killing the witch. He thus expressed how clearly he felt that the "bad mother" was to blame for the situation and that she wanted to be rid of her child. The boy identified himself strongly with the baby and it was possible to explain this to him. It is clear that many of the children identify themselves with the new baby and thus show their motive for not wanting to the kill the baby. This was most marked in those children whose mothers were most aggressive towards them.

Another little boy of 5 had shown very marked aggression in trying to kill three younger siblings ever since the arrival of the first when he was 18 months old. He was a child who had suffered from celiac disease which had inhibited his growth so that two of his younger siblings were already larger than he. His jealousy of his siblings was open and dramatic. He said that he hated his mother for having so many children and that he hated the little brothers and sister and wanted them to die. He tried to push them out of the window, he put them on their tricycles and tried to push them in the streets in front of cars, he threw out their food; he tried to choke them. He admitted these things when he first came to the hospital, but showed no aggressive tendencies toward the children on the ward and in a few days would no longer discuss his feelings towards his siblings and his mother.

He enjoyed the show about Casper in Africa enormously, especially the parts which showed the alligator and the monkey. He seemed equally delighted when the alligator was showing his aggressiveness and when the monkey was fighting the alligator. He liked to play with the alligator himself, and said: "Now I can eat everybody up." He pretended that another puppet was his mother, and ate her up. He showed the greatest excitement when the monkey was killing the alligator. He would jump up and down and shout, "Bing zoom; hit him Charlie; look out; run this way; hit him for me." He said he would like to be the monkey because a monkey was big and could steal bananas and hit the alligator. He also liked the fight between Casper and the cannibals. He said if he were Casper he would kill them: he would take a knife and cut their heads off.

On the other hand, when *Rock-a-bye Baby* was shown he became very subdued, inattentive and sullen. He did not want to watch it. When the mother rushed off to the hospital with the baby, he said, "It is dead." Afterwards, he was unwilling to discuss the play, and started crying. He began to play with some small toys and after a few minutes it was observed that he had arranged a funeral with a baby in a wagon, and finally buried the baby. He was asked later, with a group of children, what he would have done if Casper had called him instead of the witch and he said, "I would have been the witch and I would have killed the baby." When asked what a witch would do if she had babies of her own he said, "She would kill them with hocus-pocus." This child saw the presentation of this play several times and thus obtained considerable emotional release until it was possible to discuss the problem more frankly with him. He was finally asked if he would like a new home with a new mother and new brothers and sisters and he said "yes." When asked what kind of brothers and sisters he wanted, he said, "All big ones," and then, after a minute's thought, added, "It will be all right to have little ones, too. I won't do anything to them." He made a good adjustment to a boarding home where he was the only child, and did well in the public schools. He also received thyroid which seemed to stimulate his growth.

Other plays are produced with more complicated mechanisms and more symbolism and fantasy. One such play is entitled *How Casper Becomes a Man*.

In this play Casper is a lonely orphan without a mother, father or home. He comes to a house where there is a woman who is obviously the good mother symbol and he asks if he can work there. The woman agrees after some pleading on the part of Casper. Whenever he is left alone to do his work he is always caught daydreaming about his mother, for which the woman scolds him and calls him a sissy.

At noontime the woman calls her son Bill, who is a bad boy. Bill scolds his mother and orders her about and bullies Casper. Casper asks the children if a child should treat his mother that way and if he deserves such a good mother. The children revile Bill throughout the play. Bill reads in the paper that a beautiful girl is lost in the forest and he decides to go and find her and marry her so that he can have a wife as well as a mother to look after him and wait on him. Casper wants to go too, but Bill refuses his company, saying Casper is a sissy who talks about his mother all the time and who has to do house work. Bill's mother admonishes Bill to be good and kind to everyone, but he sneers at this. Casper decides to follow secretly.

Bill goes into the forest and sees a little monkey who asks him for food. Bill hits the monkey and drives it away, complaining that he has come into the forest to find a beautiful girl and not an ugly monkey. The children scold him, call him bad names and tell him not to mistreat Charlie. (It is to be remembered in this connection that the monkey is always the children's friend Charlie.) Then Bill runs into the alligator and has a hard time to escape being eaten by him. He cries loudly for his mother and shows that in time of trouble he is not so very brave himself.

Then he meets the witch and is defiant towards her; he even hits her. She declares that he is a very bad boy and she will turn him into stone and throw him to the bottom of the river, where he will never find the girl or see his mother again. The witch asks the children about this and they heartily agree. Bill is turned to stone with a hocus-pocus by the witch, and thrown to the bottom of the river with a loud thud. Then Casper appears in the forest and the monkey comes out and asks for something to eat and Casper shares what he has. The monkey tells Casper that if he ever needs help to call "Charlie" and the monkey will help him. Casper meets the alligator and is frightened and considers calling for Charlie but decides he wants to prove he is not a sissy, and fights and kills the alligator himself. The children encourage him in this.

Then he meets the witch, and the witch threatens to turn him into stone because he killed her alligator, but the children say, "No, No," and tell Casper to get his stick and to call for Charlie. Casper succeeds in killing the witch himself. He decides to call Charlie to help him find the beautiful girl and when he does, the beautiful girl herself appears and says that she was turned into the monkey by the witch and released when Casper killed the witch. Casper says she is as beautiful as his own mother who is dead, and asks the children if he should marry her. They agree. Then there is a loving dance with many kisses.

This play was planned for the homeless child who goes through life seeking an ideal mother and never able to adjust in boarding home or institution; but it has proved equally valuable for many other types of problems.

One example can be given which will show what the reaction is when the child is preoccupied emotionally with some very specific problem different even from that for which the play was planned. Calvin was a 6 year old boy who came to us with his 5 year old sister Mary. The history showed that both of them had been misused sexually by the father, especially the little sister Mary who, as a result, had become completely preoccupied by problems of genital sexuality. She also tried to carry on her sex play with her brother who was older and brighter. Calvin was very much bewildered by the whole situation but showed a deep aversion to his father and a deep devotion to his sister. When he was asked about this play he retold it as follows: "And the father got killed and the witch turned the father into stone. Because he was going to find the little girl and the monkey. Then he put a banana there and Charlie come and took the banana and we said Charlie took it. Then he put another banana and he got a stick and hit Charlie and then he asked the children if he should feed Charlie and the children said yes and he gave Charlie a banana and he ate it. The father wanted to marry her first but Casper got the girl and married her and was kind to her. Casper was reading the paper and the father hit him just for that. I think Casper should have the girl because I like him best, because when somebody wants to kill him, he kills them first. So he is good. (What is the worst thing that the father could do to her?) Maybe the father would marry the girl and make her do every kind of hard work; maybe he could get a gun and shoot her or maybe he could get a stick and kill her. (Suppose he might do the same thing to her that your father did to Mary?) Yes, he might hurt her that way and she would die."

Of course Calvin has combined this play with Casper in Africa, which he had also seen. The child's reaction to the play shows clearly how the children project their own problems. He identifies himself with Casper, his sister with the beautiful girl, and his father with the bad character. He also expresses the infantile idea that a sexual assault is bad because it may kill his sister. He looks upon the sexual assault as an act of aggression. It shows that the child believes that the father wants to marry in order to make his wife work but that if Casper—that is, the boy himself—could marry the girl he would be kind to her and kiss her.

The value of the use of puppet shows to determine the psychological mechanisms in the emotional problems of children and for psychotherapeutic purposes are summarized by the response of this 6 year old child. We note how the child says he would like to be Casper because Casper was good and killed only those people who wanted to kill him. He clearly expresses his opinion in the omnipotence of aggression as a threat against the child and as his justified defense. He expresses his disapproval of a cruel father who hits a child for insufficient reasons and makes a little girl do hard work, threatening to hit and kill her. His concepts about sex problems are apparently far from clear and are understood in terms of aggression. He believes that the good people will be kind to those they love and they will kiss them. He shows his fascination with the repetitious play between Casper and Charlie with the banana and the stick, when the children encourage Casper not to hit the monkey so that they can become friends in order to find food together, thus acknowledging the right of the animal drives to be satisfied. It is also shown how this boy gives expression to most of the problems which concern him.

The puppet shows readily lend themselves to identification processes with all sorts of characters, and permit the children to project problems into the characters and live them out. By the impersonal nature of the characters with which they identify themselves, and the fact that they are puppets and cannot really be hurt, the children are able to express their emotions freely and without guilt, anxiety or apprehension. The only danger of punishment for free expression is from another child in the audience who may have an opinion different from his. As a matter of fact, it is undoubtedly one of the greatest therapeutic factors that the child learns that other children about him are experiencing the same feelings that he is, and he is aided and abetted in the expression of his aggressive tendencies by the fact that all the others about him are loudly acclaiming his own feelings.

It will be noted that Calvin's recitation of the play includes the statements that Casper asked the children if the monkey should be allowed to eat the banana and the children said, yes. In retelling a play a child always emphasizes the part which the children take. Such experiences as this lead us to conclude that group therapy is not only more economical but is actually in some ways more satisfactory than individual treatment, at least in the release of primitive emotional responses and in relieving anxiety and guilt. There is also clear evidence in our puppet experiences of the tendency of children in all of their activities to depend upon rhythmic repetitions, with slight variation, that finally reach a solution. It is particularly important to realize that it is not enough for the children to be allowed a free expression of their aggressive tendencies but that there should always be a solution of the problem with equally free expressions of love.

An extremely revealing device for the study of children's reaction to the puppet show is what we called the "half-show." The children see only half of a show, that is, they see the presentation of a problem which in true dramatic fashion becomes involved and demands a solution. When the conflict is at its height, the show is stopped with the promise that it will be continued at some other time. For example, in *Rock-a-bye Baby,* the show is stopped when the mother in distress has taken the sick baby to the hospital. Then the group of children or an individual child are asked what should happen. What kind of a solution would they propose to the problems of the puppets? This technique of course is not possible unless the children have been accustomed to seeing puppet shows regularly and have complete confidence that Casper always wins,[4] and that the problem which the play presents can have a satisfactory solution. This confidence comes from the experience of having seen sufficient shows which have solved problems satisfactorily. We have found however that one or two children who have never before seen one of the puppet shows can be added to a group of children and see a half-show which stops at a critical point without these children suffering from the overwhelming anxiety that might otherwise take place, just because they are a part of the group, and the other children around them are evidently undisturbed and freely express their confidence that things will turn out all right.

The various solutions proposed by the children are colored by their own problems and their ability to understand intellectually and emotionally the implications contained in the particular problems. Each child tries to unravel the conflict in terms of his own constitution, background, emotional involvement, and general level of maturity and he is not aware of the fact that he is talking about himself. By discussing the puppets and their problems, he is spared the embarrassment of talking about himself. In this fashion relevant material, disclosing the dynamics of the child's personality development and deviations and attempts to work through his own conflicts, is easily brought to the surface. Children who block in individual interviews talk freely in a group discussion. Once the ice has been broken the transition from the problems of the puppets to the child's own conflicts can readily be made. The mere fact that children are encouraged to seek solutions to problems has a great therapeutic effect because it makes clear to a youngster that his own particular maladjustment is not a hopeless mess leading to doom and complete failure, and that there are not one but several possible solutions. Such insights are encouraging and further the process of re-education.

Casper and the Devil[5] was a play which was developed in order to consider many of the problems of asocial behavior that concern children referred to the children's ward from schools or social agencies. It also dealt with some of the fantasy material that is a part of the culture, especially the religious culture, with moral and ethical values, that concern the children. This is also

---

[4] The factor of the continuity of a character which can be trusted to solve problems satisfactorily is very important in fantasy experiences of children. It contributes to the positive values of the comics with characters like Superman, and of radio programs, with The Lone Ranger.

See Bender, Lauretta: *The Psychology of Children's Reading and the Comics.*

[5] See discussion of Billy's reaction to *Casper and the Devil,* p. 101.

See also Yarnell, Helen: *Fire Setting in Children* for fantasy material concerning the devil and its symbolic meaning.

a particularly good play to illustrate the use of the half-show and the subsequent group discussion of the children.

As the curtain opens Casper's father, after having had his breakfast, says goodbye to Casper's mother. There is a great deal of affection and many demonstrations of love between this married couple and also an understanding of their child, Casper. The mother is very proud of the father's good working record and expresses the wish that Casper will follow in his father's footsteps. The father laughingly reassures her that Casper is still a child. The father leaves for work. The mother awakens Casper and tells him that it is time for him to get up and go to school. While the mother is busy off stage Casper appears on the stage and informs the children that he is sick and tired of going to school. In his opinion a 12 year old boy has gone to school long enough and that it is now time for him to lead the life of an adult. Casper plans to play hookey; he runs off, leaving his school books at home. The mother finds the books and goes to the school with them, thinking Casper was in such a hurry that he forgot to take them along.

The second act shows a street scene with Casper alone on the stage. He is dissatisfied with playing hookey; he has no money and therefore cannot go to the movies. He curses his own lack of foresight. It would have been very easy for him to take a dime out of his mother's purse. A girl appears on the stage telling the children that she is excused from school for the day because she received a good mark in arithmetic, that her mother gave her a dime and that now she is going to the movies. Casper tries to take away the money from the girl by force but is defeated by her. He feels very lonesome and sends the whole world to the devil. No sooner said than the devil appears and offers his services to Casper. In order to avoid the penalties for playing hookey (not being promoted in school and punishment at home) Casper succumbs to the devil's wily promises. Casper can now wish for whatever he likes. After much deliberation Casper decides to become a king.

The third act finds Casper dressed in royal robes in a castle. Having all the power in the world he can now create a social order completely to his liking. He asks the children to help him in making proper decisions. Casper remembers that when he played hookey he had no money to go to the movies. He therefore declares that from now on all children will be admitted free of charge to every movie house in the kingdom. His second order proclaims that candy stores and ice cream parlors are to be available to the children whenever they so desire. Determined to change the existing social order and to make the world happy for the child, Casper now asks the children what should be done with schools, teachers, hospitals, doctors, nurses, policemen and parents. The children's decisions which Casper orders to be carried out result in revolution. Casper's life is threatened. Crying for help, the devil appears prepared to take Casper down to hell but at the crucial moment he is rescued by his parents.

After presenting this show to a group of children 5 to 15 years of age, from various racial and cultural backgrounds and suffering from a diversified number of problems, the following reactions were noted: When Casper asks the children whether to play hookey or not, on all occasions the majority of our audience encourage him to do so; the older children especially are very much in favor of this idea. Since Casper has never played hookey before he asks the audience for suggestions. Some of the children tell him to go to Coney Island, others tell him to spend the day in the movies or to go to the park. They assure Casper of their loyalty and promise not to "squeal" on him. On one occasion a 6 year old boy told Casper's mother when she finds Casper's books that Casper planned to play hookey. The group immediately out-shouted the boy and told the mother, "Don't believe him. He is nuts." "He don't know what he is saying." Some of the older boys quickly moved up front in order to beat up the child and only the quick protective gesture of a nearby nurse saved him.

When Casper appears at the beginning of the second act the children quickly tell him that his mother went to school to bring him his books. Casper does not know what to do. Very often the older children offer a way out by suggesting to Casper that he tell his mother that she either went to the wrong school or that Casper was transferred to a different school, therefore she could not find him.

Casper asks the children what they think about "swiping" money. Almost all of them tell him that it is bad; it would be right only if Casper would go out the next day shining shoes and return the money. To Casper's remark "I don't think that taking only 10 cents is stealing," the children tell him that even the taking of a penny is stealing, and that stealing is bad and therefore one should not steal.

The incident with the little girl becomes very interesting when judged by the children's reactions. Both boys and girls are on Casper's side. In many cases the children do not want to believe that the girl has been excused from school. They tell Casper "Don't you believe her; she is lying. She is playing hookey too. She stole the dime from her mother. Take it away from her." When Casper is defeated by the girl he has the children's sympathy on his side.

The appearance of the devil and his wheedling suggestions are viewed with a feeling of ambivalence. Some of the children warn Casper: "Get a stick and kill the devil. He is going to kill you. He is going to eat you." "Don't listen to him. He is telling you a lie. Don't go with him. He'll cook you in a pot and eat you up." "He is going to stick you with his pitchfork and take you down to hell. You are going to get burned." Other children encourage Casper by saying, "Go ahead, Casper, and try it." "Go with him, take all you can and then run away." When Casper is allowed to make a wish most of the younger children tell him to wish for a dime and go to the movies.

The third act is the most important in this play because it offers an opportunity to our children to create a world of their own making. When we first presented this show we received inadequate and childish responses due to the fact that most of our children did not grasp quickly enough the opportunities which such self-government offered. The first two wishes about free movies and candy are therefore suggested by Casper and not by the children. By permitting Casper first to suggest ways and means whereby conditions could be changed, the children, when confronted with the problems of disposing of schools and teachers, etc. were ready to participate.

The children's reactions towards schools and teachers were not complimentary. In all instances Casper was told that school houses should be burned or torn down. To Casper's question, "What shall I do with the school teachers?" the following answers were elicited: "Kick them out on their ears." "Fire them!" "Cut their throats!" "Kill them!" "Shoot them!" The police department fared no better. Casper was told to take all the "cops" to the East River and drown them; to shoot all of them down with a machine gun. On one occasion these answers were responsible for a fist fight among older boys. It so happened that one child's father was a policeman. This boy got up and shouted, "Stop saying that to Casper. You are insulting my old man." Most of the children are equally hostile toward the hospital, the doctors and the nurses. The smaller children are in favor of having the hospitals destroyed and the doctors killed. Very often the older children remind the rest of the audience that such a procedure would not be a very wise one. As one child said to the group, "Don't kill all the doctors. You might get sick in the middle of the night and then there is nobody to help you." Other children try to compromise by telling Casper, "Kill Dr. X. just a little bit."

Casper is also told to leave the parents alone. Some of the children even threaten him openly if he dares be aggressive towards parents or siblings. Only a few cases of intense hatred of parents or siblings have been noted. A 10 year old boy told Casper, "Go ahead and kill my mother. Kill her." Another boy of a similar age who was being treated for sibling rivalry exclaimed, "Go ahead and kill the baby." Most children inform Casper that he should give good jobs and automobiles to their fathers and money and jewelry to their mothers. The revolution is just as much of a shock to the children as it is to Casper. They tell him that they believe in him and still think he is a good king.

We draw the curtain when Casper is knocked unconscious by the devil. The problem for the children to solve is: "What will happen to Casper? Will the devil take him down to hell or can Casper be saved?" The following stories are solutions offered by some of the children:

> Harry (age 12): "I think the cops that was around the house will come in and they are going to capture the devil and kill the devil and then they are going to go home and tell his mother all about the adventure he was in and that the cops surrounded the devil and killed him. (*How did the cops get down to hell?*) They were playing craps so they heard him down there so

they thought he went down to hell so they went down after him. Then they saw Casper but they didn't see the devil. Then they went home and teachers hollered at Casper and the cops beat up Casper and the teachers and doctors operated on Casper's head to see if he was dumb. Then his mother was looking for him and his father and mother took his books to school."

In spite of the fact that Casper gave orders that all policemen be killed it was a policeman who rescued him. Casper's return from hell to the every-day world was not a very pleasant one. As some kind of retaliation for his previous behavior the school teacher hollers at him, the policemen beat him up and the doctors operate on him. In other words, this boy identifies himself with Casper and projects his own experiences into the story, namely, maladjustment in school, contact with the police department and his present hospitalization. No mention is made of Casper's (read Harry's) emotional responses and reactions.

Peter (age 14): "Casper becomes a bad king because then the devil is helping him. He will tell the kids, 'Don't go to school.' He will give the money to go to the show. He will say to them, 'If you go to school, you will go to school for nothing because they will leave you back like the devil told me.' The devil will make him do bad things and he will get in trouble and all the people will hate him. Maybe the people will put him in jail and he says, 'What bad things I did!'   He says to himself, 'If I am going to be good and tell the kids to go to school' and then the devil finds out and the devil says, 'If you do one more of those things, I am going to kill you.' He tells the kids to go to school and he tells them not to worry about it and he will get the devil and then he went home to his mother and father. (*Does Casper get punished for killing the devil?*) No, he tells the people that he thought the devil was helping and all the people understand and they forgive him. And he tells the little girl, 'I am sorry,' because he started up and the little girl hit him and then he falls in love with her. Then they married. That's all."

This story is of interest because it reveals a conflict. Casper regrets his foolish orders. He tries to repair the damage but is prevented from doing so by the devil. Casper has the choice of either conforming to the wishes of society and suffering the threats of the devil or giving free expression to his desires and having society against him. Casper would rather suffer than be an outcast of society. He overcomes his evil impulses and asks society for forgiveness. The conflict is resolved and a happy ending is the result. In other words, this boy also projects his own situation into the conclusions of the story.

Violet B. (age 8): (*What would you do if you were queen?*) "I'd be a good queen. I'd give the poor people some money and give them something to eat and build a house and tables and chairs. (*What would you do to boys and girls that are bad?*) I would make them good. I would get Casper to make them good. (*Who is Casper?*) The king. (*Is he married to you?*) Yes, we were married last year ago. (*What would you do to little girls that are bad?*) Spank them all day and night until she became good. Then I would put her in a dark cellar for a couple of nights. (*What would you do to her hands?*) I would tie her hands and legs and put all wood around the windows. (*Supposing you were that little girl, would you like to be treated that way?*) Not unless I was bad. (*Is that the right way to treat a girl?*) Yes, that's bad. . . . Ask me some more questions. (*What questions do you want me to ask you?*) Will I treat my mother good? (*Will you?*) You bet."

Violet identifies herself partly with Casper. By marrying him she would share his power. The punishment that she would mete out to naughty little girls is described in such a realistic manner that it makes one believe that personal experiences are intermingled throughout the story. In general, Violet bears no grudge against the world. Since her problem was an emotional and not a social one, we get no further indications as to what she thinks about the society she lives in.

The children interpret these social situations in the light of their own experiences, and by their answers expose social or anti-social tendencies, show remorse, fear or anxiety and express their desire to be helped. In group discussions of a general nature, we ask the children what they think about playing hookey, stealing money, lying to their parents, what schools are good for, why children should go to school, what policemen are good for, are they needed and could we do without them. The children often complain that policemen spend too much time watching children and not enough time apprehending crooks and gangsters. One 10 year old boy expressed it thus: "It seems to be the cop's business to stick his nose into your business."

In discussing the various reasons the child might have for absenting himself from school and becoming a truant, some of the following responses revealed the children's point of view towards the school situation: "Sometimes the children don't do their homework and then when they go to school the next day they get hollered at." "Some children play hookey because they don't like their teacher." "Some children cannot do their work. It is too hard for them and then the other children laugh at them." "Some children have no money to buy books and they don't like to tell the teacher in front of the whole class." These remarks were gathered from a group of pre-adolescent girls who, in another part of this group discussion, suggested that it would be better if the children had to go to school only three days a week or if the school time were cut from eight years to four. One girl in this group had been sent to us for snatching pocketbooks out of baby carriages. She resented discussing *Casper and the Devil* with the rest of the group. When we came to the "snitching a dime out of the pocketbook" incident in the show, Mary became very much excited and shouted, "I don't know what stealing is and neither do the rest of the girls know it." Her hatred towards the school system was expressed in the following manner: "I feel like tearing down my school. I put it on fire once last year. If I could, I'd put it on fire again with my teacher in it. The school is too old and the teachers smell. They even stink on ice."

Through the medium of puppet shows, the child has ample opportunity to react to various emotional and social situations, and these shows stimulate participation which results in the revelation of the child's attitudes towards his conflicts and problems. Through the medium of the puppet speedier access is gained to interrelated problems of an emotional, social and economic nature. Children who respond inadequately to the direct method of questioning do not mind discussing these problems in the impersonal terms of puppets.

The puppet shows, as an experience in themselves, have a definite therapeutic value to the child, even if that is the whole of the experience. But it has been found that the show can also be used by the physician as excellent material for further discussion. It may be used in the same way that dream material is used; first, by simply asking the child to retell the story, and then by asking pertinent questions in terms of what Casper thinks and feels and does rather than in terms of what the child himself has done and thought and felt.

Besides this, however, we have organized puppet classes which are conducted by the puppeteers, in which the children are taught to make puppets, write their own puppet plays and produce them. These have all of the usual advantages of occupational therapy, dramatics and group activities. They have the additional advantage that they may be consciously used for psychotherapeutic purposes by directing the interest of the child toward the solution of his own emotional problems through the medium of the clay used to model the heads of the puppets, by drawing puppet characters, by witnessing or producing puppet plays or by the free discussions. In the course of these puppet classes the children are led to discuss the problems brought out in the puppet plays by responses to a questionnaire which is worked out with the help of the psychiatrist. These discussions on all sorts of vital social problems are often extremely illuminating. Again, we are convinced that the value of group discussions lies partly in the fact that the children discuss more freely in groups than they will alone. They often show that they are encouraged by the presence of other children with mutual experiences and they sometimes find it especially easy to discuss their problems with the puppeteer whom they have come to know as Uncle Casper and whom they undoubtedly identify closely with his handiwork "Casper" and, therefore, with their own best ideal of themselves.[6]

---

[6] See also Woltmann, Adolf G.: *Further Contributions on Puppet Plays as a Psychiatric Technique for Children.*

❧ 16 ❧

CREATIVE DANCE[1]

DANCE is the expression of human fantasy and emotion using as its medium the motility of the body passing through space and time. This process of formulation of movement concerns itself not only with the form and action of the joints and muscles, but also with the subjective concept of the body, and with the body as seen and interpreted by an observer.

The dancer's idea of his own body is fantasy based partly on reality and partly on his emotional and intellectual make-up. This can be called the "body image"[2] and must constantly be revised and re-established. Through experimentation it has to be brought in line with the form or body appearance which is seen by the observer. Since the dancing individual can never see his entire body exactly as it is seen by others, but can see only parts at any one time and never can see certain parts at all without the aid of a mirror, he must become conscious of his own body image and learn to visualize as well as to feel its form. He must also acquaint himself thoroughly with the fundamental structure of the human body, its physical make-up and function, in other words with its anatomy, physiology and mechanics as he studies them on his own body during his dance activity. How does he conceive the body image to look? What is its relation to his physical body? What is its relation to the body appearance? Does the concept of his body image change through the influence of different emotional states and fantasies? Does it change when he moves through space at varying speeds? Does it change when he takes different positions in relation to space?

Put the head of an individual in a different position in space and you have changed the world of that individual. The new born child cannot sit or stand. However it reacts to changes in the position of the head in relation to the body and also in relation to space. One may speak of righting reflexes and postural reflexes which are in connection either with the neck righting reflexes or with the labyrinthine postural and righting reflexes. There are also body righting reflexes acting upon the head. An asymmetrical stimulation of the body surface, for instance, influences the posture of the head. There are

---

[1] Prepared by Franziska Boas as an enlargement and consolidation of two articles: Bender, Lauretta and Boas, Franziska: Creative Dance in Therapy, *American Journal of Orthopsychiatry*, *11*:235-244, 1941; and Boas, Franziska: Psychological Aspects in the Practice and Teaching of Dancing. *Journal of Aesthetics and Art Criticism*, 2:3-20, 1941-42.

[2] Schilder, Paul: *Image and Appearance of the Human Body.*

also body righting reflexes acting upon the body, and optical righting reflexes. These reflexes are not always obvious in the human individual after infancy, unless there are lesions in the central nervous system.

Everything which disturbs or changes the relation of the individual to the vertical plane (gravitation) affects the motor mechanism of the entire body. The whole system of postures is fundamentally different when an individual is lying on the ground, or when he is standing. Even when one is standing upright the muscle tone is very different according to whether the head is turned forward or to the side. The whole distribution of tone changes with every change in the position of the head, as has been described by Magnus and de Kleijn, Goldstein, Hoff and Schilder. Voluntarily turning around the longitudinal axis in play or on command stimulates the semicircular canals and causes a great number of changes in postural responses in connection with the vestibular irritation. Such turning may also occur involuntarily under pathological conditions. Turning around the longitudinal axis and rolling on the floor have very different effects, since the tone when lying on the floor is changed by the body righting reflexes. There is a further change in the tone since the head has a different position in space.

Dance routines of the usual type are rhythmical motions which keep the individual in an upright position. In these many of the fundamental physiological activities are neglected, thereby limiting the possible variety of postural experiences. The child is constantly exploring his body and experimenting with its relation to space. It is of the greatest importance to allow him to continue in this without restriction. By observing this activity the instructor gains not only an evaluation of the pupil's physical co-ordination, but also insight into his thought processes and fantasies. Without such knowledge it is impossible to know what direction should be taken in teaching and what results may be expected.

Walking on all fours is a primitive impulse. The posture itself probably brings with it a great number of primitive attitudes.[3] Jumping also is among the fundamental primitive impulses. It is obvious that important psychological changes take place when physiological mechanisms of this type are brought into play in the dance. Physiological considerations have been particularly stressed, but it should not be forgotten that they will be especially effective when combined with the well known forces of rhythmical movement, and particularly when all of these factors are integrated purposefully with the fantasy life. Bouncing, rolling, crawling, swaying and swinging, climbing, jumping, turning and tumbling are all elemental experiences in the dance. Both the child and the adult must learn to place their bodies in unaccustomed positions and to engage in unaccustomed movements. All types of variations of these movements should be encouraged. This experiment in

---

[3] Compare with Hrdlicka, Ales: *Children Who Run On All Fours.*

placing the body in strange positions in relation to space and then resolving those positions into habitual postures, establishes assurance of the reality of a fundamental body image. It is by these experiments that the child learns the mechanics of his body and explores space and time. Through motility the individual learns to establish and expand the concepts of his body image, thereby gaining confidence in the reality and control of his body.

Most adults have to be led back to this experience since it forces them to take into account their physical body and re-awakens in them the consciousness of their fundamental body image which may have been repressed. The following is an example of the relation between movement of this type and the concept of the body image. A schizophrenic boy in the children's ward when asked to turn a back somersault obeyed the initial impulse but stopped each time before his back touched the floor and before his legs went over his head, to ask, "What will happen to me? Will I die?" He had to watch someone else a few times before he dared do it at all, and then at first had to be helped. After that he repeated it with all signs of enjoyment and pleasure. The action of turning upside down and putting his legs over his head brought out his insecurity in space and his uneasiness about the reality of his body (unclear body image due to pathological processes) and made him fear that he would lose his body during the activity. The normal individual, through self-observation, knows that distortions and activity, short of injury, do not affect the limbs in their relation to each other or the body in its entirety.

With respect to posture the following points are important: Whether the body is in the horizontal, vertical or inclined plane; what relation the position of the head has to the posture of the body; whether the body is or is not supported on one surface; and the rotation and speed of rotation of the head on the body.

Fundamental changes in postural motility take place in relation to these four possibilities. It must be borne in mind that with these variations in motility, significant modifications in sensory experiences are also perceived. The orientation of a body is completely altered when various postural and righting reflexes occur. Changes in one's perception of the outside world take place while turning around the longitudinal axis. One also gets a completely different picture of one's own body. The vestibular irritation leads to important changes in the vasovegetative system. The man who is lying down and the man who is standing up are different in their somatic reactions. There are also important changes in mood and in total personality, depending upon the posture.

In applying these data to the modern creative dance in its use with children, it is to be expected that they will have an important influence on the psychological attitudes of the child. During experimentation with activities of this sort the teacher may play the active role and change the position into a passive one for the pupil by exaggerating it through his intervention. For instance, with the small child who tries to turn a forward somersault but cannot move beyond the point where his head and feet are still on the floor, the teacher may step in and turn him over. Or with an older child who wishes to stand on his own shoulders, the teacher may pick him up by the legs until only his hands still touch the floor. To be passively set in motion, to be carried, swung, turned and rolled by an adult is important to the child in extending his confidence beyond himself. In the case of the larger child and the adult where these things are not possible without the aid of rings or bars which can bear the person's weight, the pupil must be urged to use his ingenuity with occasional steadying help from the instructor. The degree of proficiency and the number of positions that will be taken depend on the age of the pupil, his muscular co-ordination, and on his fears and anxieties.

If children at a very early age are allowed to experiment with rhythmic movement without interference, they may outgrow this type of movement as mere self indulgence and chaotic behavior, and be able later to use the control and body quality gained through such experimentation for the formulation of fantasies. This type of investigation and learning should be allowed to continue to the point of saturation, when the disorganized movements and chaotic themes begin to form themselves into rhythmic repetitions and recognizable fantasies. In other words, the primitive animal-like impulses may furnish material for sublimation into an art expression. During the transition period it will be necessary for the teacher to direct the movement toward a subconscious sublimation. Those children who have been blocked in the process of sublimation will either remain in the infantile type of movement or will develop gestures which are escape patterns:

David was a very bright 10 year old boy who was entirely unable to control his infantile exhibitionism. His usual reaction to the stimulus of the dance situation was to run wildly through the room, roll on the floor, turn somersaults and crawl in such a manner that he was always in the path of the other children. Then he would lie with his head under a chair and suck his thumb. At home he used the narrow hallway to practice climbing up to the ceiling like an Alpine climber in a crevice. Occasionally in the dance hour he showed excellent co-ordination and rhythm far beyond that of the other children. These were only flashes of the sublimated form. Here was a case of overindulgence in chaotic movement. From the point of view of dance the block had occurred during the process of the formulation of motility impulses into sublimated dance material.

The natural dynamic development of the primitive type of motility is the process beginning with the simplest crawling and rolling and continuing through complicated somersaults, headstands, handsprings, back-bends, cartwheels, to passive and finally active suspensions in jumps and leaps from various heights. Thereby the pupil investigates all space levels, the ground, middle space and the air, always with the attraction to depth.

When the attraction to height begins to take shape one is confronted with the problems and rhythms of walking, running, leaping and their variants, also with the relation of the torso, arms, head and neck to the lower extremities. Whereas in the first type of movement the body remained comparatively compact, arms and legs serving as supporting points, now there are only the legs as supports. The control of the body begins to fall apart; many movable segments have to be co-ordinated—ankles, knees, hips, pelvis, chest, shoulders, elbows, wrists, fingers, neck and head.

In every movement made in the standing position there is the question of balance of these parts on a narrow base which becomes even narrower when one foot is raised from the floor. It is therefore necessary to re-establish the body as an entity, such as it was during the action on the floor.

This can be accomplished if the pupil becomes sufficiently sensitive to feel himself surrounded by a "zone of extension of the body image."[4] The peripheral nerve endings all over the body act as antennae to receive impulses from without when another object approaches. They transmit to the body image the necessity of change in contour or change in its place in space, beyond its zone of extension.

This is a concept similar to that which applies to sculpture. Open spaces are not holes but are substance which is enclosed or surrounded by the solid parts of the sculptured form. The figure holds the space within its form. In sculpture there are single space forms which are made visible, while in dance there is a constant re-grouping and re-establishing of space forms which accompany the moving figure.

It is therefore not enough merely to train the muscles and joints in physical co-ordination and strength. The sensitivity of the entire body and the mind must be trained to register "the body image with its zone of extension." This has to become automatic so that the body will react by itself in movement related to any given situation. The mind must look on and choose that which is most relevant to the idea to be expressed. It is like a dream in which the dreamer actively participates and at the same time watches the action from without. The difference is that the dreamer is a helpless bystander, while the dancer can direct and plan his actions.

The relationship of the single dancer to other dancers in the group must also be considered. There is the problem of the direct contact between two bodies, as for instance, when one is riding on the back of another. The form and duration of contact may determine the difference between frankly sexual and only latently sexual contacts. The contact will in turn be dependent upon factors of aggressiveness and body curiosity.

---

[4] Schilder, Paul: *Image and Appearance of the Human Body*, p. 211.

All these actions take place not only in a specific group but also in a definite space which determines the movement of the single individual. In dancing the relation to space is psychological not merely in the ordinary sense. Optic impressions have a definite influence on postural reactions. The situation will be fundamentally altered by the optic experience of the moving bodies of the other dancer or dancers which invite imitations and reactions. In addition to the physiological problems there is also the relationship to the leader of the group, as well as the relations of the members of the group to one another. These will depend upon the life history of the individual participants.

Dance is fundamentally a social art. Except for the young child and isolated instances of older persons, the average individual does not dance for or by himself. There is always some other person present either as a participant or onlooker. Dance is basically narcissistic.[5] If there is no outside observer there is always the self as audience. Part of the pleasure of dance is in the self-observation of changes in one's body image and appearance. In group dance each dancer tries to influence others by these changes and is in turn affected by the changes he sees in them. Aside from the relation of individuals to each other there is also the relation to space and to the objects which divide and fill space. In group dance these space shapes are constantly changing and the speed at which they move varies. If there is a direct meeting of individuals the relation between the two determines whether there is antagonism or co-operation. The character of the individuals determines whether one will change and follow, whether both will change to create new movement, or whether neither will change. If neither changes there may be active conflict, turning away to continue the individual pattern, or spacial co-ordination, i.e., movement through space in the same direction with unrelated tension, rhythm and gesture because of insistence on separate body movement patterns. The dancer must be extremely sensitive to be able to make use of each new space shape and body mass, as well as of the speed and rhythm at which they move and change.

The space in which the dancer moves is always three-dimensional. It is circumscribed by the four walls, three real, and one imaginary, the floor and the ceiling of the room in which he works. It is divided into three levels, high, middle and low, which are experienced by the individual as he passes from the floor through the standing position to the tip toes or to the jump. When moving from one place to another the dancer may pass through space from low to high in an inclined plane. When passing through all planes and taking into account all directions, front, diagonal, side and back, a spiral movement or a turn is created. These direction concepts are projections of the body direction, ventral, lateral, dorsal and diagonal, i.e., oblique, 45° between middle, ventral or dorsal, and the middle lateral, when the individual

---

[5] See Arnheim, Rudolf: *Psychology of the Dance.*

is in a standing position facing the imaginary front wall of the room. Such concepts are permanently fixed in space just as the body directions are permanently fixed within the body. However the relation of the body direction to the space direction is variable. For example, one of our children, Larry, because of unsatisfied curiosity as to what was behind curtains or in corners of the room and as to what the assistant was writing, suddenly began to walk quickly through the dance space from corner to corner, across the back of the room, around the sides and from wall to wall, always in straight lines, sometimes forwards and sometimes backwards.

Since space has volume it is also divided into smaller cubic forms depending on the distribution of groups of individuals and isolated individuals. These cubic forms shift and change shape as the dancers move. Different densities and tensions are created by these forms causing attraction or repulsion, and passage ways may be created which have a tendency to cause a desire to go from one place to another.

Recognizable rhythmic and dynamic patterns grow out of tension in the individual and tensions in the group or groups, as well as in the space forms that are created. Most of these patterns demand externalization in sound. Some require a rhythmic drum beat, others a mellow gong tone or a sharp cymbal crash. A musical accompaniment of the sounds related to the tension and movement has to be created.[6] The sounds emerging from percussion instruments in themselves have specific qualities which relate to space, time and tension. The drum bounces its listeners in space and creates a desire for rhythmic action. The cymbal softly played cuts space and spreads out in all directions horizontally. The gong fills space and suspends the hearer in it. Sharp sounds produce strong tension and penetrate space. Soft sounds produce weak tension and fill space. Regularly reproduced sounds produce repetition of movement and activate space. Crescendos produce increase in tension and fill space with activity. Decrescendos decrease tension and quiet the space. Accellerandos increase speed of movement and activate space. Retardandos decrease speed of movement and empty space of action. Sounds fill space with substance. If there is no sound, space has to be filled with the dancer's thoughts, emotions and fantasies. Without these, space would be empty, a vacuum.

The sounds which the dancer hears and the space forms and body appearances of the other dancers which he sees and feels, create in him specific reactions which manifest themselves in his movement patterns. A case in point is a modern dance dealing with the concept of forces under water. The accompaniment was gongs, cymbals and drums. The theme was the activation of two persons, conceived as bodies suspended in water, by the aggressive force of a central figure which disturbed the quiet of the space in which all

---

[6] See Boas, Franziska: *Notes on Percussion Accompaniment for the Dance.*

three were floating. The force and weight of the moving body created currents of motion in the space substance which carried the other bodies out of their original positions. Through repeated attacks and activity at great speed, the two figures were forced into conscious action to preserve their equilibrium. There resulted a transmission of power to the formerly passive forms. In dance human emotions must always be reckoned with. In this case the activity of the central figure created annoyance of unrest which resulted in concerted aggression against the disturbing force, driving it into passivity. From this situation the central figure emerged on an emotional level with the other figures so that the final solution could be a unification of effort.

Any arbitrary group of children moves in a world of everyday life experiences. Accordingly, they have resistances to primitive types of experience and it is necessary to overcome these inhibitions in order to allow for the breaking through of the deeper lying impulses of rhythmic action and dance. The use of percussion instruments is a decided help in provoking reactions and re-enforcing them when they start to appear. It is advisable to establish a basic metric beat on some instrument or to continue with a repetitious dynamic pattern. Sooner or later the pulse of the rhythm dominates the group and impels the children to rhythmic or dynamic movement. The influence of rhythmic sound very soon has a noticeable effect on the motility of the child since every sensory impression carries with it a command to specific action. It is possible that percussion instruments which seem to be felt all over the body, may have a particularly deep psychophysiological influence.

Helga was a child of high intelligence who had been constantly surrounded by adults. She had been taught extreme orderliness and cleanliness. She was told that she had no right to her own opinion because she was a child. Her fantasied stories had been criticized as falsehoods. At the age of 4 she had a bedtime ritual of carefully folding her clothes and holding a clean handkerchief in her hand. A year later she developed what seemed to be a fear of bed wetting which never actually occurred.

At 8 years she was very excitable and had facial tics. She was blocked in her fantasies. She considered herself unimaginative. She disliked playing with clay because she dirtied her hands or might spot her clothes. She thought that any person who liked her drawings or anything that she made was "crazy." She was easily distracted, asked irrelevant questions during class, had very little originality in movement when dancing with open eyes, but when dancing with closed eyes showed good co-ordination, grace and ease. She was fundamentally musical, imaginative, and rhythmically co-ordinated, but at that time was concerned with externals such as hair, clothes, fingernails. The clay figure which she modeled consisted of a child's head with curls and a hair ribbon; it had no arms and no body, but a dress with long legs was fastened directly to the head. Helga's most outstanding feature was her ability to dance freely when her eyes were closed. The externals which as a rule were her center of attention then became temporarily eliminated. A sensitivity toward her body which she usually disregarded became manifest. A psychological block was overbridged for a time. By using the closed eyes during dancing as one device she could have been guided towards a consciousness of inner values.

Another device used with Helga was persistent repetition of sound. The child responded to the continuous playing of drum rhythms, first with her usual distraction, asking questions, getting a drink, cleaning her hands, looking out of the window—then suddenly with 15 minutes of continuous dancing in the form of crawling, rolling, turning and arm and hip gestures. In response to continuous repetitious gong melodies, she gradually softened her tone of voice and muscle tension until on two occasions the complete relaxation of her emotional tension was expressed by her lying on the floor and falling asleep.

In 1940-41, the following experiment was undertaken on the children's ward of the Psychiatric Division of Bellevue Hospital: Groups of six to eight children 12 years old and younger and representing all types of behavior disorders and psychiatric problems were utilized. They included underprivileged children of New York City with a wide range of characteristics determined by race and environment. They were unselected except that boys between 6 and 12, or girls of the same age, or mixed group of boys and girls of 6 years or under, made up the separate groups. On some occasions these groupings were ignored.

Here are brief case histories of six children making up a group, with examples of their dance experiences:

Patsy, a 9 year old boy, could never accept the fact that he was not wanted by his inadequate and alcoholic parents. Although abused in his own home, he was miserable in the Catholic institution to which he was sent after frequent attempts at running away from home. In the Home he developed a severe anxiety state with numerous phobias reactive to his compulsive masturbation, and colored with religious lore.

Carrol, a 9 year old American Negro boy of almost unknown antecedents, lived with an aged couple variously referred to as grandparents or uncle and aunt. He had been exposed to most of the social traumas—gross abuse, neglect, poverty, alcoholism and sexual attacks. He displayed a distressing hysterical anxiety and believed, both when asleep and awake, that he was being chased by the devil. He could readily be thrown into a state of hysterical terror by the simple suggestion that the devil was behind him. Terror was associated with feelings of guilt for past sexual experiences, many of which were probably fantasied. He was capable of ecstatic as well as terrifying experiences but was apparently equally afraid of both.

Ralph was a 9 year old Puerto Rican Negro boy who was too wild for public schools. While hitching on a car he had fallen off and injured his head, and the question had been raised as to whether a brain injury did not account for his hyperkinesis. However, there were equally serious social factors. The father had deserted the family and the mother had moved from Puerto Rico to New York only two years before. Ralph had none of the supervision and help he needed in adjusting to a new social situation, as his mother worked away from home. His quick responsiveness to the training and socializing influences on the children's ward argued against any serious brain damage.

Fred, a dull 10 year old Italian boy, lived on the lower east side of New York City and was a member of a gang. He was caught stealing with the gang and was sent to the children's court. Because it was evident that he was the dullest, most passive and suggestible member of the gang he was sent to the children's ward for study. He had a vivid but confused fantasy life colored with the lore of the underworld.

Benjamin was a 5 year old boy from a boarding home, where he had been placed by one of the child-placing agencies. He was very bright but had been the source of a great deal of trouble in several boarding homes where he had lived. Abandoned by his mother when a baby, he had never stayed in any home long enough to feel he belonged to anyone, nor did he have the ability to make himself part of any home. For that matter, he did not seem to feel that he belonged to any social situation, either in a home or in a school, or among a group of children. His emotional reactions all seemed of the negative sort. He was always unhappy and at odds and even spoke of suicide or turning on the gas to kill others in the home. At best he was reckless in dangerous situations, such as entering traffic. What the child actually needed was the love and attention which neither his mother nor any substitute had ever given him.

Jerry was a bright 9 year old boy whose home had been made unhappy by a father who deserted, and a mother who could not carry the burden of supporting and caring for a large family. She was both too busy and unhappy to give Jerry anything but a sense of futility. Such children often find satisfaction and human warmth in schools. But in school, Jerry was doomed to failure because he had a severe reading disability in spite of being bright. He spent weeks away from school, living in an empty shack he had located. He was a precocious child, sadly aware of his problems and with an almost adult hopelessness in regard to any happy solution of them.

The group was dancing to the even, steady beat of the drum. Two boys sat in the corner weeping because they did not want to dance but wanted to go out of the room. Patsy, who always seemed to take the part of the negativistic group, supported them by beating against the door with his fists and feet and throwing his shoes at it. The two boys joined him and suddenly all three started to march in a circle, chanting: "We want to go home! We want to go home!" Their feet moved in time with the drum beat (Fig. 50a). When they were convinced by looking through the dance leader's purse that she had no key and could not let them out, Patsy began to work with the group and the other two sat quietly watching the dancing.

Ralph was always active. He was proficient at turning cartwheels and somersaults, and turning around his own axis. He had no fear unless he was

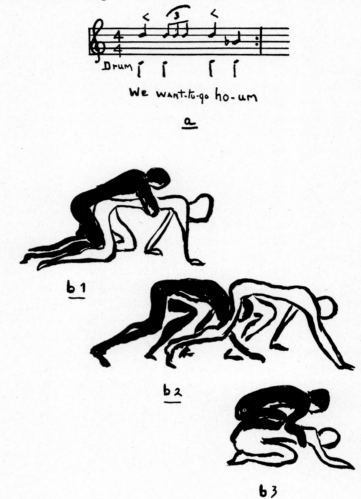

Fig. 50a. We want-to-go ho-um, music score.
Fig. 50b. Double Animal, dance positions of Carol.

being held or carried by someone. On this day, a steady pulse with a repetitious pattern was being beaten on the drum. The children were crawling and rolling on the floor. Ralph rolled over Carrol, grasping him around the neck. Carrol became frightened and, losing control of himself, attacked Ralph. Both became extremely upset and Carrol had to be taken from the room. The steady rhythm of the drum began again. Ralph gave himself up to an orgy of cartwheels and turns. When he fell to the floor, he continued his movement by rolling and turning somersaults without interruption for at least 10 minutes. When the class was dismissed Ralph stayed behind and, taking the drum, began to tell the story of *King Kong* which he had seen in the movies. He punctuated his words with drum beats and occasional explosive sounds and gestures of his whole body. When the next group of children came he participated in the work in a much less spectacular way.

The class was playing "Indians," dancing around in a circle to the steady beat of the drum. Fred decided to be the fire and sat in the center of the circle making hissing sounds and darting movements with his arms and hands. When the class left, Fred was asked to stay. His fire dance was praised and it was suggested that he repeat it and let the fire spread. The drum beat was resumed. He started his fire dance as before, sitting in the middle of the room, twisting his arms and legs and darting them out from his body. Gradually he began twisting and swaying more in his torso and the fire spread through the room with rolls and cartwheels. Fred became dizzy and tried to stop, but he must have felt the movement continuing for he said, "The house is going up." Following this, he rose from the floor, stretching up as far as he could until he was on his toes. Then he started to jump, always reaching up toward the ceiling. He became tired from the jumping, and rested. Suddenly he found a small toy pistol with wooden cartridges that one of the boys had hidden under a radiator and began shooting the doctor and the dance teacher. When they had been killed he danced a dance of triumph and then killed himself. His next game was to throw the cartridges at the wall and pretend he had blown up the building. He acted out very realistically and dramatically the collapsing of the walls and his being buried under the debris. He dug himself out again, only to place the cartridges between his toes and blow up his feet.

A gong was being played with slow, steady beats, producing a swinging tone. The children began to sway back and forth. Patsy who no longer resisted the work, began to swing his arms and legs. As the gong tone became more insistent and faster, Patsy turned slowly first to one side, then to the other, rising on his toes, then dropping his body onto the whole foot with knees bent. The gong beat increased in speed to a steady tremolo. He swung his arms more violently and turned very fast around his own axis, so lightly that his feet seemed to leave the ground.

The following notes on Carrol were taken over a period of about one month. On his first day in class when Ralph grasped him around the neck Carrol became terrified. He lost complete control of himself, screamed and kicked and tried to get at Ralph. He had to be held by the nurse who finally took him out of the room. Later he was brought back in a much quieter condition.

The group was playing at being animals. Several children began to ride on the teacher's back. Carrol was very much amused but did not take part. He played at being a buffalo and butted the children and the teacher. Then he tried to make a double animal by putting his arms around the waist of a crawling boy and crawling behind him (Fig. 50b).

Benjamin was a chicken attacking children. The chicken was killed by a child; it came alive and was killed again. Finally it was really "dead" and should be buried. The children "dug" a grave and "covered" him up. They all wanted to step on the "grave" and then left him. Carrol did not take part until Benjamin was buried. Then he crouched next to him, closed his eyes and performed a kind of sorcerer's dance. He had a slight vibration in his body and passed his hands back and forth over Benjamin's head and body. When the children came back he pushed them away. Finally he slid away of his own accord when the chicken decided to come alive again and attack.

Diary notation: Carrol made another double crawling animal, this time with his head between another boy's legs (Fig. 50b-2).

Diary notation: Today Carrol is more active. He tries cartwheels. He started a very good Indian skip. He is very self-conscious and must be coaxed into working. For the first time he really tried some of the stunts. He allowed the teacher to take him by the arms and swing him around parallel to the floor. He was extremely thrilled by the flying sensation when his feet left the ground. He kept urging the other boys to try it. He also jumped up and sat on the teacher's haunches, letting himself down to the ground backward until he could walk on his hands between the teacher's legs. It is characteristic of him that he works for short periods only. He sits quietly in a corner or on a bench between working periods and dreams. He knows he is dreaming but says he does not know what it is about. He has many impulses to start dancing but stops himself.

Diary notation: Carrol alone. An animal that "can walk through walls." He crawled around the room at the very edge, so that his body touched the walls at all times. The third time around he closed his eyes, dropped his head between his arms and felt the ground with his "fore paws" before moving ahead.

Sitting with his legs curled up under him: "Oh! I am sinking in the water, way down! Now I am down on the bottom." This was accompanied by a great many changes of facial expression; then he closed he eyes and lay down.

As a result of the cymbal sound, Carrol was an airplane. He landed in the water and became a hydroplane, moving on his abdomen, legs held quiet, the arms pulling him forward.

He was reminded of his "sorcerer's" dance. He asked for one of the boys to dance with, since he said he could not conceive an imaginary companion. While waiting for the other boy he played with the cymbal and listened to its undertone. He accompanies everything with facial expressions and sounds. Many expressions are like African masks.

Jerry came. The boys played lions; they were sleeping lions, dreaming. Carrol: "I am in a strait-jacket. I am wild." He lay perfectly still, arms at his sides making faces. He crawled around and then lay in the straight-jacket again, sleeping, dreaming. To Jerry: "You'd better watch out when I wake up. I'm wild." He began to talk of being a buffalo, then turned into a rooster. "I'm a rooster laying eggs in my nest. It is a very big nest." He climbed on Jerry's back and stayed there quietly while Jerry tried to crawl, protesting that he was no nest (Fig. 50b-3).

Jerry played the cymbal as Carrol lay on his back on the floor. He asked Jerry to hold the cymbal so close to his face that it was practically touching it. He lay still, listening and making faces. Suddenly he said: "Oh! where does that sound come from? I wonder where it is! I must find it." He looked at the teacher and smiled about his joke. Before this he had said the same thing after he had been dancing for some time to the sound of the drum. He is perfectly conscious of the origin of the sound, looks at the teacher to see whether she takes him seriously or knows he is playing.

"I am a monkey. See, I am climbing on you. You are a tree." With that he pretended to climb, holding on to the leader's clothes. He gave up very soon and lay down.

Carrol alternates activity with sitting or lying down with closed eyes, making faces and saying all kinds of things, sometimes snatches of stories, sometimes just sounds. He is full of fantasies, any one of which would be good dance material. He plays good rhythms on the instruments, not for noise, but for quality. His periods of activity are merely short fragments of his prolonged fantasies. The animal crawling throught the walls was continued for the longest period.

The atmosphere created by the repetition of sound and the quality of tone provokes movement reactions. It also causes group reactions which seem to force even the more difficult children into participation. The feeling of unreality also seems to be established since an aggressive activity is rarely carried to its realistic conclusion. If the rhythm is discontinued the group begins to fall apart. If one of the children takes the drum and plays there is a tendency for the dance activity to change into rivalry over the instrument. Only when a child is able to play well and steadily, will his accompaniment be tolerated by the other children. Sooner or later, however, they will demand their turns at the instrument. So far, the problem of having the children accompany themselves has not been solved, since playing the instruments is an attraction far greater than dancing.

The intensity of activity may be regulated through the use of the crescendo and accelerando or the diminuendo and retardando. Sometimes especially susceptible children will develop their own dynamics to the accompaniment of a steady quiet bass, or they may create all kinds of dramatic situations. The gong and cymbal may be used to quiet an especially unruly group and hold tensions at a soft or medium level. This is accomplished by playing a steady low tremolo. The crescendo of the cymbal may be used to heighten tensions to an intolerable point of suspense which is broken by a tremendous crash and muting of the cymbal. This leads to jumping or falling, usually accompanied by vocal outbursts. The gong may be used to create a swinging impulse which causes swaying of the entire body and leads to pendulum movements of the torso and arms and legs, finally to a feeling of suspension in which the child allows the body to be carried through space in curved sweeping lines, and to spin and turn.

Creative dance activity in children may also be released by using a circular formation with a rhythmic or dynamic activity such as skipping, leaping, running, and "Indian steps." Another method is to place the children on their backs on the floor and proceed with stunts. From these exercises the usual development is into animal fantasies with their characteristic movements of crawling on all fours, propelling the body across the floor without the use of the hands or feet, rolling over one another, jumping like frogs. Certain children prefer to retain their human character. This leads to dramatic dance games of shooting animals or of animals attacking humans, or horse and rider games.

From the activity on the floor the children begin to climb on one another, first on the backs of crawling children, then riding "piggy-back." Finally they attempt to ride on each other's shoulders or climb three high on one another's backs. There seems to be no consciousness of the necessity of a small child's climbing upon a larger one. Often a very large boy tries to ride on the shoulders of a very small boy. When this is frustrated through the interference of the leader or through failure of the experiment, there is usually a reaction of disinterest and a break in the continuity of group work. Soon the climbing activity is taken up again in relation to objects about the room, with the development of all kinds of jumps from various heights with different resulting fantasy activities, such as diving into water and swimming, animals jumping from trees onto people, etc. Also various jumps from the ground onto and over objects and each other are undertaken. These are soon combined with more complicated rhythms such as cartwheels and somersaults remembered from the work on the floor.

The children soon begin to feel the need of help in these more difficult activities and look to the leader for technical aid. Here, then, is the opening for the leader to place the children in unaccustomed positions in relation to space. They are encouraged to lie on their backs and are lifted by their feet so that they have to put their hands on the floor. They are then told to look between the legs of the leader and walk through on their hands. Their final position is lying flat on the abdomen. Usually the child is so astonished and pleased that this has to be repeated over and over. Or, the child jumps and sits on the haunches of the leader. Then, holding by his feet, he drops over backward and crawls through between the leader's legs. Or, the child lies on his back on the floor with his arms outstretched above his head. In this position he is swung around the leader who holds him by the hands and turns around his own axis. As the momentum increases, the feet leave the floor. This usually results in outbursts of pleasurable excitement and verbal descriptions of the sensations felt while "flying" through the air. Since all of these activities require two persons, often one or two of the stronger, more courageous children imitate the leader, and again the relation of child with child is established.

Usually in early dance training each individual is primarily concerned only with himself. The awareness of others creeps in very gradually. Then the dancer is concerned with preserving his own identity. He must slowly be led to the point where he will dare to have contact, to compete and to create with others.

The feeling of his own physical strength and the ability to control and direct it is a stage the dancer reaches after having freed himself from anxiety and fear over the dynamic violence of primitive motility and its associated emotions. For the dancer, anxiety and fear of dynamic movement spring from insecurity in the concept of his own body image and from resistance to consecutive changes in himself. Exploration of the dynamic power of movement brings to the fore instincts of self preservation, destructive and constructive drives and through their mastery brings about an understanding of these elements. In the case of successful sublimation it should lead to a feeling of security through a knowledge of the emotional sources underlying these drives, and therefore to their control. The Hindu and Balinese dance,[7] particularly that of men, is tremendous in the projection of controlled power. The difficulty in teaching this to present day adults in our civilization is the conventional rejection and fear of the "animal in man."

The ability to manipulate the body on the floor has to be learned. It is partly a technical problem; it is also a purposeful reversal to infantile movement. Often the greater part of this type of movement is resisted by the adult and even by the child because they have been taught at some time that such activity is not proper. In permitting this activity on the dance floor one block or resistance is removed and the path is open for acceptance of the psychological content through sublimation in dance form.

If, however, the person is still unable to enjoy this state of reversal, if he has learned technically to perform leaps and falls and rolls without experiencing pleasure, then a further block has been encountered. Such a person will reject this type of movement and will exclude it from his dance, or he will go through the external motions of technically controlled gestures but will avoid clarifying the content. An observer sensitive to movement forms, or a teacher who is aware of the psychological factors, will recognize in such a performance a substitution of form for content. Often a definite block becomes apparent again and again. Of course this may not be constant and the intended sublimation is able to assert itself for moments during an improvisation. However such blocks can be eliminated only by a therapeutic approach.

---

[7] Boas, Franziska (Editor): *The Function of the Dance in Human Society,* New York, Boas School, 1949.

This therapeutic approach must be handled from many angles. Physical and mental relaxation in movement, combined with the use of rhythm and sound accompaniment, provide one way. The use of drums, gongs, cymbals and rattles as accompaniment for the dance activity concentrate the pupil's attention on the rhythmic pattern and the quality of the atmosphere so that his attention is diverted from the actions of his physical body. The concentration on sound and the repetition of the same kind of sound activate the body in spite of itself; muscle tone and balance become more homogeneous and the fear of physical injury is lessened. The mind is freed from this particular worry and movement fantasy is set in motion.

This dissociation of mind and body exists to a high degree in some schizophrenic children. It appears to be a suspension, a complete physical balance in an unbalanced emotional state. One such child could, in a standing position, perform a deep back bend with apparently no effort. Another example, in an adult schizophrenic, is a complete wide circular swing of the torso. Dancers can acquire such use of body dynamics, an uninterrupted flow of movement through the entire body, only after extensive training. The mechanism enabling the schizophrenic to do this is still a matter for research, and the reason for spontaneously starting such movements is not as yet clarified. Sometimes the movement can be induced in the schizophrenic; at others there is no reaction. The particular patterns described resulted not from a verbal demand but came as a reaction to rhythmic sound.

The process of learning to be aware of the body image and its appearance, the anticipation and reaction to the movement of others, and the consciousness of space shape and the changes that occur in the body and in space, are primarily on the sensory level. Each part of the body becomes an entity in itself with its own sensitivity and desires, so that it is possible to speak of the body of an individual as the co-ordination of many different parts, each with its own personality. Certain parts of the body may be sensitive and alert and react to inner and outer stimuli while other parts may be dull and unconscious of their own existence. These parts may not react because they were neglected when motor impulses were given, or because there was not sufficient sensitivity in the muscles to respond to the message they received; or they may refuse to react because they have been immobilized by a conscious or subconscious inhibitory message due to some physical or psychological block. Such conditions will result in imbalance and poor co-ordination.

To stimulate the sensitivity to minute movements in the different parts of the body, the dancer sometimes works with closed eyes either in silence, or in the state of suspension created by the soft playing of gong tones. He is then told to move whatever part of the body seems to feel like moving regardless of the gesture which may result, or the relation of one movement to another. Usual beginnings may be scratching the nose, pushing the hair back, shifting of weight, pulling at clothes, twitchings of muscles, etc.—indications of self-consciousness; or stamping of feet, collapse of body, rubbing of hands together, shrugging of shoulders,—indications of irritation, despair, disgust. The leader points out these uncontrolled subconscious movements and discusses their significance. The pupil is urged to do exactly what he feels as soon as he feels it. In this way the body is set in motion. Gradually more and more movement is experienced and larger gestures are made. The body begins to respond to the various shifts of weight and begins to travel through different space levels following the laws of inertia, impulse and momentum. Emotional reactions become manifest and changes in tension begin to create a dynamic and rhythmic flow of movement. During these activities the instructor is constantly encouraging by words and sounds the externalization of gestures and movements which begin to make their appearance. Eventually only the percussion sounds are continued, and the body moves by itself.

There is a logic in the development of one movement into another both in the body and in the use of space. To the trained observer any interjection of an arbitrary movement can immediately be discerned. This is a sign of a break in concentration and usually takes the form of some habit movement pattern which the pupil considers "safe," i.e., either it covers up the externalization of a "forbidden" fantasy or sensation, or it prevents exploration into the unknown.

After such experimentation with the dance, the student is sometimes asked to create a figure of himself in clay. These figures invariably show, as was seen in the case of Helga, how much of the body is included in the consciousness of the body image. Sometimes a medium such as clay, paint, wood, charcoal or chalk is used to resolve a block which is apparent in dance. It has been interesting to see the correlation between the problem in dance and the new medium which is chosen.

For example, one adult enjoyed wallowing on the ground, using the body sensuously. In such a case the presence of physical pleasure observed in the student is to be used as a positive factor. Its translation into an art form can be gradually induced by indirect methods which will change the tone of the muscle tension, increase the amount of passivity or relaxation in the movement. The student must be made conscious of the audience outside herself in order that the movement may be dissociated from self-indulgence and may attain a more direct release from the original tension. This woman was immediately fascinated by clay as a medium of expression. She enjoyed the feel of substance, enjoyed mashing the hard lumps of clay and kneading the clay in preparation for the actual modeling. After a few awkward attempts at manipulation of the material she quite suddenly was able to mould it and create objects which gave expression in an objective form to her preoccupation with her body and her inner self. It happened that she had been in an accident which had distorted her face. All her figures displayed broad flat noses. The handling of the clay, the tactile element, was an adequate performance during the phase this individual was in. By concentrating the pleasure sensation which had been distributed over her whole body in her hands and fingers, she could free her fantasies and give them form in a medium removed from herself. It seemed that the sensuous feeling enjoyed while working with clay enabled her to formulate what she could not express in her own body. Her dance movement began to change and she was better able to create in both media.

To sum up, the teaching of modern creative dance offers a great many facets for the projection of physical and psychological problems. The process of mastering the elements and techniques of dance parallels closely the processes followed by a patient in psychoanalysis. The mastering of dance techniques and the formulation of emotions and fantasies in dance improvisations may clarify subconscious material and bring it to the surface of consciousness. Careful study of dance movement can become a valuable diagnostic instrument particularly for children who constantly accompany their dance activity with verbalizations expressing their fantasies.

～ 17 ～

SPECIAL SCHOOL ROOM ATTITUDES AND ACTIVITIES FOR THE PROBLEM CHILD[1]

BEFORE beginning a discussion of the school conducted within the Bellevue Psychiatric Hospital, it might be helpful to review briefly a few of the changes in ideology, attitude and method of working with the maladjusted child in the New York City school system, as revealed in the annual reports of the Superintendent of Schools.

These reports throw light on the early beginnings of what is now known as Public School No. 618, Manhattan. As far back as 1898 the educational system had recognized that there were what we now call maladjusted children, and was seeking methods of dealing with them. Today these early efforts may appear to us to have been fumbling and founded upon some amusing if not tragic misunderstandings.

"Incorrigible" was a favorite word of the time. Frequently these so-called "incorrigibles" were sent to truant schools, where they were confined 24 hours a day and subjected to a program which was calculated to inculcate a better "outfit of habits." It was the notion of the times that these "incorrigibles" must be made to acquire a "new outfit of habits" if they were to avoid becoming hardened criminals.

Emphasis was placed upon physical labor and industry; personality development was ignored. At no time during this early period is there evidence that there was an awareness of the need for security. One report which advocated establishment of a parental school contained this statement: "These incorrigibles will most certainly become criminals if they are not furnished before the years of adolescence with an entirely new outfit of habits. For such as these a truant school—a place of confinement and a place of labor—will always be necessary."[2]

---

[1] By Wanda Wright. Board of Education Teacher on the Children's Service, Psychiatric Division, Bellevue Hospital since 1935; Principal of Public School 618, Psychiatric Division of Bellevue Hospital since 1948.

This chapter was compiled from papers written by Wanda Wright and presented at staff conferences at Bellevue Hospital to acquaint the hospital staff of psychiatrists, psychologists, social workers, nurses, etc., with the aims, problems and experiences of the school rooms in the hospital, and presented also at conferences of Board of Education teachers to acquaint them with methods of caring for the problem child which had been developed in the special class rooms for problem children in the Hospital.

[2] First Annual Report of the City Superintendent of Schools to the Board of Education, for the year ending July 31, 1899.

Such was the picture at the turn of the century. During the next 24 years several special schools, in addition to the Parental School, were established. In 1905, when Public School 120 came into being as the first special school, it was realized that "tactfulness, sympathy, patience and personal magnetism on the part of a teacher are the first essentials for success in this work."[3] The reference to "success" implied success in acquiring desirable habits. It was not until much later that account was taken of the degree to which the teacher compensates for the inadequacies of the home by supplying affection, understanding, and in general a feeling of being wanted.

The Superintendent's annual reports continued to recommend procedures for the children attending the Parental and special day schools. When new subjects were added to the curriculum they were designed to assist in instilling the habit patterns required by the industrial world instead of supplying new experiences out of which the child would derive satisfactions and achieve a greater realization of his abilities and potentialities. Among the subjects emphasized were manual training, gardening, farming and practical trades.

However, despite the concentration on habit formation, the report of 1908 included a statement to the effect that there can be no academic achievement without having acquired the ability to read. The importance of reading was stressed, and it was obvious that the writer was aware that reading was essential in helping a child adjust to a school situation. Also of interest was a report on a statistical study which sought to trace the relationship of poverty to maladjustment, but which failed to make the present-day point that teachers must compensate for the inadequacy of their pupils' homes.

There were instances showing that some educators were aware that something was lacking in the formal teaching approach. The reports continued to stress the need for academic subjects, physical training, industrial or vocational training, and moral training. The last was considered of great importance.

In 1922 it was suggested that provision be made for examinations by psychologists and psychiatrists before pupils were admitted to the probationary schools. By 1924 there was evidence that a new era was approaching. The boys were no longer considered "incorrigibles." Truancy began to be explained in terms of parental incompetency. Placement in foster or boarding homes was suggested. It was also pointed out that "only by careful examination—educational, psychological, psychiatric and social in character—can the problem of truancy be understood and managed. In practically all of these cases it was found that the picture is a complex one. The examination revealed a picture of faulty mental or personality development, poor environment, serious physical defects, forced promotions and wrong classification in

---

[3] Seventh Annual Report, *Ibid.* 1905.

school. It would seem in the light of our present knowledge that the truancy problem must be approached from the remedial and not from the disciplinary point of view."[4]

The report appears to have aroused the exponents of remedial reading techniques, for in 1929 the point was made that remedial measures should be undertaken in all cases of reading retardation. By 1930, then, educational and psychological theory in regard to problem children had undergone a drastic change. The emphasis on habit training no longer existed. In its place was the realization that truancy was the result of certain known causes. From this point forward great strides were made. The now well-known Bureau of Child Guidance was established in 1931.

The opening of Public School No. 37 in Manhattan was an important milestone in the advance of education for the problem children of New York City. This school, to which all other schools in the city sent their most serious problem boys, was the laboratory out of which grew the new "600-schools division."

This new division, established in 1947, embraces about a dozen schools, some of them regular day schools and others special schools operated in city psychiatric hospitals and in institutions housing disturbed children. Whatever the type of 600-school, the fundamental approach is a therapeutic one, based on providing affection and insight.

The school in the Psychiatric Division of Bellevue Hospital became part of the 600-schools division, thereby becoming "a special school within a special school." It is now known as Public School 618, Manhattan.

While P.S. 618 has the same guiding principles and philosophies, it functions somewhat differently from other schools in the division. The time element is mainly responsible for the differences. In the Bellevue school, children rarely remain more than a month, and for this reason long-term planning is out of the question.

After this brief history of schools for problem children in New York City, let us turn to a consideration of methods and attitudes in this "special school within a special school" in Bellevue Hospital.

It may be worth while to set forth briefly the reasons for there being a school at all in a children's psychiatric ward. First is a basic theory of democracy that all children, regardless of aptitude or ability shall be afforded an opportunity to attend school. Second, it is generally recognized that an important aspect of adjusting the maladjusted child consists of enabling him to get into a school. A very large part of the life situation of a child must necessarily involve attending school and as long as schooling presents difficulties for him he remains but poorly adjusted. Hence it is essential that while he is in the hospital every effort should be made to assist him in adjusting to class-

---

[4] Twenty-Sixth Annual Report, *Ibid.* 1924.

room situations. Obviously to assist him in adjusting, the classroom situation in Bellevue is a modification—and sometimes a very great modification—of the ordinary classroom situation, the need for which is apparent. It must be remembered that nearly all of the children who come to Bellevue have been found unable to profit by attending schools designed for normal or near-normal children. It should also be noted that the teachers and principals with whom these children have been in contact have worked earnestly to help many of them. When we receive a child's school records we learn more often than not that for years the child has had grave difficulties in one or more ways in school. In other words, these children are maladjusted not merely in the home or in their social group; they are maladjusted in school.

Not so many years ago reading, writing and arithmetic were regarded as the essential elements of a school, and there are people today who still appear to think that schools should be judged by their success in teaching the use of these tools. But education has come to be much more all-embracing. Education in any real sense implies preparation for dealing with the vast complexity of life situations. Important as it is for the child to learn to read, write and do arithmetic, it is equally important for him to learn how to live as a social being; frequently it is necessary for him to learn or unlearn many things before he is capable of or willing to tackle reading, writing and arithmetic. That is why it has been found necessary to provide classrooms in Bellevue, which are in many respects quite different from those to be found in the neighborhood schools.

There are times when if one looked in on one of the class sessions, one might well wonder what subject if any was being taught. One child might be working on arithmetic, another might be reading comics, a third writing, a fourth engaged in a quarrel which might turn into a brawl, and others variously occupied listening to a record, idly or intently watching the tropical fish, daydreaming in the arm chair, rocking in the rocker, playing checkers or cards or sitting painting at the easel. One might not even notice the boy seated close to the teacher's desk laboriously struggling with a pre-primer, the simplest of all readers. He is the boy who two, three, or even four weeks earlier came into the hospital so convinced that he would never be able to read that he would go into a violent tantrum at the very mention of reading. He is the boy who has overcome some of his earlier anxieties toward failure and is developing healthier attitudes toward school. He is the boy who, having arrived at this stage, should, if he returns to his old school, be ready to receive the help which he has rejected in the past. It might be asked why he suddenly has consented to attempt reading. The answer is that it was not sudden; it was merely a result of the operation of the program to which we subscribe.

The first and most important step in this program is the development of a warm teacher-child relationship. In the development of such a relationship the child dominates every situation. The teacher must maintain a casual and only mildly interested attitude toward the unusual behavior and unreasonable demands made by the child. The children do not accept the passive role of the teacher without suspicion. Over and over again they test her loyalties by trying, in a deliberate and calculating manner, to break her down. Some of them go so far as to ask for punishment. Each time a session like this has been lived through, the bond between child and teacher is strengthened and the child has come a little closer toward the desired goal.

In striving to reach that goal, frictions, pressures, tensions and punishments cannot exist. Extreme patience and a willingness to allow whatever time is necessary to obtain results are essential. There are wide variations in the amount of time it takes a child to become oriented, but sooner or later almost every child becomes ready to receive help. Much has been gained if a child arrives at this point before he leaves Bellevue. If in learning a few words he has gained the knowledge that he is able to learn, he has made great strides. From this point forward, he should be returned to his school or placed in a special school, with recommendations.

Another reason for establishing a school in Bellevue is to afford an opportunity for the observation of the children in a situation somewhat similar to that of a classroom. Such observations tend to confirm the notations on the pupils' record cards, which usually do not arrive until sometime after our hospital observations have been made. How the schools managed to keep some of these disturbed children for years is difficult to comprehend. Some of the children are constantly in a state of flight and assuredly schools cannot be expected to accommodate children on the run. It has been found possible to classify children into groups, displaying behavior traits peculiar to their respective group. The schizophrenic child is more fleeing than any of the other groups into which these children fall. The epileptic has an entirely different set of values from the neurotic, who in turn is quite different from the psychopath, and so on. However, occasionally a child enters the class who defies classification. Here it may be noted that children are not adversely affected by the unusual behavior of other children. Regularly someone visits the classroom who shows concern over mixing so many complex personalities together. Our experiences have made us feel that no child suffers as a consequence of association with the other children. To the contrary, many children profit as a result of associating with children equally unfortunate and in some instances less fortunate than themselves. They begin to look upon their difficulties as somewhat commonplace.

If a child indicates that he wants to talk about his particular problems, he is encouraged to do so. A group shapes up very quickly and no child has been found to express shock at the statements, confessions, admissions and weird tales of another child. What it usually amounts to is an undramatic pooling of experiences. The teachers in a psychiatric hospital where children are studied and treated by psychiatrists, psychologists, nurses and social workers, have found that it is not necessary to know the backgrounds or family histories of these children in order to help them. The non-reader usually has factors other than his inability to read which have played an important role in his admission to Bellevue, but if his reading difficulty is concentrated on, he becomes sufficiently well adjusted for the assumption to be made that his other problems have diminished in intensity. In other words, it has been found that a child who has arrived at the point where he is willing to learn to read and then receives private coaching or special remedial help from some source makes a better adjustment to a difficult home situation than before he learned to read. This is so even when the home situation has remained essentially the same.

It is possible to ease these children into situations from which they will derive satisfactions sufficient to enable them temporarily at least to be somewhat removed from the stresses and strains life has placed upon them. Malcolm H. Finley has discussed the stresses and strains that such problem children must deal with in the group situation of the usual school room.[5] Such children, in spite of essentially normal and above normal IQ's have failed to acquire certain fundamental knowledge although they have attended school from four to six years. For obvious reasons it would be unwise to reconstruct a typical school situation. Activities have to be planned which provide experiences which will lead to the desired goals.

During the school year the amount of time spent in preparation for festive occasions is not small. Halloween, Christmas, St. Valentine's Day, Easter and the June party receive all-out attention and effort. In addition to these, a number of other occasions arise which warrant a party. A party project is, however, not without its heartaches. Pleasurable experiences are not wholly pleasurable for these children. Both positive and negative qualities are brought into sharper focus during a party activity. It seems to put a keen edge on their emotions; one does not need a magnifying glass to detect the most infantile child in the group, the most destructive, the most co-operative, the most creative and gifted, the most withdrawn, the greatest chatterer, the least productive, the one most in need of assurances that his production is worthwhile and should be preserved, the most stable, the one least able to concentrate, and so on. One could go on indefinitely mentioning personality traits which manifest themselves and seem to stand out in bold relief during one of the hectic sessions leading up to a gala occasion.

The approach to a party, too, is quite different from that which would prove successful with normal children. It is possible with normal children to set a goal and encourage them to work toward that goal. With the children

---

[5] See Finley, Malcolm H.: The Classroom as a Social Group and Its Reaction to the Problem Child, with discussion by Wanda Grutzner (Wright). *American Journal of Orthopsychiatry,* *11*:21-33, 1941.

in the school, long-time planning serves only to annoy them and to make them impatient or out of sympathy with the whole idea. They must have concrete evidence of an end result before they will direct their energies in any one direction. To be more specific: to try to interest them on a Monday morning in preparations for a Halloween party to be held on the following Friday afternoon would be a waste of time. They would respond either by being disinterested or by wanting the party immediately. A gradual and indirect approach is far more effective. For instance, it would be better to say, "If anyone would like to make a pumpkin, here is paper and crayon." If at least one child responds, the program is launched. From this point forward, the teacher receives suggestions from the children and subtly serves as a guide and as a protector of their creations.

To keep the children from destroying their own work and the work of other children is a big task. Even after the children have displayed their enthusiasm and have given evidence of deriving satisfaction in whatever they happen to be doing at the moment, the project does not go forward without interruption. It regularly happens that the entire preparations are threatened by one child or another. The recent Halloween project may serve as a typical illustration. The children worked feverishly at the drawing and coloring of cats, witches, pumpkins, bats, autumn leaves and many other symbols of the Halloween season. However, many more productions were destroyed by children who were dissatisfied with their own work. The children usually do not serve notice that they intend to destroy their work but very impulsively and in an explosive manner bring about complete destruction. This behavior is mainly limited to and typical of the behavior of schizophrenic children. The schizophrenic child has been observed to work diligently with interest and concentration on something that promises to be a very worth-while production when suddenly he seems driven by an inner force completely to eradicate any evidence of the existence of the piece of work before him. On the other hand, there is the type of child who takes the time to threaten to destroy his work. This is quite often an obvious indication that he wants his work admired; with a little encouragement he then returns to it with greater interest.

There are children who cannot tolerate the competition of other children. They will tear or mark over another child's work. This motive occurs less frequently than any other reason for destruction. When a boy destroys another boy's work, it is quite often as a result of a quarrel entirely unrelated to the piece of work involved. If the recipient of the attack happened to have a toy with him instead of a piece of his work the toy would be destroyed. It has been found that children more often are proud of another child's work rather than envious of it. Very often they call attention to the other child's art work and are very generous in their praise of him. It is not unusual for one boy to sit by and with interest watch another boy at work. If a boy's art is defaced, it is because the boy is unpopular in the group. Last spring, there was a boy (Donald) in the class whose art was enjoyed by all the children; however Donald's personality was so very offensive and objectionable that the children's only resource was to smear his large murals when he was not around. The same behavior carries over to other subjects. For example, if an arithmetic paper, a spelling or a composition paper of a child is put on the bulletin board, it is rarely removed by another child. With much greater frequency it happens that the child himself in a fit of anger tears his work off the board and destroys it.

To return to the Halloween project, it is a fact that a large amount of work is not wilfully destroyed but finds its way to the floor or the trash can because it is not complete.

These children tire of things very quickly. The fact that they are full of enthusiasm and make bold statements about what they plan to do means nothing at all. They are apt to leave their work unfinished and move on to something else. When asked if they would not like to complete what promises to be a nice piece of work, they flatly refuse, say they are tired and quite often suggest that someone else finish it. Another large portion of the work is destroyed, not by violence or failure to complete it, but merely because they do not seem to be able to preserve it. In general, these children cannot keep themselves intact and their inability to take care of their work or of their things seems to be part of the whole picture. For example, if they go to the bookcase for a book, they regularly arrive back at their destination, which may be no further away than the other side of the room, without it. On the way something has happened to the book; at all events, they do not have it.

Another feature to be mentioned is the amount of material expended or what might commonly be termed wasted in developing a project like the Halloween project.

These children consistently feel that they are making mistakes. They are just as uncertain of themselves and just as easily frustrated when they are attempting to do something specific as they are in their relationships with other people. Therefore, it is not difficult to understand that great quantities of paper are consumed. Such expenditure of material could not be tolerated in every school but in this special set-up it is justified; it is justified because to try to avoid it would defeat the very purpose that is being sought. It would be placing restrictions upon the children, refusing them the free use of materials and subjecting them to routine check-ups. These would serve to activate the child to rebel and he would again relive situations reminiscent of unpleasant past experiences. Since it is one of our primary functions to afford him the luxury of a permissive atmosphere wherein he can enjoy new and pleasant experiences, sacrifices must be made in order not to restrict him. If the children were in the hospital school for a longer period, they would be expected to arrive at a point where their adjustment was such that their careless extravagance would diminish and they would assume a sense of responsibility. As it is, improvement is seen in individuals, but because of a daily turnover the entire group never shows progress as a group.

With so many problems growing out of an activity of this sort, one might question the value of the activity. There are times when it would be easier to stop all preparations and to transfer to something less enervating. For example, when Cosmo went on a rampage and ripped from the window a work of his which was the center of interest, it required real effort to encourage the other children to fill in the gaps. It is only the knowledge that the values derived from a project of this sort are immeasurable that gives the teachers the strength to see it to completion. Over a period of years, some very interesting data in reference to these parties have been accumulated. First of all it is a group activity in which sooner or later almost every child takes part. Upon completion the children are extremely proud of their work. They admire it, they want others to admire it, and in general their finer qualities come to the fore. To see the vigor with which they throw themselves into the spirit of the party itself is to be convinced that the hard work put into it was well worth while. It is always refreshing to learn that these children who seem to have been deprived of the refinements of life never fail to express their appreciation. Quietly and individually a great many children at some time during the festivities take time to give expression of their happiness often in a very touching manner.

Of greater significance perhaps is a situation which occurs regularly. Many of the boys who leave the children's ward return to Bellevue sometimes years later and become patients on the adolescent ward. We sometimes meet these boys and men on the elevator, and in trying to help us identify them they may say something like this: "Don't you remember me? I was in your class when we had a Christmas party. I made the big Christmas picture, etc." An even more striking example is that of the boy who returned every year at Christmas time to help decorate. He never sent word in advance, but just appeared every year. One year he was employed as a truck driver; that time he drove his truck to the hospital, brought his helper up with him and put him to work. He returned even the year after he came back from overseas. Since then he married, and last year he sent an announcement of the birth of his baby.

Another very important aspect in working with the children in the school is to surround them with an atmosphere in which it will be possible for them to relax and create. These children are very easily over-stimulated. It is often advisable to give them a good letting alone. They have in the past been talked to, lectured to, advised, scolded, threatened and in general subjected to a variety of attempts made by persons in the hope of bringing about changes. Every effort is made to avoid this approach. First, they are surrounded with a good physical set-up. The part that an attractive room containing carefully chosen materials play cannot be overrated. The attempt is made to have materials which will appeal to children of all levels of interest and intelligence. While academic procedures are not stressed, every opportunity must be afforded the child who is capable of acquiring knowledge to seek it. If children are ready for it, they need no motivation other than accessible materials and the freedom to help themselves. As an example, one boy, William, spent most of his time absorbed in the encyclopedia which was at hand. Occasionally he would call attention to something he had found of special interest thereby stimulating other children to ask questions.

In order to have readily available material which will appeal to the many interests of the children, the custodial job becomes tremendous. These children differ from normal children in that they have no sense of preservation of materials. They are themselves messy and everything they come in contact with is doomed for a transformation. They have been termed "fluid" and this word well describes what happens to the things about them. They drop, lose or misplace materials without intent or effort. At that point they move on, and someone must clear up the mess and salvage what can be salvaged. That someone else is usually the adult in charge. It has been found that the morale of the group is in no small measure dependent upon the cheerfulness and attractiveness of the room. The fact that the children enjoy and give voice to their enjoyment of pleasant surroundings in no way imbues them with a sense of pride in preserving the harmony of the room.

These ideas are not entirely new nor do they belong solely to this era. Many people believe in and support similar practices and as a result the child as an individual gets more attention than he formerly did. We are not dogmatic in prescribing procedures for dealing with the problem child today nor do we wish to make definite predictions as to the ultimate outcome of the various practices employed.

THE THERAPY OF A CHILD[1]

CHILDREN approach life with zest. Driven by instinctual impulses which demand release in motor activity, they are continuously attempting to understand and master the world they live in. To do so they make endless experiments involving the physical, social, and emotional realities which confront them. The specific nature and patterning of these experiments are normally determined by psychobiological levels of maturation. Direct experimentation however inevitably comes up against limitations for the child in his constant striving to live out his impulses. The natural laws of the physical world and the prohibitions of culture force him to supplement his direct approach to life with fantasy, where no problem is too difficult to solve and no forbidden sexual or aggressive impulse impossible to experience either in direct or symbolic form. Paul Schilder has stated that symbols appear when the experimentation process belonging to a specific maturation level has been interrupted by danger or threat.[2] The symbolic act or fantasy can thus be seen to serve simultaneously the dual purpose of fulfillment and protection. That is, fulfillment of an instinctual impulse in a safe form which serves as protection from the danger and threats imposed by the environment. The manifold problems of sexuality in childhood very often express themselves in symbolic rather than in direct form, inasmuch as direct experimentation as an approach to these problems is culturally forbidden.

Regardless of the primary nature of the problem being dealt with, however, the symbolic fantasy is normally not an aim in itself. Although it stems from and points towards a dangerous reality situation which the child seeks to master, the tendency is to redirect it towards approved goals which permit of direct experimentation, thus utilizing it ultimately as a constructive approach to reality. In doing this the child ceaselessly and actively strives to establish a relationship between his self-made inner world of fantasy and the external reality which he must face. When he succeeds in establishing this relationship in a socially approved constructive manner, he gains additional mastery of himself and his environment. A continuous flow of creative activity thus occurs, within which the successful completion of each individual step frees the child to try for new levels of integration, levels of self-fulfill-

---

[1] Published in part as: Bender, Lauretta and Montague, Allison: Psychotherapy Through Art in a Negro Child. *The College Art Journal*, Autumn 1947.

[2] Schilder, Paul: *The Child and the Symbol*, 1938.

ment which are limited only by the stage of psychobiological maturation which has been reached.

One can observe this process in the behavior of any child who, unlike the adult, needs little encouragement and few special external conditions in order to express himself creatively. Art materials are convenient tools of expression to place in the hands of a child whom one wishes to observe in action. Many children with emotional conflicts are driven to greater productivity and special kinds of artistic experimentation by the very nature of their problems.

The value of art work in psychotherapy with children has been emphasized.[3] It has been shown that the process of production in itself is a valuable experience whereby the child gains release of accumulated emotional tension through expressing problems related to aggressive and sexual impulses. For the therapist the art work of the child is a means of gaining an insight into his fantasy life, thus affording a record which often contains key answers to emotional, social and intellectual problems.

The above considerations will be illustrated by presenting in some detail the therapeutic process in a child whose art work was an integral part of the treatment she received for her emotional problems.

Jean Cannon[4] was a Negro girl just 6 years old when she was abandoned in a children's shelter in September 1943. She was sent to a child-caring institution after a month and to the children's ward of the Psychiatric Division of Bellevue Hospital three months later with a letter stating that Jean "had been taken (to the children's shelter) by a Mrs. Carper with whom she had lived since she was 5 months old. Mrs. Carper claimed that she was a financial burden and that her behavior was annoying and that she no longer wanted to assume responsibility for her. There was some hint that Mrs. Carper might have been the real mother, but this was never verified. Since leaving the child, Mrs. Carper has moved and her whereabouts are unknown. Nothing is known about the father.

"Since she has been at (our institution), she has been completely unresponsive both in the school room and in the cottage. She shows no change in expression and speaks very little. She is enuretic and has trouble both in the day and at night. There is a possibility of placement in a foster home . . . but we feel it extremely important that the child have a period of observation before such placement is made as we do not know whether she is mentally deficient as well as having emotional difficulties."

It was in this condition that Jean was admitted to the children's ward of the Psychiatric Division of Bellevue Hospital.

At first she showed depression and emotional blocking, but with encour-

---

[3] See Chapter 13.
[4] All surnames used are fictitious.

agement she joined in the various group activities, and during the course of individual psychotherapeutic interviews with her psychiatrist[5] she became very responsive and productive. She particularly enjoyed expressing herself through art work which she was encouraged to do both with the group art classes, in the school room, and when she was alone with the psychiatrist. Seventy-five sheets of her art production were preserved of which Figs. 51, 52, 53 (Color Plate IV), and Fig. 54 are representative. Simultaneously her memories were further explored by means of direct interviews and telling of dreams. The material of her interviews with the psychiatrist will be given in full.

Jean was admitted to the children's ward on December 31, 1943. On January 6, 1944, one week later, she said to her psychiatrist, in response to questions as to how she liked it in the hospital and why she had come: "I like it here. My mother took me to the shelter because my hair is this way— too short. She cut it short." Jean was a dark skinned well developed, essentially healthy Negro girl with the short kinky hair typical of her racial constitution. It was certainly improbable that her hair had been cut. But in this brief introductory statement Jean expressed her concern over her body image problems related to her racial characteristics, the negative relationship with the rejecting "mother," her own feelings of guilt and inadequacy, possibly a castration problem, and her positive attitude toward her psychiatrist and her new environment. All of these problems recurred in subsequent material. Her only physical defect was a "pot-bellied" posture which is typical in depressed children, especially girls of this age. It improved with her general emotional progress under psychotherapy.

(Suppose you had three wishes what would they be?)[6]
"First, to be here. Second, because I like it here, it is a nice place. Third, they treat you nice here."

(Better than at home?) "Yes at home my mother and brother hit me all the time."

(Whom do you love most?) "My brother, he is 4 years old."

(Who next?) "My father."

(What is your mother's name?) "Hilda Quinn."

(What is your father's name?) "Herman Carper."

(Are they married?) "No."

---

[5] Dr. Allison Montague.
[6] The questions of the psychiatrist, often abbreviated, are in parentheses and italicized.

(Is your father married?) "Yes, to my mother, Mrs. Carper."

(You said your mother's name was Quinn?) "Well, she has too many names."

(Do you have more than one mother?) "Yes, two. First was Mrs. Carper. But she was not my real mother. She is dead now—a long time. I used to live with her and another father. I forgot his name. Then I came to Miss Hilda and my father and my brother."

(Whom do you love most?) "Mrs. Carper. She is dead."

(How about Miss Hilda?) "Not so much, she don't look so good. She is a little bit blacker than I am."

(Why did your mother hit you at home?) "Because I was bad. I didn't do what she told me to do. I like it here because they treat me nice."

(Tell me a dream.) "Once I dreamt I went into the bathroom. I coughed and then I had to vomit. A round little thing came out. And then a string came out and a bigger thing. I was scared. I don't like to tell dreams, I'd rather play."

(Tell me another dream.) "I dreamt I saw another girl and I said 'hello' to her. She said, 'Get out of here, I don't know you.' Once I dreamt I had a bad headache and I went to the hospital to see what was wrong. The doctor said, 'Let's see.' Another time I dreamt I had a bad pain in my stomach and my side."

(Do you hear voices?) "No." *(Maybe sometimes?)* "Once in a while."

(Whose voice?) "My own, saying 'Don't bother me.' "

(Where does it come from?) "I don't know. I didn't mean my own voice, I meant the voice of the Boogey man. Sometimes I hear him talking out of bathrooms—says, 'I'm coming to get you.' "

(Is it real or imagination?) "It's real."

(What would he do?) "He would take his nails and stick it into me—into my stomach and my legs, too."

(Did you ever see him?) "In the show—he's dressed all in black."

(Does he talk to you here?) "No, only at home."

(What's inside of you?) "Food, spinach and fruit."[7]

In the interview, the child was quiet, soft-spoken, over-polite, but very responsive. She stated emphatically that she liked it better in the hospital than at home "because my mother hits me." She was greatly mixed up as to the family circle. She spoke of two mothers whom she constantly confused; she was consistent only in stating that her father was not married to her "real" mother. She said she did not like her "real" mother but loved her "first" mother who she stated was dead. This "mother" had the same name, Carper, as the "father." This was the name given by the woman who left the child, at the children's shelter, and about whom there was some hint that she might be the real mother.

Jean's dreams and fantasies were concerned with bodily harm, especially penetration and there was some indication of an oral fixation.

She showed good capacity for object attachment. She was not at all enuretic or lacking in responsiveness as she had been in the child-caring institution. It seemed probable that her behavior was reactive to a rejecting if not actually abusive foster mother. It was prognosticated that after a period she would be a good candidate for a good foster home.

On January 12th, when she was 6-4 years she was tested with the Stanford-Binet intelligence test. She scored a mental age of 6-6 and an IQ of 103. She obtained a basal age of 5 years and scattered through the 7th year level. While extremely cooperative, she seemed blocked and inhibited, which may have lowered her IQ to some extent. Her mental age on the Goodenough drawing test was 6 years. Educationally there was no achievement except that she could write her name, and recognize letters and numbers. Her gestalt drawings were carefully done, but showed spatial disorientation, and difficulties in all diamond formations. They were discrete and well organized.

Her Rorschach showed that she was apparently brighter than the IQ on the Stanford-Binet indicated. She gave a high percentage of well seen forms including animals and human figures, but one ghost. There was evidence of blocking, insecurity, and emotional deprivation.

On January 19th, in a psychotherapeutic interview, she was asked to play and no direction was given to her. Her play showed certain obsessive features, that is, orderly re-arranging of wooden numbers and letters according to size, shape, and color, counting them, stringing beads, counting them, etc.

---

[7] Paul Schilder and David Wechsler found that normal children believe that their insides are full of food, while Jack Rapoport pointed out that fantasied introjected bodies are indicative of more serious emotional problems. Our experience with schizophrenic children shows that such introjected bodies, especially symbolic of bad parents, are often present. Also the type of auditory hallucinations that this girl experienced have been found by Lauretta Bender and H. Lipkowitz to occur in normal children suffering from inadequate parental relationship and attention.

She was then given clay to play with. She called one flat mass a "body" and when further questioned she said "my body." Then she made a pie and again returned to the body, making head, arms, legs, and long red hair (everything else was grey). She stated as she finished, "I don't like my hair this short and my father doesn't either." When asked who cut it, she would not say, instead she told the following story:

"My father was beating up my other father and he was all bloody and fell on the bathroom floor. After that I was afraid to go to the bathroom, especially after dark. But I don't think he is lying there bloody any more." *(When did the boogeyman start talking to you?)* "Right after that."

(Why did your father fight?) "My other father was standing near the stove— he wanted some food. My father and mother were there. My father pushed him away and they had a fight."

(Tell me a dream.) "Last night I dreamt I was reading some comic books and all of a sudden I saw some snakes. I felt afraid."

(Why afraid?) "They might eat me up and then I wouldn't have any body."

This dream of Jean's confirms our experience that snakes in the dream and fantasy life of children are not penetrating phallic symbols as they often are in adults. They represent rather a devouring animal and are usually experienced by those children who have had anxiety relative to aggressive or sadistic parents or parent substitutes.[8]

(Tell me another dream.) "I had some red chalk in my mouth. The doctor came and said I would have to go to the hospital and have an operation. It was the chalk I love."

(What kind of an operation?) "On my mouth and on my stomach to get the chalk out."

(Tell me another dream.) "No." *(Sure.)* "One more. I was in the hospital and had a stomach ache. The doctor took my temperature. I was afraid." *(Why afraid?)* "He might stick the thermometer way down my throat."

Jean's dreams from the first were largely concerned with oral sensations and fear of being attacked and injured orally or in her stomach. This is a concern for the well-being of her insides and for a little girl it is also related to her genitals. These dreams may also be said to represent thinly disguised

---

[8] See Chapter 14 for discussion on symbolism of snakes, also Chapter 11 for children's drawings of snakes, and Chapter 15 for the meaning of the alligator in puppet shows.

fantasies of oral impregnation. In the last dreams it was evidently her physician whom she feared would attack her, injure her and impregnate her.

At this point she was started on benzedrine therapy.[9] We have given benzedrine to children who are anxious, blocked, tense, or overactive when the overactivity is related to anxiety (but not when the overactivity is related to the disorganized impulses in a brain-damaged child). Children who have had sexual stimulation or are sexually preoccupied benefit especially from this drug. We expect the child under benzedrine therapy to become less tense, less blocked, less anxious and to be able to relate better to other children and to adults whether teachers or psychotherapists, and to be able to occupy themselves with the normal interests of a latency-age child. They lose their sexual drives and fantasies and tend to forget them.

Jean had been attending school in the hospital and applied herself to the work. She was just beginning to learn to read and write and add numbers. She liked best to do art work. She also attended art classes almost daily where she was very productive. Of the 75 sheets of her art work which were produced in art classes, school room classes and in the psychiatrist's interviews we found her first work to be primitive, dreary with black or dark colors, and disorganized. It was not always possible to recognize what the child was representing. We have found that benzedrine therapy is usually reflected in the art work with more clearly expressed concepts and brighter colors and increased productivity. Fig. 51 shows some of her earliest work with dark coloring and indistinct or disintegrating forms. Fig. 52 shows clearer forms, clear concepts, and brighter colors. It will be noted however that even her earliest drawings had some of the same forms which emerged later into clear-cut concepts. A tree, a house, and a church was her chief motif.

On January 23, 1944, the physician's note states that Jean came to him in the evening after supper and said that she had just vomited.[10] (The nurse's notes indicate that this had happened a couple of times before.) However she did not seem much upset by the fact, explaining that she had eaten too much supper. She then proceeded to get silly, running around laughing and saying, "I'm going to vomit."

(Tell me a dream.) "I dreamt about that I wanted to go to sleep and then I was so sleepy I couldn't wake up."

(Tell me a dream.) "I dreamt that I was with a doctor. This doctor wasn't

---

[9] See Bender, Lauretta and Cottington, Frances: *The Use of Amphetamine Sulphate (Benzedrine) in Child Psychiatry*. The usual dose for a child is 20 mgm. on awakening in the morning, although it is usual to start with 5 mgms., increasing 5 mgms. daily to 20 mgms., to rule out sensitivity.

[10] Vomiting in the morning after taking benzedrine may indicate a toxic response to the benzedrine. Vomiting in the evening has no such significance.

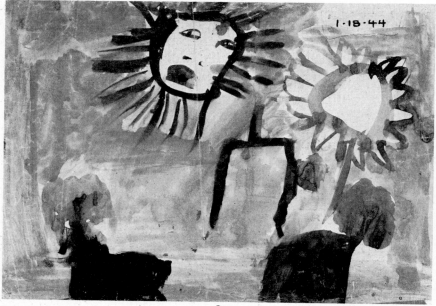

a

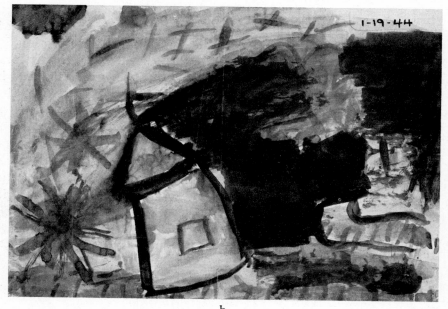

b

Fig. 51a, b. Early scenes with the indistinct emergence of form and color, by Jean (*water color*).

coming back and I cried and woke up. I couldn't go back to sleep again because I was crying."

(*Another dream.*) "I dreamt I was in a doctor's room. He asked me why

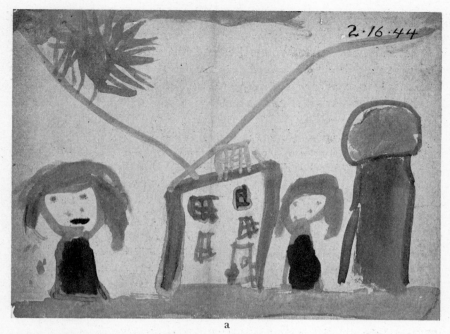

a

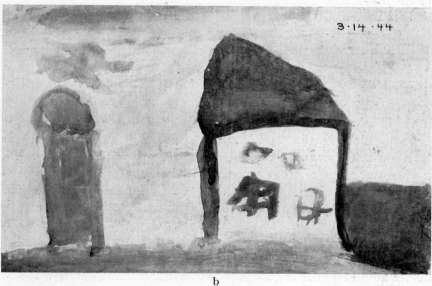

b

Fig. 52a, b. Later scenes in which form is more distinct and colors clear and pleasant, by Jean (*water color*).

my mother brought me here and I said, 'Because I have knobby hair.' Then he asked me if my mother sent me out on the street to play and I said, 'No.' "

These will be recognized as transference dreams; the last one re-experiences and clarifies the first interview with the psychiatrist. In the dream the child expresses her feeling of being rejected by the mother because of her short knobby hair, or her racial characteristics, although in the actual interview Jean had stated that her mother had cut off her hair. It will also be recalled that on one occasion Jean said she did not like this mother because she was a little bit darker than she was. Furthermore in the dream the child admits that her mother did not treat her well at home.

(Does your mother have any boy friends?) "Two."

(Soldiers?) "Five, if you count the soldiers."

(Do they pay her?) "Sure they pay her—she has to buy food."

(What does she do with the men friends?) "I don't know, they close the door."

(Whom do you sleep with?) "With my mother—no—alone on the floor."

(Whom does your mother sleep with?) "My brother."

(Whom does your father sleep with?) "He sleeps alone."

(Does your mother sleep with anyone else?) "My father."

(Anyone else?) "First with my brother. Then with my real father—then with my other father—then with all the rest of the soldiers."

(How many soldiers?) "Two."

These questions by the psychiatrist are justified because it is necessary to get Jean to clarify her problems, and her own feelings of guilt and rejection. Meanwhile our social service department had attempted to learn more about Jean and had so far discovered that Mrs. Carper, the alleged foster mother whom the agencies suspected of being Jean's real mother had had over 25 addresses during the previous five years. It was thought that undoubtedly she had been running a house of prostitution. It was also learned that she had taken Jean to the children's shelter because some neighbors complained about the house and the child's presence in it and she feared that she would be taken to court. Afterwards, the agency found this woman's new address but before they could reach her, they learned that she had entered a hospital ill, and had died.

February 4, 1944. *(Tell me a dream.)* "I dreamt that Caroline (another girl—white—on the ward) was coming back from home. We were asleep and didn't know she was coming. I woke up and she wasn't really there."

(Another dream?) "I dreamt someone was in my bed." *(Who?)* "Jean." (Another white girl on the ward.) "I asked her why she was there and she said she was getting my clothes to fix them. Then she asked me, did I want her to give me a drink of water and I said, no."

Jean dreams of other little girls with increasing frequency. It will be recalled that the second dream she reported in the first interview was of seeing another little girl to whom she said, "hello" but was answered with the unfriendly statement that "I don't know you." These dreams reveal the process of identification in the latency period through projection into other girl figures and through their experiences. These processes are especially important in a child who has had such confusing and negative experiences in her infantile period.

(Tell me another dream.) "I went to a hospital for eating a marble up. The doctor bust my stomach open and got it all out." *(How did he do it?)* "He did it with a big black knife. I dreamt I was in a box. I was sleeping. Some girls came and moved me and they woke me up and put me in my bed."

(How do you feel?) "I get stomach aches—bad ones."

(Did you have them before?) "Yes, at home—not bad though."

(When?) "Sometimes." *(When?)* "When they do those bad things."

(Who?) "My mother and father or the soldiers."

(Did you see it?) "Yes, my mother is bad. She does bad things with women and men. Sometimes they all do bad things together."

(How many?) "Five. My brother and I watch it sometimes. It's bad. It makes me feel sick in the stomach."

(Do you feel happy or sad?) "Sad."

(Why?) "Because I'm bad and I don't want to be."

(How are you bad?) "Those bad things I told you about before. I did it once with my brother."

(Anyone else?) "My father did it to me twice."

(Whose idea?) "Mine. No, it wasn't anybody's idea—it just happened."

(Tell me a story.) "Once there was a little girl and her name was Shirley. She went to the store and asked for some food—potatoes and rice and jelly.

So she came back and everything was messed up in her house—somebody had messed it up and she guessed who it was—a girl named Jean. She looked all around and almost found her. So she gave her a good spanking and she never did it any more. Then she looked in the house to see if it was fixed and she did it once more so her mother said, 'I'll give you just one more chance.' "

February 18, 1944: Jean was drawing in her psychotherapeutic session. As usual she drew a house, a tree and a church (see Figs. 53-b and 54). She and her psychiatrist were talking about the picture.

(What does the tree remind you of?) "My house."

(Something inside or outside?) "Somebody—the devil—is telling me to say 'inside.' Is the devil a man and why does he have to tell us to do bad things?"

(Where is he?) "In the sky and in us'es—in all the boys' and girls' stomachs."

(What does he say?) "He tells us to do all those bad things—to my mother and my brother."

(What are you drawing?) "A tree, a house and a church. That is what I always draw. Only sometimes I forget." "Is God still up there?" (Points to the sky.) "Somebody said He's not there any more."

(When does the devil talk to you?) "When you're round me. He tells me to pay you no mind. And then he says to do bad things with you."

(What else?) "Sometimes when I am with Miss F. (social service worker) he say I should kiss her backside."

(What does the devil say your drawings mean?) "He says to pay you no mind with that question."

(What does the devil say the tree is?) "My father's thing."

(The church?) "A God damned pussy."

(The ladder?) "Ass hole."

(The door?) "Pussy."

(Church?) "I'm not supposed to say anything bad about the church."

This remarkably simple but explicit interpretation of her art work and fantasy life was due to the kind of experiences that she had lived through, at the age of leaving early childhood for the latency period, the psychothera-

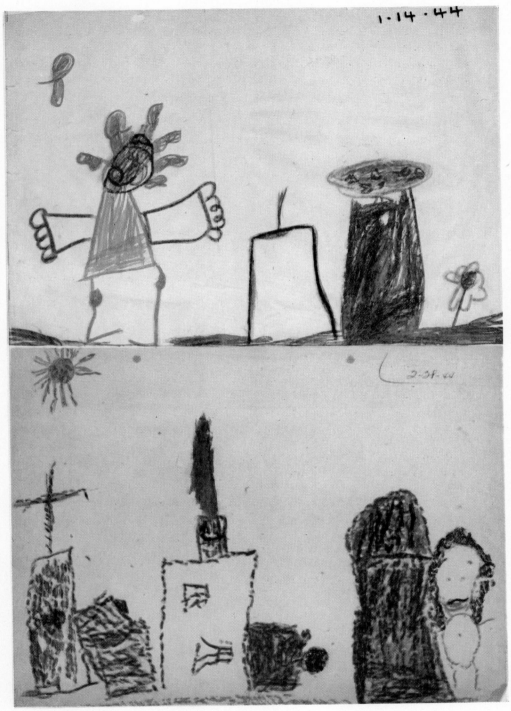

FIG. 53a (*top*). A Self Portrait with a House and a Tree, by Jean (*crayon*).
FIG. 53b (*bottom*). A Church, A House, and A Tree, by Jean (*crayon*).

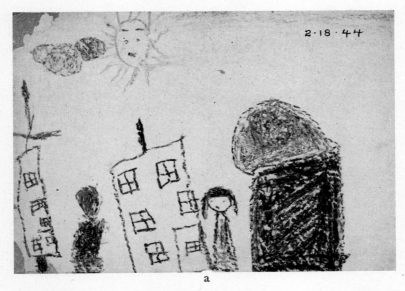

a

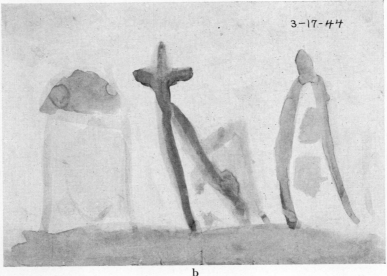

b

FIG. 54a, b. A Tree, A House, and A Church, by Jean (*water color*).

peutic relationship with her psychiatrist (perhaps facilitated by the benzedrine) and the felicitous use of techniques of drawing and talking through the intermediary of the devil.

March 9, 1944: (*Tell me a dream.*) "My mother was sleeping. I was sleeping. She got up and started looking for me. Then I got up and started looking for her. Then she started crying and I started crying. Then both of us said 'good-bye' and that was the end."

This dream indicates Jean's effort to give up her past life and her mother.

March 10th: *(Dream.)* "A nasty one. The devil said when I get married to play those nasty things."

March 14th: Jean is drawing and talks as she does so. "It's a little girl's house. Her name is Caroline. It's something like new houses. It looks new but it is old. You can make black smoke out of gray smoke. I always make old houses." *(Why?)* "I don't know how to make them straight."

(What's inside?) "Ladies, men, dogs. Fathers—mothers." (This of course is another meaning for a house—a place where people live together or a home.) "There's a moon inside that's something like an airplane on the side. You go inside through a door. It's warm inside. You come out and climb down a long ladder. It's cold outside. It's nice inside. You play around with games and have a good time."

(This might be interpreted as a more regressed fantasy of returning inside her mother.)

"Why does God make us this way—with hair like this?"

"Why is colored people? You know colored is better than white. That's what Joan (a colored child on the ward) said. I used to think that white was better than colored. I like white—No, I like them both."

Thus with the help of another little girl on the ward, Jean is able to deal with her problem of racial inferiority.

During her hospital stay Jean showed progressive improvement, and after three months she was prepared for placement in a foster home. The disturbance in her inner life had quieted considerably as shown in her fantasy material during an interview near the time of her discharge.

When asked for a dream, she stated: "No, I don't dream anymore. I just think. One night I thought my mother was here and she was coming to take me home. I was mad and I was crying. She went back home. Then she came back and asked me do I feel O.K. and I said, 'Yes.' Then she asked my brother if he missed me and he said 'Yes' and he said 'ain't it a shame for little people to be alone like that?' He said to me do I really love him and I said 'yes' but he didn't believe me. One night when I was going to bed I thought I was talking with my doctor. Someone waked me up and said there was a ghost after me. Someone else asked why I woke up and I said, 'someone said there was a ghost' and they said 'Don't worry, that was wrong. There ain't no ghost.' "

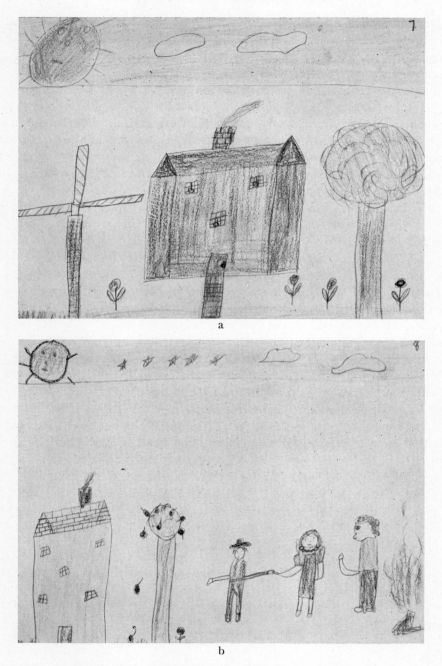

FIG. 55a, b. Drawings three years later, by Jean (*crayon*).

These dreams indicate her readiness to give up the old family relationship and the last one shows that she is ready to terminate her therapy and give up her therapist, also.

Jean entered a foster home in April 1944 and has since made what has been described as a remarkable adjustment. Her school record is good and there is mutual affection and devotion between her, her foster parents, and two foster sisters.

Jean was seen again in January 1947, three years after her initial referral to the hospital. She was 9½ years old. She had forgotten all but a few details of her life in her original home, and these were inaccurately remembered in a direction that made them relatively harmless. She remembered her hospital experience pleasantly, and when showed her original art work, recalled having done some, but not all of it. She was no longer aware of the symbolism. Her spontaneous drawings (Fig. 55) at that time followed the same general pattern as her earlier ones but in form and execution were appropriate to her age level. They were done with less facility, however, and showed a rigidity which was lacking in her earlier works. The verbalized fantasy material which accompanied them remained at a symbolic level and kept the deeper instinctual material well covered at all times.

In the first of the latter drawings the sign concerning the cross now appears on a windmill and she states: "That's to keep you cool." The tree is realistically portrayed. In the last picture there is a girl standing by a fire with hand outstretched towards her parents who are hand in hand. Beyond the parents is a tree reminiscent of her earlier ones. It has apples falling from it. Concerning this picture she states: "The little girl saw the apples falling off the tree. She told her mother and her mother came out and picked them up. Then the father came home from work and the little girl told him what had happened. The mother told her to go outside to get out of her way and the little girl looked up at the sky and made a fire and stood by it. The mother said the apples were no good because they were in the dirt and were rotten. The little girl looked at the sky to see if the sun was shining."

Thus the last drawing might be said to recapitulate and condense into a single, fleeting, mobile, pictorial pattern the entirety of Jean's life experiences which have been emotionally meaningful to her so far. Is this not also true of any spontaneous creative production?

~ 19 ~

THE ART OF CHILDREN AND THE PROBLEMS
OF MODERN ART[1]

THE STUDY of the art of children and especially of problem children helps in the understanding of modern art and the problems of modern life. Indeed, the problems of human life and of human art find such a clear expression in these children that their consideration leads to the discussion of problems of general concern, as well as to an approach to the problems of modern art.

THE FORM OF THE HUMAN BODY IN RELATION TO
GEOMETRICAL FORMS

The human body has always been one of the main concerns of art. Human beings are inclined to think that the human body is familiar to them and that they have a clear picture of their own bodies and of the bodies of others. Many schools of psychology are even inclined to believe that the child from the beginning has a clear cut knowledge and experience of its own body and sees the world in comparison to its own body. However, it has been shown clearly in Paul Schilder's writings and our experience with the graphic and plastic art of children that the child has to gain the knowledge of its own body in the same way that it learns to know the world. Franziska Boas has considered this problem also in relation to dance.

In the gradual constructive processes the child builds up the knowledge of its own body as the body image. This body image is in no way an experience which is stabilized. It undergoes continuous change. If human beings were able to have a clear conception of their own bodies there would be no need for mirrors. Persons learn about their bodies by their continuous contact with the outer world. The bodies of others have to be seen, human beings have to look at themselves and at others. The body image continually changes its shape. It is built, dissolved, remodeled and reconstructed. One is never sure; one has to gain this knowledge by continuous effort. This is the basis for the continuous curiosity mankind has concerning the body. Naked or covered, it is mysterious and incomplete. One's own body is more familiar to one than that of others. The human form is seen everywhere, the body images of other human beings are perceived but animals and even plants are also graced with

---

[1] Written by Paul Schilder as the concluding chapter in *Art of the Problem Child*. (See Foreword.)

303

the dignity of body images. One might even go so far as to see such images in stones and in the forms of inanimate nature.

This is a world not only of curves, circles, ellipses and straight lines; it is also one of the human organic forms which are strictly incomparable with geometry. Wherein the actual difference between these human forms and geometrical forms lies is the great riddle. After all, the soft curves of the breasts and the buttocks are also geometrical lines. One is not sure where the borderline lies between geometry and the body image. Sometimes the body image is seen everywhere and seems to substitute for geometry. On other occasions geometry progresses into the body. Inanimate and animate nature retain, at first, something of the appearance of human forms in the struggle against geometrical tendencies but finally triangles, circles, rectangles, curves, angles and straight lines invade and substitute for the body image. In *Cubism and Abstract Art*[2] there is quoted the letter written by Paul Cezanne to Emile Bernard which reads: "You must see in nature the cylinder, the sphere, the cone." Pablo Picasso's *Head of a Woman* is symmetrically broken in facets like a cut diamond but the form is still sculptural. The paintings and bronzes of this period of cubism are closely related to Negro sculptures. But this so-called "analytical cubism" of Picasso and Georges Braque is soon replaced by so called "synthetic cubism," in which the tendency to an extreme, almost geometrical severity is outstanding. Similar tendencies can be found in the work of Fernand Leger. In one of the early works of Picasso, *The Studio* (1928), geometry is dominant. From this point of view it is stimulating to study Theo Van Doesburg's *Aesthetic Transformation of the Object* in which a cow and a person are finally transformed into a rectangular pattern. These painters and sculptors reveal the geometry both in nature and in the human body.

Body image and geometry are eternal enemies. The body image can be pushed aside but it still remains, and it tries to come back. In the later work of Picasso, organic forms crept back; and some of his pictures of the latest period so far as they are not strictly classical in style, are bone-like and show forms which are of "organic type." One picture by Max Ernst in which embryonic forms prevail is entitled *The gramineous bicycle garnished with bells, the pilfered graybeards and the echinderms bending the spine to look for caresses.* One of the pictures of Yves Tanguy is entitled *Heredity of Acquired Characteristics.*

It is interesting to compare these developments with the work of children who at first draw the human body as an incomplete circle supported on two lines; at about three years vertical configurations replace horizontal ones. The drawings of defective children often consist mostly of geometrical patterns and the relation of these geometrical patterns to the human form is not always obvious. Our most valuable material in this respect is offered in

---

[2] Barr, Alfred H.: *Cubism and Abstract Art.*

the drawings and paintings by Francine (Frontispiece and Figs. 17, 20 and 21) who drew figures with studied symmetry, reminiscent of some of the work of Henri Rousseau. Afterwards she descended to completely abstract patterns similar in many respects to Orphism, and to designs in which there are only vague hints of organic form (Fig. 20). The whole problem of body image and geometry also reflects itself, then, in the productions of our children. From this point of view it is very important to study some of the sidewalk drawings (Fig. 3a), the drawings of the encephalitic children (Fig. 27) and of the schizophrenic children: Joan (Fig. 22) and Marty (Fig. 43), in which the bodies appear in more or less geometrical patterns.

THE MEANING OF THE DISTORTION OF THE BODY IMAGE IN ART

We have stressed the relation between the body image and geometry. We have seen similar trends toward experimentation with body images and geometry in modern art and in the drawings of our patients. The body image can also be changed in very different ways. In some of the pictures of Amedeo Modigliani (in the collection of George Gershwin, 1937), not only are the necks elongated but other parts of the body as well. The curves of the cheek in a man's portrait are exaggerated and in a woman's portrait the curves of the breasts and the buttocks are emphasized. In the picture of *Anna de Zoorowska* the face is not only slanted but also distorted in the direction of the slant. In Georges Rouault's pictures the figures are often sturdy and quadrangular, as if they had been artificially shortened and compressed from head to foot so that they are broadened. It is remarkable that this painter so frequently chooses to draw dwarf clowns. It is as if he had a particular pleasure in experimenting with the space of the body image and changing it almost arbitrarily.

In plastic art the possibilities for distortions of the space of the body are still greater. One sculptor arranges mother and child in nearly cubic form. Other sculptors prefer to shorten the third dimension so that the figures almost resemble a bas-relief; as, for example, in many of the sculptures of Isamu Noguchi. If the depth dimension is decreased, the figures are elongated; the postures especially of the neck stiffen out and the front view of the figure gains paramount importance. One might say that it is almost as if the human figure had been exposed to a definite pull in one direction or in the other, or as if in some of these pictures the influence of the gravitational forces on the body had been decreased or increased. Similar distortions are indeed subjectively experienced in individuals in whom the organs of equilibrium are affected as if by the vestibular apparatus and its central connections.[3]

---

[3] Schilder, Paul: *Vestibular Apparatus.*

In our material we find characteristic distortions in the human figure as drawn by Julius (Fig. 32), who was interested in the funny side of human experiences. Here the distortion does not follow a general principle but is the expression of the individual problem of the patient and his particular way of looking at the world. Also with Francine, the far-reaching distortions of figures merely served her need to cling to at least one outstanding part of reality as in the facial distortions of "Bender" (Fig. 21c). In both cases caricature is an expression of helplessness concerning reality, and an attempt to keep to reality by seeing its single features in distortion.[4]

The schizophrenic child may draw an eye or a face separately outside of the head as Joan does (Fig. 22). In their drawings, pieces of bodies are strewn all over the world. This is true not only of schizophrenic patients but also of some patients with organic damage to the brain. Everyone, as a child, is confronted with the problem of building up the image of his own body. These patients have returned to the primitive mode of experience.

The modern painter, the schizophrenic artist and the child who draws, go back to the fundamental problem of gaining knowledge of their own body. In order to know it, they have to experiment again and again, and one has no right to say that the seemingly finished product which classic art and conventional drawing offer is a final solution. When one sees the famous picture of Duchamp, *Nude Descending a Staircase,* one wonders which is the staircase and which is the nude. The nude has become almost a geometrical motif. Is this arbitrary? Indeed human beings have to learn about themselves. This is only one of the many phases of the experimental approach of human beings to their own bodies. Accepted and conventional forms make one forget that the organism and human life are in a continuous process of construction and reconstruction. The immense value of modern art lies in its renewed approach to these fundamental form problems. Schizophrenic artists may handle these problems in a way which allows a deeper understanding of them.

EXPERIMENTATION WITH SPACE AND GRAVITATION

The child obviously struggles to bring objects into the proper spatial relation. Marty, the schizophrenic boy, when he was most disturbed moved his figures about in the air but was able to orient them better as he became more controlled (Fig. 43); so also did Nat (Fig. 33). Jean was not schizophrenic but when she was disturbed by emotional problems her figures were also in the air (Fig. 53).

Modern artists, however, experiment in a much more energetic way with

---

[4] The five following paragraphs are reprinted from Schilder, Paul: *Theoretical Aspects of the Art Work in Bellevue Hospital, in Direction,* Vol. 2, #2, pp. 2-3, 1939.

the distortions of space. In the picture by Man Ray, *Observatory Time—the Lovers,* an object in the form of a vulva or a pair of lips of gigantic size is suspended in the air. These artists attempt energetically to overcome the fetters of gravitation. The whole problem of the vertical line and the vertical direction in general is a problem which is of the greatest importance for physiology. It is very probable that a vertical line is perceived as such, not merely by the eye, but also by the vestibular influences and by the whole apparatus for equilibrium. Paul Cezanne, for instance, in some of his landscapes stresses the perpendicular line, thereby exaggerating the importance of gravitation. In other pictures he reverts to a compository form which already played an important part in the work of Leonardo da Vinci and of Nicholas Poussin. It is a tendency to use the triangle as a scheme for the organization of human hopes. However, Dominiko Theotokopoulous (El Greco) was much more radical in this respect. The faces of his figures are oblique, asymmetrical and distorted. Pseudo-physiological reasoning has been employed by some critics who surmised that the man was astigmatic, and therefore, distorted the world. This reasoning is preposterous, since one would have to see the canvas astigmatically also, and the picture drawn after nature therefore would not show any distortions. If El Greco was astigmatic in one eye he must have had a reason for choosing the so-called distortion.

Faces and objects which have been brought from the vertical into the oblique line indeed have another meaning. A new symmetry and asymmetry has to be invented and the pictures, less earth-bound than before, acquire a new spiritual meaning. Max Weber's picture *Invocation* is an example of this principle. The fight against gravity has become a religious struggle. The oblique line is in some way more appropriate to the ascetic than the perpendicular line.

Boccioni's *Unique Forms of Continuity in Space,* in the Museum of Modern Art (New York), is an attempt to catch movement in space with rather abstract forms. Modern art is fundamentally interested in problems of space, movement and gravitation. In some pictures of Chagall, figures float in the air head down. The individual is no longer earth-bound. Objects and persons fly and float. The individual is liberated from the laws of gravitation. Our patients, too, seek escape from these laws. All human beings feel that they are too closely bound to the earth. It is one of the oldest dreams of mankind to get rid of this constraint.

In early childhood man learns that he has a great enemy. This is the force that makes him fall down and hurt himself. By standing upright gravitation is overcome. The vertical is a direction of fundamental importance. The vertical is not merely an optical experience but one's whole body participates in determining what it is. Such biologically important experiences inevitably affect painters and artists. When orientation is changed from a vertical to an inclined plane some measure of freedom from gravitation is gained. This can be seen in some pictures of Weber and Picasso. In various pictures of Cezanne which treat the motif of the bathers, the human body is seen on an inclined plane and no doubt the deep impression which is received from these pictures is due in part to the freedom from gravitation which the artist has gained.

So art comes into close relation with the dreams of flying which belong to the deepest inheritance of mankind. Both the child and the artist want to fly. So does the primitive man. Man's dreams, the day dreams of the child, the artist and the primitive come first. Second comes the inventor, the engineer who translates these dreams into some sort of reality. Artists are forever experimenting with space, with gravity, with inclined and vertical lines. Superman and many of the figures in the comics deal with the same problem. Similarly, people who have lost contact with everyday life or who are confronted with difficult situations can no longer be satisfied with small conventional concepts. The value of our patients' pictures lies in the fact that they are the expression not of people who are satisfied but of human beings who strive anew. They have been thrown back to a more primitive world and now have to experiment and build up a new world all over again.

Art should be seen as one of the experimental and constructive drives of human life. Whenever new principles in art occur, whether it be surrealism, dadaism, or cubism, they will in some way be connected with the spiritual movements of the times. The fundamental problems of form which are of importance to the modern artist are also the problem of the primitive man, of the child and of the mentally sick. In order to handle a new problem in the complex world of today, one has to go back and reduce the problem to its simplest, most primitive terms. Then one can determine its true significance. If one wants to know whether a new movement in art has a definite value one should go back to the art of the psychiatric patient and find out whether the patient tries to solve similar problems. If he does, then we may be sure that the new art tendency deals with fundamental experiences. The art of the patient and the creative artist will always be a disturbing element. In creative art one is forced to go back to primitive experiences and wage again the fight for the conquest of the world. In the art of the mentally ill is thus found the germ from which richer experiences can originate. The creative artist attempts the fulfillment of the deep urge to form and order which manifests itself also in the pictures of our patients.

OTHER APPROACHES TO REALITY

The drawings of almost all of our children indicate that even somewhat complicated proportions in the outer world are comparatively well perceived. It would be easy to relate any apparent distortions to the technical difficulties involved. It is at least probable that the emotional attitude of intense interest towards the human body is a factor in the perception of both the human form and the outer world.

Children in their drawings mostly refrain from distorting reality in such a far-reaching way as Gino Severini, for instance, does when he mixes the different parts of reality together so that they look like pieces of a jig saw puzzle which are not brought into the proper order. In an artist like Severini, reality is not merely a structure consisting of units and wholes but also of parts. Obviously there is a great satisfaction in seeing these parts as such, with the knowledge that by renewed effort the jig saw puzzle of reality can be put together again. Such principles indeed are to be found in free imagination and it is characteristic that in one of the pictures by Severini the life of a dancer appears in different sectors emanating from the eye. Such experimentation is not generally found in children. They cling more to what they can reach and what can be expressed in comparatively primitive form. Only when there is a severe dissociation, as in schizophrenic children, may reality be seen in pieces or the inner relation of the body may be distorted completely, as by Marty (Fig. 43); or in emotionally disturbed children, such as Jean, may a distortion of reality be shown due to an inner confusion (Fig. 51).

On the whole children also want to reach reality in their drawings. If they cannot reach reality in developed form, they choose primitive rhythmical forms and geometrical designs, as post-encephalitic children (Fig. 27) or mentally defective children do, or they seek a simplified reality. In the human figure the child may cling to one outstanding trend, as in the characteristic faces of Francine (Fig. 21) and Julius (Fig. 32) and the human figures of Joan (Fig. 22b). However none of these attempts are rigid. The child not only clings to reality, but when it playfully appears to give up reality it is for the purpose of new play, new experimentation and renewed contact with reality. Nothing is so false to the child as the impressionistic way of drawing, if impressionism is considered as the basic theory that the world consists of single sensual impressions and that reality is built up of single impressions which are called sensations. In some way the impressionists believe implicitly in the theory of Condorcet, that at first there is nothing in the mind and that the sensations enter, one after another, until a picture of the world appears. Newer psychology shows conclusively that sensations are far from being primitive units of experience, but are rather products of a complicated process of abstraction.

COLORS

If any new proof were necessary, the drawings of children would show conclusively that they see objects and configurations, and do not have any "sensations." Accordingly the child is not interested in colors independent of the object. Only when the dissociation and the regression have gone very far, as with Francine, are the colors bound to primitive form (Frontispiece). In the language of psychology one can say that the child usually draws the object with the color the object has, or what Ewald Hering[5] called "Gedaechtnis." The child is generally not interested in what it sees in the atmosphere or in space but in the colors of the object. It is true that the child may be more or less arbitrary in the choice of colors. These colors find expression in the primitive pleasures in the saturated primary colors used by some Puerto Rican, South American and Negro children under emotional strain (see Plates II, III, and IV). The colors not only express the memory of the object color but also the mood of the individual; even then the color is not experienced as something going on in the subject but as a part of the object. Jean's earliest paintings were confused in form and dark and depressive in coloring; later the forms and colors became clear and distinct; finally as the fantasy material became less important, the colors became delicate and faded together with the forms. Hymen and Emelio who were so much interested in the details of forests and animals naturally used lively and vivid colors for their absorbing objects (Fig. 39, and Plate III).

The color techniques of these children is that of classical painting, and not the technique of impressionism and surrealism. It is in connection with this that the child usually prefers to have clear contours of the objects, which is a principle foreign to impressionism. In most of the children's art work the colors are strong and direct. More delicate features occur in the landscapes of Joseph (Fig. 25). In the light of these experiences the impressionistic principle of painting seems more or less an interesting experimental principle which has very little relationship to any of the developmental stages of drawing and to any developmental disturbance.

THE CONTENT OF DRAWINGS

What is the content of drawings which interest the child and especially the problem child? According to Meyer Shapiro,[6] there can be no question that every special art technique prefers special objects. The early stage of cubism showed an interest in human faces; later on, the mandarin, guitar, etc., became more and more important. In the later phases the distorted human figures assumed greater importance, as in the latest creations of Pablo Picasso. Abstract cubism prefers inanimate nature. The surrealism of Salvador Dali has fantastic and uncanny content but he paints with the utmost care and realistic technique.

---

[5] See Hartshorne, Charles: *The Philosophy and Psychology of Sensation.*
[6] Personal communication.

In many of our drawings the children are interested in landscapes when they want to escape difficult personal situations. Many immature children are interested in boats and nautical scenes (Fig. 34). Other children with difficult relationships within the family draw animals (Figs. 36-39). The mentally deficient children prefer simple objects like houses, the forms of which they can master. A 6 year old girl, Jean, with unusual sex experiences drew mostly "a house, a church, and a tree" with symbolic implications (Figs. 51-53). A boy was interested in clowns and monkey faces (Fig. 32). Francine lived within a world of primitive forms or drew portraits in caricature. The problems of content and form always have a deep inner connection. One should keep in mind that there is always the same fundamental problem expressed in drawings and pictures as in one's attitude towards the world. It is interesting that none of the formal principles appearing in our material nor any of the content are foreign to the experiences of any normal person and any normal child. This is a problem that interested R. A. Pfeifer who studied schizophrenic art and compared it to the free creations of artists who were given the task of drawing fantastic and demoniac material. It is interesting that some of these artists produced drawings very similar to the content of the paintings of Dali. Sexual and emotional problems in general often will find a rather uninhibited expression in the psychopathic artist, child as well as adult. Hans Prinzhorn reproduces a sadistic scene of beating. Nat was interested only in the problem of fighting (Fig. 33). Sexual material appears still more openly in the clay modeling of children studied by Adolf G. Woltmann (Fig. 45).

THE EMERGENCE OF FORM PRINCIPLES

For children and adults, mentally balanced or unbalanced, art is a preliminary approach to reality. These persons try to master the primitive form principles of the circle, the wave and the straight line. They are interested in ellipses, rectangles and loops. They want to explore symmetry and assymmetry, rhythm, repetition and number. Furthermore they want to approach the objects of nature, animate and inanimate. They are interested not only in hills and stones and rivers, but also in trees, flowers, animals and human beings. The problem of form for them is closely related to that of color. Forms extend in space. All of the problems mentioned are more or less specifically connected with problems of space. The fundamental problem of which way the primitive form principles and primitive color principles are integrated into more complicated forms, especially animate forms, appear in hundreds and hundreds of variations. In the transition from primitive to developed forms, the whole cycle of human experience is gone through and all the contents of human life make their appearance. All the solutions given by art either in the normal or abnormal individual are preliminary. The lack of definiteness of final action is characteristic for art as is also the fact that one level reached may be given up again for renewed play with primitive forms and experiences.

It is the great merit of modern art that it has taken up the spirit of free experimentation which has been far too long submerged. The final aim of art is the preparation for a definite approach to reality. But to find this approach one often has to give up the preliminary gain, the crystallization of form which appears to be definite. In order to make any approach really progressive one has to regress from time to time and go back to the basic primitive approach. This is the deepest meaning of impressionism, futurism, cubism, constructivism, dadaism and surrealism.

The abnormal child and the abnormal artist have an easier access to the primitive forms. Also they are often driven by their pathology back to the primitive experience (regression) and then strive more or less earnestly to regain full reality. There is a continuous striving to reach from the primitive experience to the well-developed one and no regression is definite even in the psychotic case. There is always the allure of reality. This is a dynamic process. The art of disturbed children and the psychotic adult brings phases of this gigantic struggle more clearly into evidence. Therefore they represent the same basic human qualities which appear in every fact of art production and in its history. The dynamic approach to reality is an interplay between regression and progression in which the creative forces finally prevail. Since these creative forces are biologically determined by the urge to reality, they conquer reality.

BIBLIOGRAPHY

ABT, LAWRENCE E. (Ed.): Projective Psychology. New York, Knopf, 1950.

ALDRICH, C. ANDERSON: The pediatrician looks at personality. Am. J. Orthopsychiat., 17: 571-574, 1947.

ALDRICH, C. ANDERSON and ALDRICH, MARY M.: Babies Are Human Beings. New York, Macmillan, 1938.

ALDRICH, MARY M.: Jt. author, see Aldrich, C. Anderson and Aldrich, Mary M.

ALSCHULER, ROSE H. and HATTWICK, LA BERTA WEISS: Painting and Personality; A Study of Young Children. Chicago, Univ. Chicago Press, 1947.

AMATRUDA, CATHERINE S.: Jt. author, see Gesell, Arnold L. and Amatruda, Catherine S.

AMENT, W.: The Mind of a Child; A Comparative History of Life. New York, A. and C. Boni, 1923.

ANASTASI, ANNE and FOLEY, JOHN P. JR.: An analysis of spontaneous drawings by children in different cultures. J. Applied Psychol., 20:689-726, 1936.

ANASTASI, ANNE and FOLEY, JOHN P. JR.: A study of animal drawings by Indian children of the North Pacific Coast. J. Soc. Psychol., 9:363-374, 1938.

ANASTASI, ANNE and FOLEY, JOHN P. JR.: A survey of the literature on artistic behavior in the abnormal; historical and theoretical background. J. Genet. Psychol., 25:111-142, 1941.

ANASTASI, ANNE and FOLEY, JOHN P. JR.: Artistic behavior in the abnormal; experimental investigations. J. Genet. Psychol., 25:187-237, 1941.

ANDERSON, HOWARD H. and ANDERSON, GLADYS L. (Eds.): Projective Techniques. New York, Prentice Hall, 1951.

ANDERSON, JOHN E.: Methods in Child Psychiatry. Chap. I in Carmichael, Leonard (Ed.): Manual of Child Psychiatry. New York, Wiley, 1946.

APPEL, R. E.: Drawings by children as aids to personality studies. Am. J. Orthopsychiat., 4:93-97, 1934.

APPLETON, L. ESTELLE: A Comparative Study of the Play Activities of Adult Savages and Civilized Children. Chicago, Univ. of Chicago Press, 1910.

ARNHEIM, RUDOLF: Psychology of the dance. Dance Magazine, Aug. 1946.

AXELROD, PEARL L.: Jt. author, see Stewart, Kathleen K. and Axelrod, Pearl L.

BAKER, B. W.: The History of the Care of the Feeble-minded. Bull. Mass. Dept. Ment. Dis., 14:19-29, 1932.

BALDWIN, JAMES M.: Social and Ethical Interpretations of Mental Development. New York, Macmillan, 1913.

BARR, ALFRED H. JR. (Ed.): Cubism and Abstract Art. New York, Museum of Modern Art, 1936.

BARR, ALFRED H. JR.: Fantastic Art, Dada, Surrealism. New York, Museum of Modern Art, 1936.

BARTEMEIER, LEO H.: Concerning the Cornelian Corner. Am. J. Orthopsychiat., 17:594-598, 1947.

BARUCH, DOROTHY W.: Aggression during doll play in a pre-school. Am. J. Orthopsychiat., 11:252-259, 1941.

BARUCH, DOROTHY W.: Play techniques in pre-school as an aid in guidance. Psycholog. Bull., 36:570, 1939.

BATCHELDER, MARJORIE H.: The Puppet Theatre Handbook. New York and London, Harper, 1947.

BEAUMONT, CYRIL W.: Puppets and the Puppet Stage. London, The Studio, 1938.

BECK, SAMUEL J.: The Rorschach Test as applied to a feeble-minded group. New York, Arch. Psychol., No. 136, 1932.

BECKH, ERICA: Jt. author, see Jenkins, R. L. and Beckh, Erica.

BELL, JOHN E.: Projective Techniques: a Dynamic Approach to the Study of the Personality. New York, Longmans, 1948.

313

BENDER, LAURETTA: Art and Psychopathology. Exhibition jointly sponsored by Psychiatric Division of Bellevue Hospital and Federal Arts Project of W.P.A. Am. Orthopsychiat. A., New York, Hotel Commodore, 1939.

BENDER, LAURETTA: Art and therapy in the mental disturbances of children. J. Nerv. and Ment. Dis., 86:249-263, 1937.

BENDER, LAURETTA: Cerebral sequelae and behavior disorders following pyogenic meningo-encephalitis in children. Arch. Pediat., 59:772-783, 1942.

BENDER, LAURETTA: Childhood schizophrenia. Am. J. Orthopsychiat., 17:40-56, 1947.

BENDER, LAURETTA: Childhood schizophrenia. Nerv. Child., 1:138-140, 1942.

BENDER, LAURETTA: Gestalt function in mental defect. Proc. and Addr. Am. A. Ment. Deficiency, 41:192-210, 1932.

BENDER, LAURETTA: Gestalt principles in the sidewalk drawings and games of children. Pedagog. Seminar and J. Genet. Psychol., 41:192-210, 1932.

BENDER, LAURETTA: The Goodenough Test (drawing a man) in chronic encephalitis in children. J. Nerv. and Ment. Dis., 91:277-286, 1940.

BENDER, LAURETTA: Group activities on a children's ward as methods of psychotherapy. Am. J. Psychiat., 93:1151-1173, 1937.

BENDER, LAURETTA: Manual for Instruction and Test Cards for Visual Motor Gestalt Test. Am. Orthopsychiat. A., 1946.

BENDER, LAURETTA: One hundred cases of childhood schizophrenia treated with electric shock. Trans. Am. Neurol. A., 72:165-169, 1947.

BENDER, LAURETTA: Post-encephalitic Behavior Disorders in Childhood, in Neal, Josephine B. (Ed.): Encephalitis, a Clinical Study. New York, Grune and Stratton, Chapt. viii: 361-385, 1943.

BENDER, LAURETTA: Principles of gestalt in copied form in mentally defective and schizophrenic persons. Arch. Neurol. and Psychiat., 27:661-686, 1932.

BENDER, LAURETTA: The Problem of Anxiety in Disturbed Children, in Hoch, Paul and Zubin, Paul (Eds.): Anxiety. New York, Grune and Stratton, 1950, pp. 119-139.

BENDER, LAURETTA: The psychology of children's reading and the comics. J. Educ. Sociol., 18:223-231, 1944.

BENDER, LAURETTA: Psychological principles of the visual motor gestalt test. Trans. New York Acad. Sc., 11:164-170, 1949.

BENDER, LAURETTA: Psychopathic Behavior Disorders in Children; in Lindner, R. M. and Seliger, R. V. (Eds.) Handbook of Correctional Psychology. New York, Philosophical Library, 1947, pp. 360-377.

BENDER, LAURETTA: Techniques in Child Psychiatry. Chap. IV in Glueck, Bernard (Ed.): Current Therapies of Personality Disorders. New York, Grune and Stratton, 1946.

BENDER, LAURETTA: The treatment of aggression: Aggression in childhood. Am. J. Orthopsychiat., 13:392-399, 1943.

BENDER, LAURETTA: A Visual Motor Gestalt Test and Its Clinical Use. Research Monogr. No. 3. Am. Orthopsychiat. A., 1938.

BENDER, LAURETTA and BLAU, ABRAM: The reaction of children to sexual relation with adults. Am. J. Orthopsychiat., 17:500-518, 1937.

BENDER, LAURETTA and BOAS, FRANZISKA: Creative dance in therapy. Am. J. Orthopsychiat., 11:235-245, 1941.

BENDER, LAURETTA and COTTINGTON, FRANCES: The use of amphetamine sulphate (benzedrine) in child psychiatry. Am. J. Psychiat., 99:116-121, 1942.

BENDER, LAURETTA and CURRAN, FRANK J.: Children and adolescents who kill. J. Crim. Psychopath., 1:297-322, 1940.

BENDER, LAURETTA and LIPKOWITZ, H.: Hallucinations in children. Am. J. Orthopsychiat., 10:471-490, 1940.

BENDER, LAURETTA and LOURIE, REGINALD S.: The effect of comic books on the ideology of children. Am. J. Orthopsychiat., 11:540-550, 1941.

BENDER, LAURETTA and MONTAGUE, ALLISON: Art in Schizophrenic Children. Exhibit at 5th Intern. Congr. of Pediatrics. New York Official Program, 154-155, 1947.

BENDER, LAURETTA and MONTAGUE, ALLISON: Psychotherapy through art in a Negro child. College Art Journal, 7:12-16, 1947.

BENDER, LAURETTA and RAPOPORT, JACK: Animal drawings of children. Am. J. Orthopsychiat., 14:521-527, 1944.

BENDER, LAURETTA and SCHILDER, PAUL: Aggressiveness in children. Genet. Psychol. Monog., 18:410-525, 1936.

BENDER, LAURETTA and SCHILDER, PAUL: Art and the Problem Child (unpublished).

BENDER, LAURETTA and SCHILDER, PAUL: Form as a principle in the play of children. J. Genet. Psychol., 49:254-261, 1936.

BENDER, LAURETTA and SCHILDER, PAUL: Impulsions, a specific disorder in the behavior of children. Arch. Neurol. and Psychiat., 44:990-1008, 1940.

BENDER, LAURETTA and SCHILDER, PAUL: Mannerisms as organic motility syndrome. Confinia Neurologica, 3:321-330, 1941.

BENDER, LAURETTA and SCHILDER, PAUL: Studies in aggressiveness: II Aggressiveness in children. Genet. Psychol. Monogr. 18: Nos. 5 and 6, 410-525, 1936.

BENDER, LAURETTA and SCHILDER, PAUL: Suicidal Preoccupations and attempts in children. Am. J. Orthopsychiat., 7:225-234, 1937.

BENDER, LAURETTA and WOLFSON, WILLIAM Q.: The nautical theme in the art and fantasy of children. Am. J. Orthopsychiat., 13:462-467, 1943.

BENDER, LAURETTA and WOLTMANN, ADOLF G.: Play and psychotherapy. Nerv. Child., 1:17-42, 1941.

BENDER, LAURETTA and WOLTMANN, ADOLF G.: Puppetry as a psychotherapeutic measure for behavior problems in children. Month Bull. New York State A. Occup. Therapists, 7:1-9, 1937.

BENDER, LAURETTA and WOLTMANN, ADOLF G.: The use of plastic material as a psychiatric approach to emotional problems in children. Am. J. Orthopsychiat., 7:283-300, 1937.

BENDER, LAURETTA and WOLTMANN, ADOLF G.: The use of puppet shows as a psychotherapeutic measure for behavior problems in children. Am. J. Orthopsychiat., 6:341-354, 1936.

BENEDEK, THERESE: The psychosomatic implications of the primary unit: mother-child. Am. J. Orthopsychiat., 19:642-654, 1949.

BENEDICT, RUTH: Child rearing in certain European countries. Am. J. Orthopsychiat., 19: 342-350, 1949.

BENJAMIN, ANNE and WEATHERLY, HOWARD E.: Hospital ward treatment of emotionally disturbed children. Am. J. Orthopsychiat., 17:665-674, 1947.

BERRIEN, F. K.: A study of the drawings of abnormal children. J. Educ. Psychol., 26: 143-150, 1935.

BETTELHEIM, BRUNO: Self-interpretation of fantasy. Am. J. Orthopsychiat., 17:80-100, 1947.

BETTELHEIM, BRUNO and SYLVESTER, EMMY: Therapeutic influence of the group on the individual. Am. J. Orthopsychiat., 17:684-692, 1947.

BIBER, BARBARA, et al: Child Life in School. New York, Dutton, 1942.

BINET, ALFRED: The Intelligence of the Feeble-minded. Transl. by Skite, E. Baltimore, Williams and Williams, 1916.

BLAU, ABRAM: Jt. author, see Bender, Lauretta and Blau, Abram.

BLEULER, MANFRED: Schizophrenia; review of the work of Prof. Eugen Bleuler. Arch. Neurol. and Psychiat., 26:610-627, 1931.

BOAS, FRANZISKA: Notes on percussion accompaniment for the dance. Dance Observer, 5:71-72, 1938.

BOAS, FRANZISKA: Percussion music and its relation to modern dance. Dance Observer, 7:6-7, 1940; 10:71-72, 1943.

BOAS, FRANZISKA: Psychological aspects in the practice and teaching of creative dance. J. Aesthetics and Art Criticism, 2:3-20, 1941-42.

BOAS, FRANZISKA: Teaching the lay dancer. Progressive Physical Educator, 23:2, 1941.

BOAS, FRANZISKA (Ed.): The Function of Dance in Human Society. New York, Boas School, 1944.

BOAS, FRANZISKA: Jt. author, see Bender, Lauretta and Boas, Franziska.

BOCHNER, RUTH and HALPERN, FLORENCE: The Clinical Application of the Rorschach Test. 2nd Ed. New York, Grune and Stratton, 1945.

BORNSTEIN, BERTA: Phobia in a two-and-a-half year old child. Psychoanalyt. Quart., 4:93-119, 1935.

BORNSTEIN, STEFF: Child analysis. Psychoanalyt. Quart., 4:190-225, 1935.

BOSSARD, JAMES H. S.: Sociology of Child Development. New York, Harper, 1948.

BOWLBY, JOHN: Forty-four Juvenile Thieves; their Character and Home Life. London, Bailliére, Tindall and Co., 1946. Also in: Intern. J. Psycho-Anal., 25:19-53, 1944.

BOWMAN, KARL M.: The psychiatrist looks at child psychiatry. Am. J. Psychiat., 101:665-675, 1944.

BRADLEY, CHARLES: Indications for residential treatment of children with severe neuropsychiatric problems. Am. J. Orthopsychiat., 19:427, 431, 1949.

BRADLEY, CHARLES: Schizophrenia in Childhood. New York, Macmillan, 1941.

BREWSTER, DOROTHY and BURELL, AGNES: Adventure or Experience. New York, Columbia Univ. Press, 1930.

BROWN, ELIZABETH E.: Notes on Children's Drawings. U. of Calif. Studies, Part 2, No. 1, 1897.

BROWN, FRANCIS J.: The Sociology of Childhood. New York, Prentice Hall, 1939.

BRUCH, HILDA: Obesity in Childhood.
I. Physical growth and development of obese children. Am. J. Dis. Child., 58:457-ff., 1939.
II. Basal metabolism and serum cholesterol of obese children. Am. J. Dis. Child., 58:1001-ff., 1939.
III. Physiologic and psychologic aspects of the food intake of obese children. Am. J. Dis. Child., 59:739-781, 1940.
IV. Energy expenditure of obese children. Am. J. Dis. Child., 60:1082-1109, 1940.

BRUCH, HILDA: Obesity in childhood and personality development. Am. J. Orthopsychiat., 11:467-475, 1941.

BRUCH, HILDA: Obesity in relation to puberty. J. Pediat., 19:365-ff., 1941.

BRUCH, HILDA: Psychiatric aspects of obesity in children. Am. J. Psychiat., 99:752-757, 1943.

BRUCH, HILDA: Psychological aspects of obesity. Bull. New York Acad. Med., 24:73-86, 1948.

BRUCH, HILDA: The role of the parent in psychotherapy with children. Psychiatry, 11:169-ff., 1948.

BRUCH, HILDA and HEWLETT, IRMA: Psychologic aspects of the medical management of diabetes in children. Psychosom. Med., 9:205-209, 1947.

BRUCH, HILDA and TOURAINE, G.: Obesity in childhood: V. The family frame of obese children. Psychosom. Med., 2:141-206, 1940.

BUEHLER, CHARLOTTE: From Birth to Maturity. London, Kegan Paul, Trench, Trubner and Co., 1935.

BUEHLER, CHARLOTTE: The World Test Manual of Directions. Los Angeles, privately printed, Charlotte Beuhler.

BUEHLER, CHARLOTTE; KELLY, LUMRY G., and CARROL, H.: World Test Standardization Studies. Child Psychiatry Monographs, 1949.

BUEHLER, KARL: Die Geistige Entwicklung des Kindes. Jena, Fischer, 1929.

BUEHLER. KARL; MUSOLD, DORA and VOKELT, H.: Die Neue Psychologie. Ztsch. f. Psychiat., 99:145-154, 1926.

BURELL, AGNES: Jt. author, see Brewster, Dorothy and Burell, Agnes.

BURLINGHAM, DOROTHY T.: Jt. author, see Freud, Anna and Burlingham, Dorothy T.

BURLINGHAM, SUSAN: Therapeutic effects of a play group for pre-school children. Am. J. Orthopsychiat., 8:627-638, 1938.

BURT, CYRIL L.: Mental and Scholastic Tests. London, P. S. King and Son, 1933.

CAMERON, KENNETH: A psychiatric in-patient department for children. J. Ment. Sc., 95: 560-566, 1949.

CAMERON, WILLIAM M.: The treatment of children in psychiatric clinics with particular reference to the use of play techniques. Bull. Menninger Clinic, 5:172-180, 1940.

CARLSON, JESSIE J.: Psychosomatic study of fifty stuttering children. III. Analysis of responses on the revised Stanford-Binet. Am. J. Orthopsychiat., 16:120-126, 1946.

CARMICHAEL, LEONARD (Ed.): Manual of Child Psychology. New York, John Wiley and Sons, 1946.

CARROLL, H.: Jt. author, see Buehler, Charlotte; Kelly, Lumry G., and Carrol, H.

CHENEY, FRANCIS E.: Fernald's influence on the special class movement. Bull. Mass. Ment. Dis., 14:75-94, 1930.

CHESS, STELLA: Developmental language disability as a factor in personality distortion in childhood. Am. J. Orthopsychiat., 14:483-490, 1944.

CHILD. CHARLES M.: The Origin and Development of the Nervous System. Chicago, Univ. of Chicago Press, 1921.

CLARK, L. PIERCE: Lincoln; A Psycho-biography. New York and London, Scribner, 1933.

CLARK, L. PIERCE: Nature and Treatment of Amentia. London, Bailliére, Tindall and Cox, 1933.

CONN, JACOB H.: Children's reactions to the discovery of genital differences. Am. J. Orthopsychiat., 10:747-762, 1940.

CONN, JACOB H.: The child reveals himself through play. Ment. Hyg., 23:49-70, 1939.

CONN, JACOB H.: The play interview: a method of studying children's attitudes. Am. J. Dis. Child., 58:1199-1219, 1939.

CONN, JACOB H.: A psychiatric study of car sickness in children. Am. J. Orthopsychiat., 8:130-141, 1938.

COTTINGTON, FRANCES: Jt. author, see Bender, Lauretta and Cottington, Frances.

CRAMER, JOSEPH B.: Jt. author, see Peck, Harris B.; Rabinovitch, Ralph D. and Cramer, Joseph B.

CURRAN, FRANK J.: Art techniques for use in mental hospitals and correctional institutions. Ment. Hyg., 23:371-378, 1939.

CURRAN, FRANK J.: The drama as a therapeutic measure in adolescents. Am. J. Orthopsychiat., 9:215-231, 1939.

CURRAN, FRANK J.: Organization of a ward for adolescents in Bellevue Psychiatric Hospital. Am. J. Psychiat., 95:1365-1388, 1939.

CURRAN, FRANK J.: Value of art in a psychiatric hospital. Dis. Nerv. Syst., 1, No. 1, 1940.

CURRAN, FRANK J. and SCHILDER, PAUL: A constructive approach to the problems of childhood and adolescence. J. Crim. Psychopathol., 2:125-142, 1940; 3:305-321, 1941.

CURRAN, FRANK J.: Jt. author, see Bender, Lauretta and Curran, Frank J.

CURRAN, FRANK J.: Jt. author, see Jenkins, Richard L. and Curran, Frank J.

CUSHMAN, L. S.: The art impulse, its form and relation to mental development. Proc. Nat. Educ. A., p. 515, 1908.

DALCROZE, EMILE JACQUES: Rhythm, Music and Education. Transl. by Rubenstein, H. R. London. Putnam, 1921.

DENNIS, WAYNE: The historical beginnings of child psychology. Psychol. Bull., 46:224-235, 1949.

DESPERT, J. LOUISE: Emotional problems in children; technical approaches used in their study and treatment. Utica, New York State Hospitals Press, 1938.

DESPERT, J. LOUISE: A method for the study of personality reactions in pre-school age children by means of analysis of their play. J. Psychol., 9:17-29, 1940.

DESPERT, J. LOUISE: Psychosomatic study of fifty stuttering children. I. Social, physical, and psychiatric findings. Am. J. Orthopsychiat., 16:100-113, 1946.

DESPERT, J. LOUISE: Technical Approaches Used in the Study and Treatment of Emotional Problems in Children. Utica, New York, State Hospital Press, 1938.

DEUTSCHBERGER, PAUL: The psychosomatic component in problem behavior. Am. J. Orthopsychiat., 16:147-155, 1946.

DEWEY, JOHN H.: Art in Education, in Monroe, Paul (Ed.): Encyclopedia of Education, Vol. I, 223-225, New York, Macmillan, 1911.

DUNNETT, RUTH: Art and Child Personality. London, Methuen, 1948.

EARL, C. J. C.: The human figure drawing of feeble-minded adults. Proc. and Addr. Am. A. Ment. Deficiency, 38:107-120, 1933.

EDDINGTON, ARTHUR: Space, Time, and Gravitation. Cambridge, 1920.

EISERER, PAUL E. The relative effectiveness of motion and still pictures as stimuli for eliciting fantasy stories about adolescent-parent relationships. Genet. Psychol. Monogr., 39:207-280, 1949.

EISSLER, KURT R. (Ed.): Searchlights on Delinquency; New Psychoanalytic Studies (dedicated to August Aichorn). New York, Intern. Univ. Press, 1949.

ELIASBERG, W.: Die Veranschaulichung in der Hilfsschule, Ztschr. f. exper. Paedog., 27:134-145, 1926.

ELKISCH, PAULA: Children's drawings in a projective technique. Psychol. Monogr. 58, No. 1, 1945.

ELKISCH, PAULA: Diagnostic and therapeutic value of projective techniques. Am. J. Psychotherapy, 1:279-312, 1947.

FABIAN, ABRAHAM A.: Vertical rotation in visual motor performance—its relationship to reading reversals. J. Educ. Psychol., 36:129-154, 1945.

FINLEY, MALCOLM H.: The classroom as a social group; its reaction to the problem child. Am. J. Orthopsychiat., 11:21-32, 1941.

FIRST ANNUAL REPORT of the City Superintendent of Schools to the Board of Education, New York City, 1899.

FORD, MARY: Application of the Rorschach Test to Young Children. Minneapolis, Univ. of Minnesota Press, 1946.

FRANK, LAWRENCE K.: The fundamental needs of the child. Ment. Hyg., 22:353-379, 1938.

FRANK, LAWRENCE K.: Projective Methods. Springfield, Ill., Thomas, 1948.

FRANK, LAWRENCE K.: Projective methods for the study of personality. J. Psychol., 8:389-413, 1938.

FREUD, ANNA: The Ego and the Mechanisms of Defence. New York, Intern. Univ. Press, 1946.

FREUD, ANNA: Introduction to the Technique of Child Analysis. Nerv. & Ment. Dis. Monogr. Series No. 48, 1928.

FREUD, ANNA: The psychoanalytic study of infantile feeding disturbances, in: Psychoanalytic Study of the Child. 2:119-132, 1946.

FREUD, ANNA: The Psychoanalytic Treatment of Children. London, Imago Pub. Co., 1946.

FREUD, ANNA (Ed.): Child analysis; a symposium. Psychoanalyt. Quart., 4:1-2; 15-24, 1935.

FREUD, ANNA; HARTMANN, HEINZ and KRIS, ERNST (Eds.): The Psychoanalytic Study of the Child. Vol. I, 1946; Vol. II, 1947; Vols. III & IV, 1949. New York, Intern. Univ. Press, Vol. V, 1950.

FREUD, ANNA and BURLINGHAM, DOROTHY T.: Infants Without Families. London, Medical War Books, 1944.

FREUD, ANNA and BURLINGHAM, DOROTHY T.: War and Children. London, Medical War Books, 1943.

FREUD, SIGMUND: Analysis of a Phobia in a Five Year Old Boy (1909). Collected Papers, Vol. III, London, 1925.

FREUD, SIGMUND: Beyond the Pleasure Principle. London, Intern. Psycho-Analytical Press, 1922.

FREUD, SIGMUND: Collected Papers. Vol. VIII, London, Hogarth Press.

FREUD, SIGMUND: General Introduction to Psychoanalysis. New York, Boni & Liveright, 1920.

FREUD, SIGMUND: Inhibitions, Symptoms, and Anxiety. London, Hogarth Press, 1936.

FREUD, SIGMUND: Interpretation of Dreams, in: Brill, A. A. (Ed.): The Basic Writings of Sigmund Freud. New York, Modern Library, 1938.

FREUD, SIGMUND: Introductory Lectures to Psychoanalysis. New York, W. W. Norton & Co., 1926.

FREUD, SIGMUND: Three Contributions to the Theory of Sex, in Nerv. & Ment. Dis. Monogr. Series No. 7, 4th Ed., 1930.

FREUD, SIGMUND: Totem and Taboo. London, Kegan Paul, 1931.

FRIEDLANDER, KATE: Psycho-analytic Approach to Juvenile Delinquency. New York, Intern. Univ. Press, 1947.

FRIES, MARGARET E.: Play techniques in the analysis of young children. Psychoanalyt. Rev., 24:233-245, 1937.

FRIES, MARGARET E.: Value of a play group in a child-development study. Ment. Hyg., 21:106-116, 1937.

GATES, M. F.: A comparative study of some problems of social and emotional adjustment of crippled and non-crippled girls and boys. J. Genet. Psychol., 68:219-244, 1946.

GERARD, MARGARET W.: Child analysis as a technique in the investigation of mental mechanisms. Am. J. Psychiat., 94:653-663, 1937.

GERARD, MARGARET W.: Direct Treatment of the Child in: Orthopsychiatry 1923-1948. New York, Am. Orthopsychiat. A., 1948.

GESELL, ARNOLD L.: Infant and Child in the Culture of Today. New York and London, Harper and Bros., 1943.

GESELL, ARNOLD L. et al.: Biographies of Child Development. New York, P. B. Hoeber, 1939.

GESELL, ARNOLD L. et al.: The First Five Years of Life. New York and London, Harper, 1940.

GESELL, ARNOLD L. and AMATRUDA, CATHERINE S.: Developmental Diagnosis. New York and London, P. B. Hoeber, 1941.

GESELL, ARNOLD L. and ILG, FRANCES L.: The Child from Five to Ten. New York and London, Harper, 1946.

GESELL, ARNOLD L. and ILG, FRANCES L.: Feeding Behavior of Infants; a Pediatric Approach to the Mental Hygiene of Early Life. Philadelphia, Lippincott, 1937.

GESELL, ARNOLD L. and THOMPSON, HELEN: Infantile Behavior; its Genesis and Growth. New York: McGraw-Hill, 1934.

GITELSON, MAXWELL: Direct psychotherapy of children. Arch. Neurol. and Psychiat., 43:1208-1223, 1940.

GITELSON, MAXWELL (Chairman): Play Therapy. Am. J. Orthopsychiat., 8:499-524, 1938.

GLUECK, BERNARD (Ed.): Current Therapies in Personality Disorders. New York, Grune and Stratton, 1945.

GOLDFARB, WILLIAM: The effects of early institutional care on adolescent personality. J. Exper. Educ., 12:106-120, 1943.

GOODENOUGH, FLORENCE L.: Children's Drawings. Chap. XIV in Murchison, C. (Ed.): Handbook of Child Psychology. Worcester, Mass., Clark Univ. Press, 1931.

GOODENOUGH, FLORENCE L.: A new approach to the intelligence of young children. Pedagog. Seminar, 33:185-211, 1926.

GOODENOUGH, FLORENCE L.: The Measurement of Intelligence by Drawings. Yonkers, World Book Co., 1926.

GOODENOUGH, FLORENCE L.: The Measurement of Mental Growth in Childhood. Chap. IX in Carmichael, Leonard (Ed.): Manual of Child Psychology. New York, John Wiley and Sons, Inc., 1946.

GOODENOUGH, FLORENCE L.: The psychological interpretation of children's drawings. North American Teacher, 11:112-115, 1928.

GOODENOUGH, FLORENCE L.: Studies in the psychology of children's drawings. Psychol. Bull., 25:272-283, 1928.

GREENE, R. A.: Conflicts in diagnosis between mental deficiency and certain psychoses. Proc. and Addr. Am. A. Ment. Deficiency, 38:127-143, 1933.

GRIFFITHS, RUTH: A Study of Imagination in Early Childhood. London, Kegan, Paul, Trench, Trubner and Co., 1935.

GROOS, KARL: Das Spiel als Katharsis. Ztschr. f. Paedagog. Psychol., 1911.

GROOS, KARL: The Play of Animals. New York, Appleton, 1898.

GROOS, KARL: Play of Man. New York, Appleton, 1901.

GUILLET, C.: Retentiveness in children and adults. Am. J. Psychol., 20:318-352, 1909.

GUREWICZ, SAUL: Beurteilung Freier Schueleraufsaetzen und Schuelerzeichnungen auf Grund der Adlerschen Individualpsychologie. Zurich, Rascher Verlag, 1948.

HALL, G. STANLEY: Adolescence. New York, Appleton, 1905.

HALL, G. STANLEY: The contents of children's minds on entering school. Pedagog. Seminar, 1:139-173, 1891.

HALPERN, FLORENCE: Jt. author, see Bochner, Ruth and Halpern, Florence.

HAMILTON, GORDON: Psychotherapy in Child Guidance. New York, Columbia Univ. Press, 1947.

HARMS, ERNST: Child art as aid in the diagnosis of juvenile neurosis. Am. J. Orthopsychiat., 11:191-209, 1941.

HARMS, ERNST: Kinderkunst als diagnostisches Hilfsmittel bei infantilen Neurosen. Ztschr. f. Kinderpsychol., 6:129-143, 1940.

HARMS, ERNST: The psychotherapeutical importance of the arts. Occup. Therapy, 18:235-239, 1939.

HARMS, ERNST (Ed.): Handbook of Child Guidance. New York, Child Care Publications, 1947.

HARTLAUB, G. F.: Der Zeichner Josephson, Genius. Ztschr. f. bildende Kunst, 21:175-177, 1910.

HARTMANN, G. W.: Gestalt Psychology. New York, Ronald, 1935.

HARTMANN, HEINZ; KRIS, ERNST and LOWENSTEIN, RUDOLPH M.: Comments on the formation of psychic structure. Psychoanal. Study of the Child, 2:11-38, 1946.

HARTMANN, HEINZ: Jt. editor, see Freud, Anna; Hartmann, Heinz and Kris, Ernst (Eds.).

HARTSHORNE, CHARLES: The Philosophy and Psychology of Sensation. Chicago, Univ. of Chicago Press, 1934.

HASSALL, JAMES G.: The serpent as a symbol. Psychoanalyt. Rev., 6: 1919.

HATTWICK, LA BERTA WEISSS Jt. author, see Alschuler, Rose H. and Hattwick, La Berta Weiss.

HAWKINS, MARY O'N.: Psychoanalysis of children. Bull. Menninger Clin., 4:181-186, 1940.

H'DOUBLER, MARGARET: Dance: A Creative Art Experience. New York, Crofts, 1940. (This book contains an annotated reading list.)

HEALY, WILLIAM: Twenty-five Years of Child Guidance: An Appraisal. Studies from the Institute for Juvenile Research, Chicago, Series C. No. 256, 1944.

HEALY, WILLIAM and BRONNER, AUGUSTA F.: Criminals and Delinquents: Their Making and Unmaking. New York, Macmillan, 1926.

HENRY, JULES and HENRY, ZUNIA: Speech disturbances in Pilagá Indian children. Am. J. Orthopsychiat., 10:362-369, 1940.

HENRY, ZUNIA: Jt. author, see Henry, Jules and Henry, Zunia.

HEWLETT, IRMA: Jt. author, see Bruch, Hilda and Hewlett, Irma.

HILDEBRAND, ADOLF: Problem of Form Painting and Sculpture. New York, Stechert, 1932.

HINRICHS, W. E.: The Goodenough drawing test in relation to delinquency and problem behavior. Arch. Psychol., No. 175, 1935.

HOFF, HANS and SCHILDER, PAUL: Die Lagereflexe des Menschen. Vienna, Springer, 1927.

HOMBURGER, ERIC: Configurations in play—Clinical notes. Psychoanalyt. Quart., 6:139-214, 1937.

HORNEY, KAREN: The Neurotic Personality of Our Time. New York, W. W. Norton & Co., 1937.

HORNEY, KAREN: New Ways in Psychoanalysis. New York, W. W. Norton & Co., 1939.

HOROWITZ, R. and MURPHY, LOIS B.: Projective methods in the psychological study of children. J. Exper. Educ., 7:133-140, 1938.

HRDLICKA, ALES: Children Who Run on All Fours and Other Animal-like Behavior in the Human Child. New York, Whittlesey House, 1931.

ILG, FRANCES L.: Jt. author, see Gesell, Arnold L. and Ilg, Frances L.

INTERNATIONAL CONGRESS ON MENTAL HEALTH. International Preparatory Commission. Statement on Human Relations, 2:65-98, 1949.

ISAACS, SUSAN: Childhood and After. New York, Intern. Univ. Press, 1949.

ISAACS, SUSAN: The nature and function of phantasy. Intern. J. Psycho-Analysis, 29:73-97, 1948.

ISAACS, SUSAN: Social Development in Young Children. New York, Harcourt, 1933.

ISRAELITE, JUDITH: A comparison of the difficulty of items for intellectually normal children and mental defectives on the Goodenough drawing test. Am. J. Orthopsychiat., 6:494-503, 1936.

ITARD, J. M. G.: The Wild Boy of Aveyron. Transl. by Humphrey, George and Humphrey, Muriel. New York, Century, 1932.

JELLIFFE, SMITH ELY: Psychoanalysis and the Drama. New York, Nerv. & Ment. Dis. Pub. Co., 1922.

JENKINS, RICHARD L. and BECKH, ERICA: Finger puppets and mask making as media for work with children. Am. J. Orthopsychiat., 12:294-300, 1942.

JENKINS, RICHARD L. and CURRAN, FRANK J.: The evolution and persistence of groups in a psychiatric observation ward. J. Soc. Psychol., 12:279-289, 1940.

JENNINGS, HELEN: Jt. author, see Moreno, J. L. and Jennings, Helen.

JOHNSON, HARRIET M.: School Begins at Two. New York, New Republic, 1936.

JOHNSON, MARTIN C.: Art and Scientific Thought. New York, Columbia Univ. Press, 1949.

JOSEPH, ALICE and MURRAY, VERONICA FRAZER: Chamorros and Carolinians of Saipan. Report from the Pacific Science Board to National Research Council (in press).

JUNG, CARL G.: Psychology of the Unconscious. New York, Dodd Mead, 1931.

KANNER, LEO and SCHILDER, PAUL: Movements in the optic images and optic imagination of movements. J. Nerv. and Ment. Dis., 72:489-517, 1930.

KARSTEN, ANITRA: Psychische Saettigung. Psychol. Forschung, 10:142-154, 1927.

KATZ, DORA: Der Aufbau der Tastwelt. Ztschr. f. Psychol., 11:1-270, 1925.

KELLY, LUMRY G.: Jt. author, see Buehler, Charlotte; Kelly, Lumry G., and Carrol, H.

KILPATRICK, W. H.: Froebel's Kindergarten Principles Critically Examined. New York, Macmillan, 1916.

KINDER, ELAINE: Jt. author, see Nissen, H. W.; Machover, Saul and Kinder, Elaine.

KLEIN, HENRIETTE R.: Jt. author, see Potter, Howard W. and Klein, Henriette R.

KLEIN, MELANIE: A contribution to the theory of anxiety and guilt. Intern. J. Psycho-Analysis, 29:114-123, 1948.

KLEIN, MELANIE: A contribution to the theory of intellectual inhibition. Intern. J. Psycho-Analysis, 12:206-218, 1931.

KLEIN, MELANIE: Contribution to Psycho-Analysis, 1921-1945. London, Hogarth Press, 1948.

KLEIN, MELANIE: Notes on some schizoid mechanisms. Intern. J. Psycho-Analysis, 27:99-110, 1946.

KLEIN, MELANIE: Personification in the play of children. Intern. J. Psycho-Analysis, 10:193-204, 1929.

KLEIN, MELANIE: Personification in the play of children, in: Contributions to Psychoanalysis, 1921-1945. London, Hogarth Press, 1948.

KLEIN, MELANIE: The Psycho-Analysis of Children. London, Intern. Psycho-Analyt. Press, 1932.

KLOPFER, BRUNO and MARGULIES, M. A.: Rorschach reaction in early childhood. Rorschach Research Exchange, 5:1-23, 1941.

KLUEVER, HEINRICH: Behavior Mechanisms in Monkeys. Chicago, Univ. of Chicago Press, 1933.

KOEHLER, WOLFGANG: Gestalt Psychology. New York, Liveright, 1929.

KOEHLER, WOLFGANG: The Mentality of Apes. New York, Harcourt, 1931.

KOEHLER, WOLFGANG: The Place of Value in the World of Facts. New York, Liveright, 1938.

KOEPKE: Quoted by Lewin, Kurt in: A Dynamic Theory of Personality.

KOFFKA, KURT: The Growth of the Mind: An Introduction to Child Psychology. New York, Harcourt, 1931.

KOFFKA, KURT: Principles of Gestalt Psychology. New York, Harcourt, 1935.

KOFFKA, KURT: Problems in the Psychology of Art. In Art, A Symposium. Bryn Mawr, Bryn Mawr College, 1940.

KOFFKA, KURT and WULF, F.: Ueber die Veraenderung der Vorstellungen. Psychol. Forschung, 1:333-337, 1922.

KOPP, HELEN: Psychomatic study of fifty stuttering children. II. Ozeretsky Tests. Am. J. Orthopsychiat., 16:114-119, 1946.

KRAUTTER, OTTO: Die Entwicklung des Plastischen Gestaltens beim Vorschulpflichtigen Kinde; ein Beitrag zur Psychogenese des Gestaltens. Ztschr. f. Angew. Psychol., 50: 1930.

KRETSCHMER, ERNST: Physique and Character. New York, Harcourt, 1925.

KRIS, ERNST: Approaches to Art in: Lorand, Sandor (Ed.): Psychoanalysis Today. New York, Intern. Univ. Press, 1944.

KRIS, ERNST: Bemerkungen zur Bildnerei der Geisteskranken. Imago, 22:339-370, 1936.

KRIS, ERNST: Ego development and the comic. Intern. J. Psycho-Analysis, 19:77-90, 1938.

KRIS, ERNST: On psychoanalysis and education. Am. J. Orthopsychiat., 18:622-635, 1948.

KRIS, ERNST: Jt. editor, see Freud, Anna; Hartmann, Heinz and Kris, Ernst (Eds.).

KRIS, ERNST: Jt. author, see Hartmann, Heinz; Kris, Ernst and Loewenstein, Rudolph M.

KRUGMAN, MORRIS: Psychosomatic Study of Fifty Stuttering Children. IV. Rorschach study. Am. J. Orthopsychiat., 16:127-133, 1946.

LAMPARTER, P.: Die Musikalitaet in ihren Beziehungen zur Grundstruktur der Persoenlichkeit—Exp. Beitraege zur Typenkunde. Ztschr. Psychol., 3 Ergaenzungsband 22, 1932.

LAMPRECHT, K.: Les dessins d'enfant comme source historique. Bull. de l'Acad. Roy. de Belgique, No. 9 and No. 10: 457-469, 1906.

LEE, HARRY B.: On the esthetic states of the mind. Psychiatry, 10:281-306, 1947.

LEHTINEN, LAURA E.: Jt. author, see Strauss, Alfred A. and Lehtinen, Laura E.

LEITCH, MARY and SCHAFER, SARAH: A study of the thematic apperception tests of psychotic children. Am. J. Orthopsychiat., 17:337-342, 1947.

LERNER, EUGENE and MURPHY, LOIS B. (Eds.): Methods for the study of personality in young children. Monogr. Soc. Research Child Develop., 6: No. 4, 1941.

LESSING, GOTHOLD E.: Laocoon. Transl. by Phillimore, Rt. Hon. Sir Robert. London, Macmillan, 1874.

LEVINE, ESTHER L.: Jt. author, see Schilder, Paul and Levine, Esther L.

LEVY, DAVID M.: Attitude therapy. Am. J. Orthopsychiat., 7:103-112, 1937.

LEVY, DAVID M.: Body interest in children and hypochondriasis. Am. J. Psychiat., 12:295-315, 1932.

LEVY, DAVID M.: Hostility patterns in sibling rivalry. Am. J. Orthopsychiat., Monogr., No. 2, 52-96, 1937.

LEVY, DAVID M.: A method of integrating physical and psychiatric examinations. Am. J. Psychiat., 9:121-194, 1929.

LEVY, DAVID M.: Psychotherapy and childhood. Am. J. Orthopsychiat., 10:905-910, 1940.

LEVY, DAVID M.: Trends in therapy; Release therapy. Am. J. Orthopsychiat., 9:713-736, 1939.

LEVY, DAVID M.: The use of play technic as experimental procedure. Am. J. Orthopsychiat., 3:266-277, 1933.

LEVY, JOHN: The use of art techniques in treatment of children's behavior problems. Proc. Am. A. Ment. Deficiency, 39:258-260, 1934.

LEWIN, KURT: Behavior and development as a function of the total situation. Chap. XVI in: Carmichael, Leonard (Ed.): Manual of Child Psychology. New York, John Wiley & Sons, 1946.

LEWIN, KURT: Conceptual Representation and the Measurement of Psychological Forces. Durham, N.C., Duke Univ. Press, 1938.

LEWIN, KURT: Contributions to Psychological Theory. Durham, N.C., Duke Univ. Press, I, No. 4, 1938.

LEWIN, KURT: A Dynamic Theory of Personality. New York, McGraw-Hill, 1935.

LEWIN, KURT: Principles of Topological Psychology. New York and London, McGraw-Hill, 1936.

LEWINSKI, ROBERT J.: The psychometric pattern: epilepsy. Am. J. Orthopsychiat., 17:714-722, 1947.

LEWIS, NOLAN D.C. and PACELLA, BERNARD L. (Eds.): Modern Trends in Child Psychiatry. New York, Intern. Univ. Press, 1945.

L'HOTE, ANDRÉ: The unconscious in art. Transition, 26:89, 1937.

LIEF, ALFRED: The Commonsense Psychiatry of Adolf Meyer. New York, McGraw-Hill, 1948.

LIPKOWITZ, H.: Jt. author, see Bender, Lauretta and Lipkowitz, H.

LISS, EDWARD: Play techniques in child analysis. Am. J. Orthopsychiat., 6:17-22, 1936.

LORAND, SANDOR: Fairy tales, Lilliputian dreams, and neurosis. Am. J. Orthopsychiat., 7:456-464, 1937.

LOURIE, REGINALD S.: Jt. author, see Bender, Lauretta and Lourie, Reginald S.

LOWENFELD, MARGARET: Play in Childhood. London, Victor Gollancz, 1935.

LOWENFELD, MARGARET: The world pictures of children. Brit. J. Med. Psychol., 8:65-101, 1939.

LOEWENSTEIN, RUDOLPH M.: Jt. author, see Hartman, Heinz; Kris, Ernst and Loewenstein, Rudolph M.

LOWREY, LAWSON G.: Psychiatry for children, a brief history of developments. Am. J. Psychiat., 101:375-388, 1944.

LOWREY, LAWSON G.: Psychiatry for Social Workers. New York, Columbia Univ. Press, 1946.

LUDWIG, HEINRICH (Ed. & translator): Das Buch von der Malerei, by Leonardo da Vinci. Quellenschriften fuer Kunstgeschichte und Kunsttechnik. V. 18, 1882.

McCARTHY, DOROTHEA: Language Development in Children. Chap. X. Carmichael, Leonard (Ed.): Manual of Child Psychology. New York, John Wiley & Sons, Inc., 1946.

McELWEE, E. W.: Profile drawings of normal and subnormal children. J. Applied Psychol., 18:599-603, 1934.

MACHOVER, KAREN: Personality Projection in the Drawing of the Human Figure. Springfield, Ill., Thomas, 1948.

MACHOVER, SAUL: Jt. author, see Nissen, H. W.; Machover, Saul and Kinder, Elaine.

MARGUILES, M. A.: Jt. author, see Klopfer, Bruno and Marguiles, M. A.

MASON, BERNHARD S.: Jt. author, see Mitchell, Elmer D. and Mason, Bernhard S.

MEAD, MARGARET: From the South Seas. New York, Morrow, 1939.

MEAD, MARGARET: Research on Primitive Children. Chap. XIII in Carmichael, Leonard (Ed.): Manual of Child Psychology. New York, John Wiley & Sons, 1946.

MERRILL, MAUD A.: Problems of Child Delinquency. New York, Houghton, Mifflin, 1947.

MITCHELL, ELMER D. and MASON, BERNHARD S.: Theory of Play. New York, A. S. Barnes & Co., 1934.

MONEY-KYRLE, R. E.: Superstition and Society. London, Hogarth Press, 1939.

MONROE, PAUL (Ed.): Encyclopedia of Education. New York, Macmillan, 1911.

MONTAGUE, ALLISON: The Art of the Schizophrenic Child, in: Anderson, Howard H. and Anderson, Gladys L. (Eds.): Projective Techniques. New York, Prentice Hall, 1951.

MONTAGUE, ALLISON: Jt. author, see Bender, Lauretta and Montague, Allison.

MONTGOMERY, JOHN C.: Toilet education. Am. J. Orthopsychiat., 17:590-593, 1947.

MORENO, J. L. and JENNINGS, HELEN: Spontaneity training, a method in personality development. Sociometric Review, 1936, Report of the Research Staff to the Advisory Research Board. Hudson, N.Y., New York Training School for Girls, 1936.

MORGENSTERN, SOPHIE: La pensée magique chez l'enfant. Rev. franç de Psychoanal., 7:1-ff., 1937.

MORGENSTERN, SOPHIE: Le Symbolisme et la valeur psychoanalytique des dessins infantiles. Rev. franç. de Psychoanal., 11:39-48, 1939.

MOSSE, ERIC P.: Painting-analysis in the treatment of neuroses. Psychoanalyt. Rev., 27:65-82, 1940.

MULLAHY, PATRICK: Oedipus: Myth and Complex. New York, Hermitage Press, 1948.

MUNCIE, WENDELL: Psychobiology and Psychiatry. St. Louis, Mosby, 1939.

MURCHISON, CARL (Ed.): Handbook of Child Psychology. Worcester, Mass., Clark Univ. Press, 1933.

MURPHY, LOIS B.: Jt. author, see Horowitz, R. and Murphy, Lois B.

MURPHY, LOIS B.: Jt. author, see Lerner, Eugene and Murphy, Lois B.

MURRAY, VERONICA FRAZER: Jt. author, see Joseph, Alice and Murray, Veronica Frazer.

MUSOLD, DORA: Jt. author, see Buehler, Karl; Musold, Dora and Vokelt, H.

NAUMBURG, MARGARET: Studies of the Free Art Expression of Behavior Problem Children and Adolescents as a Means of Diagnosis and Therapy. Nerv. and Ment. Dis. Monogr., No. 71, 1947.

NEAL, JOSEPHINE (Ed.): Encephalitis, A Clinical Study. New York, Grune and Stratton, 1942.

NEUMANN, E.: Vorlesungen zur Einfuehrung in die Experimentale Pedagogik. 2nd Ed., Leipzig, Verlag Engelmann, 1911, vols. I, II and III.

NEWELL, H. WHITMAN: Play therapy in child psychiatry. Am. J. Orthopsychiat., 11:245-252, 1941.

NISSEN, H. W.; MACHOVER, SAUL and KINDER, ELAINE F.: A study of performance tests given to a group of native African Negro children. Brit. J. Psychol., 25:308-355, 1935.

OGDEN, C. K. and RICHARDS, I. A.: The Meaning of Meaning. New York, Harcourt Brace, 1923.

OLIVER, WRENSHALL A.: A state hospital children's unit. Am. J. Psychiat., 106:265-267, 1949.

ORTON, SAMUEL T.: Reading, Writing and Speech Problems in Children. New York, W. W. Norton & Co., 1937.

PACELLA, BERNARD L.: Jt. editor, see Lewis, Nolan D.C. and Pacella, Bernard L.

PASCAL, GERALD R. and SUTTELL, BARBARA J.: The Bender-Gestalt Test. New York, Grune and Stratton, 1951.

PAULSSON, G.: The creative mind in art. Scandinav. Sci. Rev., 2:11-173, 1923.

PAYNTER, J.: Jt. author, see Sheimo, S. L.; Paynter, J. and Szurek, S. A.

PECK, HARRIS B.; RABINOVITCH, RALPH D. and CRAMER, JOSEPH B.: A treatment program for parents of schizophrenic children. Am. J. Orthopsychiat., 19:592-598, 1949.

PFEIFER, R. A.: Der Geisteskranke und Sein Werk, eine Studie ueber Schizophrene Kunst. Leipzig, Kromer, 1923.

PIAGET, JEAN: The Language and Thought of the Child. New York, Harcourt Brace, 1932.

PINTNER, RUDOLF: The Feebleminded Child, in Murchison, Carl (Ed.): Handbook of Child Psychology. Worcester, Mass., Clark Univ. Press, 1933.

POTTER, HOWARD W.: Psychotherapy in children. Psychiat. Quart., 9:335-348, 1935.

POTTER, HOWARD W.: Schizophrenia in children. Am. J. Psychiat., 12:1253-1270, 1933.

POTTER, HOWARD W.: The treatment of problem children in a psychiatric hospital. Am. J. Psychiat., 91:869-880, 1935.

POTTER, HOWARD W. and KLEIN, HENRIETTE R.: An evaluation of the treatment of problem children as determined by a follow-up study. Am. J. Psychiat., 94:681-689, 1937.

PREUSS, K. TH.: Der Ursprung der Religion und Kunst. Globus 86:87, 1902-5.

PREYER, WILHELM: The Mind of the Child. 2 vols. New York, Appleton, 1888, 1889.

PREYER, WILHELM: Psychogenesis. Deutsche Rundschau, 23:198-221, 1880. Transl. by Talbot, Marion, in J. Spec. Philosophy, 15:159-188, 1881.

PREYER, WILHELM: Die Seele des Kindes; Beobachtung ueber die Geistige Entwicklungen des Menschen in den ersten Lebensjahren. Leipzig, T. Grieben, 1882.

PRINZHORN, HANS: Die Bildenerei der Geisteskranken. Berlin, Springer, 1922.

RABINOVITCH, RALPH D.: Jt. author, see Peck, Harris B.; Rabinovitch, Ralph D. and Cramer, Joseph B.

RAMBERT, MADELEINE L.: Children in Conflict. New York, Internat. Univ. Press, 1949.

RAMBERT, MADELEINE L.: Une nouvelle technique en psychoanalyse infantile: le jeu de guignols. Rev. franç. de Psychoanal., 10: No. 1, 1938.

RANK, OTTO: Das Schauspiel in Hamlet. Imago, 4, 1916.

RAPAPORT, DAVID: Diagnostic Psychological Testing. 2 vols. Chicago, Yr. Bk. Publ., 1946.

RAPAPORT, DAVID: Emotions and Memory. Baltimore, Williams and Wilkins, 1942.

RAPAPORT, DAVID: Principles underlying projective techniques. Character and Personality, 10:213-219, 1942.

RAPOPORT, JACK: Phantasy objects in children. Psychoanalyt. Rev., 31:316-331, 1944.

RAPOPORT, JACK: Joint author, see Bender, Lauretta and Rapoport, Jack.

READ, HERBERT: Education for Peace. New York, Scribner, 1949.

READ, HERBERT: Education Through Art. Pantheon Books, New York, 1949.

REICH, WILHELM: Der Triebhafte Charakter. Vienna, Psychoanalytischer Verlag, 1925.

REISE, WALTHER: Vincent Van Gogh in der Krankheit. Grenzfragen des Nerven und Seelenlebens, 75:1-38, 1926.

RENZ, BARBARA: Der Orientalishe Schlangendrache. Augsburg, Haas und Grabherr, 1930.

RIBBLE, MARGARET A.: Rights of Infants; Early Psychological Needs and Their Satisfaction. New York, Columbia Univ. Press, 1944.

RICHARDS, I. A.: Jt. author, see Ogden, C. K. and Richards, I. A.

RICHARDS, SUSAN S. and WOLFF, E.: The organization and function of play activities in the set-up of a pediatric department. Ment. Hyg., 24:229-237, 1940.

ROBINSON, J. FRANKLIN: The role of the resident professional worker. Am. J. Orthopsychiat., 19:674-682, 1949.

ROGERS, CARL R.: Clinical Treatment of the Problem Child. New York, Houghton Mifflin, 1939.

ROGERSON, C. H.: Play Therapy in Childhood. New York, Oxford Press, 1939.

ROHEIM, GEZA: Riddle of the Sphinx. London, Hogarth Press, 1934.

ROSENTHAL, PAULINE: Group studies of pre-adolescent delinquent boys. Am. J. Orthopsychiat., 12:115-126, 1942.

ROSENZWEIG, SAUL and SHAKOW, DAVID: Play technique in schizophrenia and other psychoses. I. Rationale. Am. J. Orthopsychiat., 7:32-47, 1937.

ROUMA, GEORGES: Le Langage Graphique de l'Enfant. Brussels, Misch et Thron, 1912.

ROUSSEAU, JEAN JACQUES: Emile, A Treatise on Education. Transl. by Payne, H. P. New York, Appleton, 1897.

SCHAFER, SARAH: Jt. author, see Leitch, Mary and Schafer, Sarah.

SCHILDER, PAUL: Brain and Personality. New York and Wash., Nerv. and Ment. Dis. Monogr. Series No. 53, 1931. New York Internat. Univ. Press. 1951.

SCHILDER, PAUL: The child and the symbol. Scientia (Milan), 64:21-26, 1938.

SCHILDER, PAUL: Congenital alexia and its relation to optic perception. J. Genet. Psychol., 65:67-88, 1944.

SCHILDER, PAUL: Experiments on imagination, after-images and hallucinations. Am. J. Psychiat., 13:597-611, 1933.

SCHILDER, PAUL: Goals and Desires of Man. New York, Columbia Univ. Press, 1942.

SCHILDER, PAUL: Health as a psychic experience. Arch. Neurol. and Psychiat., 37:1322-1337, 1937.

SCHILDER, PAUL: Image and Appearance of the Human Body: Studies in the Constructive Energies of the Psyche. London, Kegan Paul, 1935. New York Internat. Univ. Press, 1950.

SCHILDER, PAUL: Introduction to a Psychoanalytic Psychiatry. New York and Wash., Nerv. and Ment. Dis. Publ. Co., 1928. New York Internat. Univ. Press, 1951.

SCHILDER, PAUL: Language and the constructive energies of the psyche. Scientia (Milan), 149-158; 205-211, Mar.-Apr., 1936.

SCHILDER, PAUL: Mind: Perception and Thought in Their Constructive Aspects. New York, Columbia Univ. Press, 1942.

SCHILDER, PAUL: Psychiatry and Art. Lecture at Med. Psychol. Club, Jan. 11, 1937.

SCHILDER, PAUL: The psychological effect of Benzedrine Sulphate. J. Nerv. and Ment. Dis. 87:584-587, 1938.

SCHILDER, PAUL: Psychological implications of motor development in children, in Proc. of 4th Institute on the Exceptional Child. Child Research Clinic, The Woods Schools, Langhorne, Pa., 4:38-59, 1937.

SCHILDER, PAUL: Psychotherapy. New York, W. W. Norton and Co., 1938. 2nd enlarged edition: Bender, L., (Ed.) 1951.

SCHILDER, PAUL: Results and problems of group psychotherapy in severe neuroses. Ment. Hyg., 33:87-96, 1939.

SCHILDER, PAUL: Space, time and perception. Psyche (London), 14:124-138, 1934.

SCHILDER, PAUL: Theoretical aspects of the art work in Bellevue Hospital. Direction, 2:2-3, 1939.

SCHILDER, PAUL: The vestibular apparatus in neurosis and psychosis. J. Nerv. and Ment. Dis., 78:1-23; 137-164, 1933.

SCHILDER, PAUL: Vita and Bibliography of Paul Schilder. J. Crim. Psychopathology, 2:221-234, 1940.

SCHILDER, PAUL: Wahn und Erkenntnis. Berlin, Springer, 1918.

SCHILDER, PAUL: Yellow and Blue. Psychoanalyt. Rev., 17:123-125, 1930.

SCHILDER, PAUL: Jt. author, see Bender, Lauretta and Schilder, Paul.

SCHILDER, PAUL: Jt. author, see Curran, Frank J. and Schilder, Paul.

SCHILDER, PAUL: Jt. author, see Hoff, Hans and Schilder, Paul.

SCHILDER, PAUL: Jt. author, see Kanner, Leo and Schilder, Paul.

SCHILDER, PAUL and BENDER, LAURETTA: Mannerisms as organic motility syndrome. Confinia Neurol., 3:321-330, 1941.

SCHILDER, PAUL and LEVINE, ESTHER L.: Abstract art as an expression of human problems. J. Nerv. and Ment. Dis., 95:1-10, 1942.

SCHILDER, PAUL and WECHSLER, DAVID: The attitudes of children toward death. J. Genet. Psychol., 46:406-451, 1934.

SEARL, M. N.: Play, reality and aggression. Intern. J. Psychoanalysis, 14:310-320, 1933.

SEGUIN, EDOUARD: Idiocy and its treatment by the physiological method. Albany, N.Y., Brandow Printing Co., 1907.

SEVENTH ANNUAL REPORT of the City Superintendent of Schools to the Board of Education, New York City, 1905.

SENN, MILTON J. E. (Ed.): Problems of Early Infancy. New York, Josiah Macy Found., 1947.

SHAW, RUTH S.: Finger Painting, a Perfect Medium for Self-expression. Boston, Little, Brown, 1934.

SHAKOW, DAVID: Jt. author, see Rosenzweig, Saul and Shakow, David.

SHEIMO, S. L.; PAYNTER, J. and SZUREK, S. A.: Problems of staff interaction with spontaneous group formations on a children's psychiatric ward. Am. J. Orthopsychiat., 19:599-611, 1949.

SHINN, MARIE W.: Notes on the development of a child. Univ. of Calif. Studies, 1: Parts 1-4, 1893-1897.

SHIRLEY, HALE F.: Psychiatry for the Pediatrician. New York, Commonwealth Fund, 1948.

SHIRLEY, MARY M.: The First Two Years, A Study of Twenty-five Babies. Minneapolis, Univ. of Minnesota Press, 1931, 1933.

SLAVSON, S. R.: Creative Group Education. New York, Association Press, 1937.

SLAVSON, S. R.: The Fields and Objectives of Group Therapy, in: Glueck, Bernard (Ed.): Current Therapies of Personality Disorders. New York, Grune and Stratton, 1946.

SLAVSON, S. R.: Group Therapy. Ment. Hyg., 24:36-49, 1940.

SLAVSON, S. R.: Introduction to Group Therapy. New York, Commonwealth Fund, 1943.

SOLOMON, JOSEPH C.: Active play therapy. Am. J. Orthopsychiat., 8:479-498, 1938.

SOLOMON, JOSEPH C.: Active play therapy: Further experiences. Am. J. Orthopsychiat., 10:763-781, 1940.

SPENCER, HERBERT: Essays on Education, etc. Everymans Library No. 504. New York, Dutton, 1911 Ed., 1946 reprint.

SPERLING, MELITTA: Problems in analysis of children with psychosomatic disorders. Quart. J. Child Behavior, 1:12-18, 1949.

SPITZ, RENÉ A.: Hospitalism. Psychoanalytic Study of the Child, 2:113-117, 1946.

SPITZ, RENÉ A. and WOLF, KATHERINE M.: Anaclitic depression; an inquiry into the genesis of psychiatric conditions in early childhood. Psychoanalytic Study of the Child, 2:313-342, 1946.

SPOCK, BENJAMIN: Pocket Book of Baby and Child Care. New York, Pocket Books, 1946.

SPOCK, BENJAMIN: Preventing early problems. Am. J. Orthopsychiat., 17:575-579, 1947.

SPOERL, DOROTHY T.: The drawing ability of mentally retarded children. J. Genet. Psychol., 57:259-277, 1940.

STAPLES, RUTH: The responsiveness of infants to color. J. Exper. Psychol., 15:119-141, 1932.

STERN, WILHELM: Psychology of Early Childhood up to the Sixth Year of Age. New York, Holt, 1930.

STEWART, KATHLEEN K. and AXELROD, PEARL L.: Group therapy on a children's psychiatric ward. Am. J. Orthopsychiat., 17:312-325, 1947.

STRAUSS, ALFRED A.: Therapeutic pedagogy; a neuropsychiatric approach in special education. Am. J. Psychiat., 104:60-63, 1947.

STRAUSS, ALFRED A. and LEHTINEN, LAURA E.: Psychopathology and Education of the Brain-injured Child. New York, Grune and Stratton, 1947.

STREET, RAYMOND F.: A Gestalt Completion Test. New York, Teachers College Contrib. to Education No. 481, 1931.

SULLY, JAMES: Studies of Childhood. New York, Appleton, 1897.

SUTTON, HELEN A.: Some nursing aspects of a children's psychiatric ward. Am. J. Orthopsychiat., 17:675-683, 1947.

SYLVESTER, EMMY, Jt. author, see Bettelheim, Bruno and Sylvester, Emmy.

SZUREK, S. A.: Dynamics of staff interaction in hospital psychiatric treatment of children. Am. J. Orthopsychiat., 17:652-664, 1947.

SZUREK, S. A.: Jt. author, see Sheimo, S. L.; Paynter, J. and Szurek, S. A.

TEICHER, JOSEPH D.: Preliminary survey of motility in children. J. Nerv. and Ment. Dis., 94:277-304, 1941.

THOMPSON, HELEN: Jt. author, see Gesell, Arnold L. and Thompson, Helen.

TOURAINE, G.: Jt. author, see Bruch, Hilda and Touraine, G.

TWENTY-SIXTH ANNUAL REPORT of the City Superintendent of Schools to the Board of Education, New York City, 1924.

VAN ALSTYNE, DOROTHY: Play Behavior and Choice of Play Material of Pre-school Children. Chicago, Univ. of Chicago Press, 1932.

VAN DE WALL, WILLEM: Music in Institutions. New York, Russell Sage Foundation, 1936.

VERWORN, M.: Kinderkunst und Urgeschichte. Korrespond. Blaetter der Deutschen Gesellsch., f. Anthrop. 38:42-46, 1907.

VOKELT, H.: Jt. author, see Buehler, Karl; Musold, Dora and Vokelt, H.

VON WIEGAND, CHARMION: Prehistoric Rock Pictures. Art Front, 10:June, July 1937.

WAEHNER, TRUDE S.: Interpretations of spontaneous drawings and paintings. Genet. Psychol. Monogr., 33:3-70, 1946.

WAELDER, ROBERT: The psychoanalytic theory of play. Psychoanal. Quart., 2:208-224, 1933.

WATSON, GOODWIN (Chairman): Areas of agreement in psychotherapy. Am. J. Orthopsychiat., 10:698-709, 1940.

WATSON, JOHN B.: What the Nursery Has to say About Instincts. Chap. I, in Murchison, Carl (Ed.): Psychologies of 1925. 3rd Ed. Worcester, Mass., Clark Univ. Press, 1928.

WEATHERLY, HOWARD E.: Jt. author, see Benjamin, Anne and Weatherly, Howard E.

WECHSLER, DAVID: Wechsler Intelligence Scale for Children Manual. New York, Psychological Corp., 1949.

WECHSLER, DAVID: Psychological Diagnosis, in Wechsler, Israel: Textbook of Clinical Neurology, 6th Ed. Philadelphia and London, Saunders, 1947.

WECHSLER, DAVID: Jt. author, see Schilder, Paul and Wechsler, David.

WEISS-FRANKL, ANNI B.: Play interviews with nursery school children. Am. J. Orthopsychiat., 11:33-39, 1941.

WERNER, HEINZ: Comparative Psychology of Mental Development. New York, Harper, 1940.

WERNER, HEINZ: Die Melodische Erfindung im Fruehen Kindesalter, quoted (p. 161) by Read, Herbert in: Education Through Art. New York, Pantheon Books, 1945.

WERTHAM, FREDERIC: The matricidal impulse. J. Crim. Psychopath., 2:455-464, 1941.

WERTHEIMER, MAX: Productive Thinking. New York and London, Harper, 1945.

WERTHEIMER, MAX: Untersuchungen zur Lehre von der Gestalt. Psychol. Forschung, 4:332-337, 1923.

WHYTE, LANCELOT L.: The Next Development in Man. New York, Holt, 1948.

WINNICOTT, D. W.: Pediatrics and psychiatry. Brit. J. Med. Psychol., 21:229-240, 1947-1948.

WITMER, HELEN L.: Psychiatric Clinics for Children. New York, Commonwealth Fund, 1940.

WITMER, HELEN L.: Psychiatric Interviews with Children. New York, Comonwealth Fund, 1946.

WITMER, HELEN L. (Ed.): Pediatrics and the Emotional Needs of the Child. New York, Commonwealth Fund, 1948.

WITTELS, FRITZ: The criminal psychopath in the psychoanalytical system. Psychoanalyt. Rev., 24:276-291, 1937.

WOLF, KATHERINE M.: Jt. author, see Spitz, René and Wolf, Katherine M.

WOLFF, E.: Jt. author, see Richards, Susan S. and Wolff, E.

WOLFF, WERNER: Personality of the Pre-School Child. New York, Grune and Stratton, 1947.

WOLFSON, WILLIAM Q.: Jt. author, see Bender, Lauretta and Wolfson, William Q.

WOLTMANN, ADOLF G.: Puppetry as a Means of Psychotherapy, in: Encyclopedia of Child Guidance. New York, Philosophical Library, 1943.

WOLTMANN, ADOLF G.: Therapeutic Aspects of Puppetry in: McPhalin, Paul (Ed.): Yearbook of Puppetry, 1942-1943, Columbus, O., 1944.

WOLTMANN, ADOLF G.: The Use of Puppetry as a Projective Method, in: Anderson, Howard H. and Anderson, Gladys: Projective Techniques. New York, Prentice Hall, 1951.

WOLTMANN, ADOLF G.: The use of puppets in understanding children. Ment. Hyg., 24:445-458, 1940.

WOLTMANN, ADOLF G.: Jt. author, see Bender, Lauretta and Woltmann, Adolf G.

WULF, F.: Jt. author, see Koffka, Kurt, and Wulf, F.

YARNELL, HELEN: Firesetting in children. Am. J. Orthopsychiat., 40:272-286, 1940.

YEPSEN, L. N.: The reliability of the Goodenough drawing test with feeble-minded subjects. J. Educ. Psychol., 20:448-451, 1929.

YERKES, ROBERT M.: Jt. author, see Yoakum, Clarence S. and Jerkes, Robert M.

YOAKUM, CLARENCE S. and YERKES, ROBERT M.: Army Mental Tests. New York, Holt, 1920. Army Performance Test 6, Designs pp. 43-152.

NAME INDEX

SUBJECT INDEX

This Book

CHILD
PSYCHIATRIC TECHNIQUES

By

Lauretta Bender, B.S., M.A., M.D.

was set, printed and bound by the Collegiate Press of Menasha, Wisconsin. The page trim size is 6⅞ x 9⅞ inches. The type page is 30 x 48 picas. The type face is Linotype Baskerville set 11 point on 13 point. The text paper is 70 pound White Deep Falls Enamel. The cover is Bancroft Buckram No. 3100.

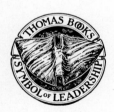

With THOMAS BOOKS *careful attention is given to all details of manufacturing and design. It is the Publisher's desire to present books that are satisfactory as to their physical qualities and artistic possibilities and appropriate for their particular use.* THOMAS BOOKS *will be true to those laws of quality that assure a good name and good will.*